Molecular Mechanisms and Therapies of Colorectal Cancer 2.0

Molecular Mechanisms and Therapies of Colorectal Cancer 2.0

Editor

Donatella Delle Cave

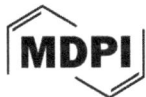

Basel • Beijing • Wuhan • Barcelona • Belgrade • Novi Sad • Cluj • Manchester

Editor
Donatella Delle Cave
Institute of Genetics and
Biophysics Adriano
Buzzati-Traverso (IGB-ABT),
CNR
Naples
Italy

Editorial Office
MDPI
St. Alban-Anlage 66
4052 Basel, Switzerland

This is a reprint of articles from the Special Issue published online in the open access journal *International Journal of Molecular Sciences* (ISSN 1422-0067) (available at: https://www.mdpi.com/journal/ijms/special_issues/F83345V1EF).

For citation purposes, cite each article independently as indicated on the article page online and as indicated below:

Lastname, A.A.; Lastname, B.B. Article Title. *Journal Name* **Year**, *Volume Number*, Page Range.

ISBN 978-3-7258-0951-6 (Hbk)
ISBN 978-3-7258-0952-3 (PDF)
doi.org/10.3390/books978-3-7258-0952-3

© 2024 by the authors. Articles in this book are Open Access and distributed under the Creative Commons Attribution (CC BY) license. The book as a whole is distributed by MDPI under the terms and conditions of the Creative Commons Attribution-NonCommercial-NoDerivs (CC BY-NC-ND) license.

Contents

About the Editor vii

Athanasios G. Papavassiliou and Donatella Delle Cave
Novel Therapeutic Approaches for Colorectal Cancer Treatment
Reprinted from: *Int. J. Mol. Sci.* **2024**, *25*, 2228, doi:10.3390/ijms25042228 1

**Solomiia Bychkova, Mykola Bychkov, Dani Dordevic, Monika Vítězová,
Simon K.-M. R. Rittmann and Ivan Kushkevych**
Bafilomycin A1 Molecular Effect on ATPase Activity of Subcellular Fraction of Human
Colorectal Cancer and Rat Liver
Reprinted from: *Int. J. Mol. Sci.* **2024**, *25*, 1657, doi:10.3390/ijms25031657 5

**Murali R. Kuracha, Venkatesh Govindarajan, Brian W. Loggie, Martin Tobi and
Benita L. McVicker**
Pictilisib-Induced Resistance Is Mediated through FOXO1-Dependent Activation of Receptor
Tyrosine Kinases in Mucinous Colorectal Adenocarcinoma Cells
Reprinted from: *Int. J. Mol. Sci.* **2023**, *24*, 12331, doi:10.3390/ijms241512331 23

**Aleksandra Sałagacka-Kubiak, Dawid Zawada, Lias Saed, Radzisław Kordek,
Agnieszka Jeleń and Ewa Balcerczak**
ABCG2 Gene and ABCG2 Protein Expression in Colorectal Cancer—In Silico and Wet Analysis
Reprinted from: *Int. J. Mol. Sci.* **2023**, *24*, 10539, doi:10.3390/ijms241310539 37

**José María Sayagués, Juan Carlos Montero, Andrea Jiménez-Pérez, Sofía del Carmen,
Marta Rodríguez, Rosario Vidal Tocino, et al.**
Analysis of Circulating Tumor DNA in Synchronous Metastatic Colorectal Cancer at Diagnosis
Predicts Overall Patient Survival
Reprinted from: *Int. J. Mol. Sci.* **2023**, *24*, 8438, doi:10.3390/ijms24098438 74

**Leonard A. Lobbes, Marcel A. Schütze, Raoul Droeser, Marco Arndt, Ioannis Pozios,
Johannes C. Lauscher, et al.**
Muscarinic Acetylcholine Receptor M3 Expression and Survival in Human Colorectal
Carcinoma—An Unexpected Correlation to Guide Future Treatment?
Reprinted from: *Int. J. Mol. Sci.* **2023**, *24*, 8198, doi:10.3390/ijms24098198 85

**Aleksandr S. Martianov, Natalia V. Mitiushkina, Anastasia N. Ershova,
Darya E. Martynenko, Mikhail G. Bubnov, Priscilla Amankwah, et al.**
KRAS, NRAS, BRAF, HER2 and MSI Status in a Large Consecutive Series of Colorectal
Carcinomas
Reprinted from: *Int. J. Mol. Sci.* **2023**, *24*, 4868, doi:10.3390/ijms24054868 99

**Da-Been Lee, Seo-Yeon An, Sang-Shin Pyo, Jinkwan Kim, Suhng-Wook Kim and
Dae-Wui Yoon**
Sleep Fragmentation Accelerates Carcinogenesis in a Chemical-Induced Colon Cancer Model
Reprinted from: *Int. J. Mol. Sci.* **2023**, *24*, 4547, doi:10.3390/ijms24054547 109

**Ryo Ejima, Hiroyuki Suzuki, Tomohiro Tanaka, Teizo Asano, Mika K. Kaneko and
Yukinari Kato**
Development of a Novel Anti-CD44 Variant 6 Monoclonal Antibody C_{44}Mab-9 for Multiple
Applications against Colorectal Carcinomas
Reprinted from: *Int. J. Mol. Sci.* **2023**, *24*, 4007, doi:10.3390/ijms24044007 118

Javier Ros, Caterina Vaghi, Iosune Baraibar, Nadia Saoudi González,
Marta Rodríguez-Castells, Ariadna García, et al.
Targeting *KRAS* G12C Mutation in Colorectal Cancer, A Review: New Arrows in the Quiver
Reprinted from: *Int. J. Mol. Sci.* **2024**, *25*, 3304, doi:10.3390/ijms25063304 . . . . **134**

Stefan Titu, Vlad Alexandru Gata, Roxana Maria Decea, Teodora Mocan, Constantin Dina,
Alexandru Irimie, et al.
Exosomes in Colorectal Cancer: From Physiology to Clinical Applications
Reprinted from: *Int. J. Mol. Sci.* **2023**, *24*, 4382, doi:10.3390/ijms24054382 . . . . **152**

Carolin Krekeler, Klaus Wethmar, Jan-Henrik Mikesch, Andrea Kerkhoff, Kerstin Menck,
Georg Lenz, et al.
Complete Metabolic Response to Combined Immune Checkpoint Inhibition after Progression
of Metastatic Colorectal Cancer on Pembrolizumab: A Case Report
Reprinted from: *Int. J. Mol. Sci.* **2023**, *24*, 12056, doi:10.3390/ijms241512056 . . . . **165**

About the Editor

Donatella Delle Cave

Donatella Delle Cave is a postdoctoral researcher at the "Institute of Genetics and Biophysics A. Buzzati-Traverso" at the CNR in Naples, Italy. In 2017, she obtained her PhD in "Biochemical and Biotechnological Sciences" at the "Vanvitelli University" in Naples, Italy, and during that period, her project was focused on the study of the antitumorigenic effects of S-Adenosylmethionine in breast cancer cells.

During her post-doc, she acquired a comprehensive and interdisciplinary knowledge of cancer biology, in particular, gastrointestinal tumors, with a specific focus on pancreatic ductal adenocarcinoma (PDAC) and colorectal cancer (CRC). By using a multidisciplinary approach and cutting-edge strategies, which combines omics analyses with cell biology techniques, three dimensional models (spheroids and patients-derived organoids), CRISPR/Cas9 technology, drug delivery nanosystems, and in vivo mouse models (both xenograft and orthotopic), Delle Cave identified specific markers which characterize the subpopulation of cancer stem cells within these tumors. Delle Cave's research has been published in several manuscripts in which she figures as both first and corresponding author. Even as a young postdoctoral researcher, the skills she acquired allowed her to win two fellowships financed by the "Fondazione Italiana per la Ricerca sulle Malattie del Pancreas" (FIMP), two fellowships supported by "Fondazione Umberto Veronesi" (FUV), a research grant financed by FIMP, several travel grants, and a best poster award.

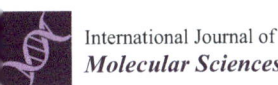

Editorial

Novel Therapeutic Approaches for Colorectal Cancer Treatment

Athanasios G. Papavassiliou [1] and Donatella Delle Cave [2,*]

[1] Department of Biological Chemistry, Medical School, National and Kapodistrian University of Athens, 11527 Athens, Greece; papavas@med.uoa.gr
[2] Institute of Genetics and Biophysics 'Adriano Buzzati-Traverso', CNR, 80131 Naples, Italy
* Correspondence: donatella.dellecave@igb.cnr.it

According to GLOBOCAN 2020 data, colorectal cancer (CRC) represents the third most common malignancy and the second most deadly cancer worldwide [1–3]. In a clinical setting, despite advances in diagnosis and surgical procedures, 20% of patients with CRC present with metastasis at the time of diagnosis due to residual tumor cells that have spread to distant organs prior to surgery, affecting the patient's survival rate [4]. Standard systemic chemotherapy, alternative therapies targeting mechanisms in cancer progression and metastasis, immunotherapy, and combination therapies are the primary strategies for treating CRC [5,6]. Unfortunately, these treatment strategies are expensive and often lack selectivity in targeting cancer cells, leading to severe toxicity in normal tissues and various side effects [7]. The main purpose of this Editorial is to provide a concise and state-of-the-art overview of novel therapeutic approaches for CRC treatment.

Mutations in different signaling pathways contribute to the initiation, progression, and chemoresistance of CRC, and among them, the overactivation of the phosphoinositide 3-kinase (PI3K)/AKT/mechanistic target of rapamycin (mTOR) signaling axis is of pivotal importance for tumorigenicity [8–10]. Although there are conflicting data regarding the effectiveness of agents directed against the PI3K axis in CRC, several studies have shown favorable results for these drugs, whether used in primary or metastatic cases. Among them, Pictilisib, a potent small-molecule class I PI3K inhibitor (PI3Ki), has shown promising results in reducing mucinous colorectal adenocarcinoma (MCA) progression; however, its effectiveness as single-agent therapy is limited due to the potential development of drug-induced resistance [11–13]. Kuracha et al. demonstrated that, in MCA cells, Pictilisib-induced adaptive resistance is regulated by the forkhead box O (FOXO)-dependent rebound activity of receptor tyrosine kinases (RTKs) [14]. The results revealed that pictilisib treatment led to an increased accumulation of nuclear FOXO1 compared to vehicle-treated CRC cells, and the authors proposed FOXO1 as a putative co-target to rescue PI3Ki single-agent resistance in MCA therapy. In CRC, as well as for the majority of tumors, cancer stem cells (CSCs) are recognized as a primary contributor to drug resistance, tumor progression, and metastasis [15–18]. Several signaling pathways are implicated in maintaining cancer stemness; consequently, targeting these pathways emerges as a feasible strategy for eliminating CSCs and potentially tumor eradication [19]. Recently, some studies have shown that CD44, a cell surface glycoprotein, and its isoforms generated from alternative splicing involving standard and variant exons (CD44v) play a crucial role in the progression of CRC [20,21]. Notably, overexpression of CD44v6 is associated with an unfavorable prognosis in CRC patients, influencing adhesion, proliferation, stemness, invasiveness, and chemoresistance [22]. Accordingly, CD44v6 emerges as a promising target for both cancer diagnosis and therapy in CRC. Ejima et al. established a novel anti-CD44mAb, C44Mab-5 (IgG1, kappa), and C44Mab-46 (IgG1, kappa), and they evaluated their applicability through enzyme-linked immunosorbent assay, flow cytometry, western immunoblotting, and immunohistochemical analyses on several CRC cells [23]. Another widely recognized CSCs marker is ATP-binding cassette superfamily G member 2 (ABCG2), a multidrug transporter that mediates the translocation of diverse physiological

Citation: Papavassiliou, A.G.; Delle Cave, D. Novel Therapeutic Approaches for Colorectal Cancer Treatment. *Int. J. Mol. Sci.* **2024**, *25*, 2228. https://doi.org/10.3390/ijms25042228

Received: 1 February 2024
Accepted: 7 February 2024
Published: 13 February 2024

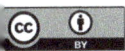

Copyright: © 2024 by the authors. Licensee MDPI, Basel, Switzerland. This article is an open access article distributed under the terms and conditions of the Creative Commons Attribution (CC BY) license (https://creativecommons.org/licenses/by/4.0/).

and xenobiotic substrates across cellular membranes in an ATP-dependent manner [24]. The expression of the *ABCG2* gene has demonstrated negative prognostic implications in various malignancies, while in CRC, its prognostic significance remains undefined [25–27]. By analyzing publicly available datasets, Sałagacka-Kubiak et al. demonstrated that ABCG2 is downregulated in colon and rectum adenocarcinomas, exhibiting lower expression levels compared to both adjacent non-malignant tissues [28]. This deregulation is suggested to be associated with the methylation level of specific sites within the *ABCG2* gene and correlated with microsatellite instability (MSI), weight, and age, whilst in rectum adenocarcinoma patients, it was linked to tumor localization, population type, and age. Furthermore, an ABCG2-centered protein—protein interaction network, constructed using STRING, revealed that the associated proteins are involved in leukotriene, organic anion, xenobiotic transport, endodermal cell-fate specification, as well as histone methylation and ubiquitination. Therefore, the downregulation of ABCG2 may serve as a marker of the activity of specific signaling pathways or protein interactors crucial for colorectal carcinogenesis. Another protein engaged in CRC progression is the muscarinic acetylcholine receptor M3 (M3R) [29–31]. Analyzing 754 surgical CRC tissue samples, Lobbes et al. demonstrated that high expression of M3R correlated with enhanced survivability, particularly in cases with lower tumor grade and a non-mucinous subtype. This association was linked to a more favorable outcome compared to cases with low M3R expression, where survival significantly decreased and higher tumor grade and mucinous subtype were prevalent [32]. Genomic instability is a hallmark of CRC, and metastatic CRC (mCRC) characterized by deficient mismatch repair (dMMR) and MSI can effectively be treated using immune checkpoint inhibitors (ICI) such as pembrolizumab and nivolumab, approved by both the FDA and EMA [12,33,34]. Alternatively, combinations of programmed cell death protein-1 (PD-1) inhibitors with ipilimumab, an antibody targeting cytotoxic T-lymphocyte-associated protein 4 (CTLA-4), have also demonstrated efficacy in this context [35–37]. Krekeler et al. described the case of a 63-year-old male with microsatellite instability (MSI-H) and mCRC associated with Lynch syndrome [38]. The patient experienced rapid normalization of tumor markers and achieved a complete metabolic remission (CMR) that has persisted for ten months. This notable outcome was observed through a sequential ICI treatment approach involving the combination of nivolumab and ipilimumab, followed by nivolumab maintenance therapy after progression on single-agent PD-1 ICI therapy. This represents the first reported instance of sustained metabolic complete remission in an MSI-H mCRC patient who initially showed progression on single-agent anti-PD-1 therapy, suggesting that individuals with dMMR mCRC may have benefited from sequential immune checkpoint regimens, even exhibiting long-term responses.

In conclusion, personalized therapeutic regimens represent the cutting edge in CRC treatment. Strategies focused on targeting patient-specific markers have the potential to augment standard chemotherapy efficacy and mitigate tumor progression.

Author Contributions: Conceptualization, D.D.C.; writing—original draft preparation, D.D.C. and A.G.P.; writing—review and editing, D.D.C. and A.G.P. All authors have read and agreed to the published version of the manuscript.

Acknowledgments: D.D.C. was supported by Fondazione Umberto Veronesi (FUV) and Fondazione Italiana per la ricerca sulle Malattie del Pancreas (FIMP).

Conflicts of Interest: The authors declare no conflicts of interest.

References

1. Xi, Y.; Xu, P. Global Colorectal Cancer Burden in 2020 and Projections to 2040. *Transl. Oncol.* **2021**, *14*, 101174. [CrossRef] [PubMed]
2. Xie, Y. H.; Chen, Y. X.; Fang, J.-Y. Comprehensive Review of Targeted Therapy for Colorectal Cancer. *Signal Transduct. Target. Ther.* **2020**, *5*, 22. [CrossRef]
3. Rawla, P.; Sunkara, T.; Barsouk, A. Epidemiology of Colorectal Cancer: Incidence, Mortality, Survival, and Risk Factors. *Prz. Gastroenterol.* **2019**, *14*, 89–103. [CrossRef] [PubMed]
4. Vatandoust, S. Colorectal Cancer: Metastases to a Single Organ. *WJG* **2015**, *21*, 11767. [CrossRef]

5. Gustavsson, B.; Carlsson, G.; Machover, D.; Petrelli, N.; Roth, A.; Schmoll, H.-J.; Tveit, K.-M.; Gibson, F. A Review of the Evolution of Systemic Chemotherapy in the Management of Colorectal Cancer. *Clin. Color. Cancer* **2015**, *14*, 1–10. [CrossRef]
6. McQuade, R.M.; Stojanovska, V.; Bornstein, J.C.; Nurgali, K. Colorectal Cancer Chemotherapy: The Evolution of Treatment and New Approaches. *CMC* **2017**, *24*, 1537–1557. [CrossRef]
7. Negarandeh, R.; Salehifar, E.; Saghafi, F.; Jalali, H.; Janbabaei, G.; Abdhaghighi, M.J.; Nosrati, A. Evaluation of Adverse Effects of Chemotherapy Regimens of 5-Fluoropyrimidines Derivatives and Their Association with DPYD Polymorphisms in Colorectal Cancer Patients. *BMC Cancer* **2020**, *20*, 560. [CrossRef] [PubMed]
8. Hua, H.; Kong, Q.; Zhang, H.; Wang, J.; Luo, T.; Jiang, Y. Targeting mTOR for Cancer Therapy. *J. Hematol. Oncol.* **2019**, *12*, 71. [CrossRef]
9. Yang, J.; Nie, J.; Ma, X.; Wei, Y.; Peng, Y.; Wei, X. Targeting PI3K in Cancer: Mechanisms and Advances in Clinical Trials. *Mol. Cancer* **2019**, *18*, 26. [CrossRef]
10. Panwar, V.; Singh, A.; Bhatt, M.; Tonk, R.K.; Azizov, S.; Raza, A.S.; Sengupta, S.; Kumar, D.; Garg, M. Multifaceted Role of mTOR (Mammalian Target of Rapamycin) Signaling Pathway in Human Health and Disease. *Signal Transduct. Target. Ther.* **2023**, *8*, 375. [CrossRef]
11. Yue, Q.; Khojasteh, S.C.; Cho, S.; Ma, S.; Mulder, T.; Chen, J.; Pang, J.; Ding, X.; Deese, A.; Pellet, J.D.; et al. Absorption, Metabolism and Excretion of Pictilisib, a Potent Pan-Class I Phosphatidylinositol-3-Kinase (PI3K) Inhibitor, in Rats, Dogs, and Humans. *Xenobiotica* **2021**, *51*, 796–810. [CrossRef]
12. Banerji, U.; Stewart, A.; Coker, E.A.; Minchom, A.; Pölsterl, S.; Georgiou, A.; Al-Lazikani, B. Unravelling the Context Specificity of Signalling in KRAS Mutant Cancers: Implications for Design of Clinical Trials. *Ann. Oncol.* **2018**, *29*, iii7. [CrossRef]
13. Vitiello, P.P.; Cardone, C.; Martini, G.; Ciardiello, D.; Belli, V.; Matrone, N.; Barra, G.; Napolitano, S.; Della Corte, C.; Turano, M.; et al. Receptor Tyrosine Kinase-Dependent PI3K Activation Is an Escape Mechanism to Vertical Suppression of the EGFR/RAS/MAPK Pathway in KRAS-Mutated Human Colorectal Cancer Cell Lines. *J. Exp. Clin. Cancer Res.* **2019**, *38*, 41. [CrossRef]
14. Kuracha, M.R.; Govindarajan, V.; Loggie, B.W.; Tobi, M.; McVicker, B.L. Pictilisib-Induced Resistance Is Mediated through FOXO1-Dependent Activation of Receptor Tyrosine Kinases in Mucinous Colorectal Adenocarcinoma Cells. *IJMS* **2023**, *24*, 12331. [CrossRef]
15. Cavo, M.; Delle Cave, D.; D'Amone, E.; Gigli, G.; Lonardo, E.; del Mercato, L.L. A Synergic Approach to Enhance Long-Term Culture and Manipulation of MiaPaCa-2 Pancreatic Cancer Spheroids. *Sci. Rep.* **2020**, *10*, 10192. [CrossRef]
16. Cave, D.D.; Hernando-Momblona, X.; Sevillano, M.; Minchiotti, G.; Lonardo, E. Nodal-Induced L1CAM/CXCR4 Subpopulation Sustains Tumor Growth and Metastasis in Colorectal Cancer Derived Organoids. *Theranostics* **2021**, *11*, 5686–5699. [CrossRef]
17. Tauriello, D.V.F.; Palomo-Ponce, S.; Stork, D.; Berenguer-Llergo, A.; Badia-Ramentol, J.; Iglesias, M.; Sevillano, M.; Ibiza, S.; Cañellas, A.; Hernando-Momblona, X.; et al. TGFβ Drives Immune Evasion in Genetically Reconstituted Colon Cancer Metastasis. *Nature* **2018**, *554*, 538–543. [CrossRef] [PubMed]
18. Tauriello, D.V.F.; Calon, A.; Lonardo, E.; Batlle, E. Determinants of Metastatic Competency in Colorectal Cancer. *Mol. Oncol.* **2017**, *11*, 97–119. [CrossRef] [PubMed]
19. Liu, Z.; Xu, H.; Weng, S.; Ren, Y.; Han, X. Stemness Refines the Classification of Colorectal Cancer with Stratified Prognosis, Multi-Omics Landscape, Potential Mechanisms, and Treatment Options. *Front. Immunol.* **2022**, *13*, 828330. [CrossRef]
20. Wang, Z.; Tang, Y.; Xie, L.; Huang, A.; Xue, C.; Gu, Z.; Wang, K.; Zong, S. The Prognostic and Clinical Value of CD44 in Colorectal Cancer: A Meta-Analysis. *Front. Oncol.* **2019**, *9*, 309. [CrossRef] [PubMed]
21. Todaro, M.; Gaggianesi, M.; Catalano, V.; Benfante, A.; Iovino, F.; Biffoni, M.; Apuzzo, T.; Sperduti, I.; Volpe, S.; Cocorullo, G.; et al. CD44v6 Is a Marker of Constitutive and Reprogrammed Cancer Stem Cells Driving Colon Cancer Metastasis. *Cell Stem Cell* **2014**, *14*, 342–356. [CrossRef]
22. Ma, L.; Dong, L.; Chang, P. CD44v6 Engages in Colorectal Cancer Progression. *Cell Death Dis.* **2019**, *10*, 30. [CrossRef]
23. Ejima, R.; Suzuki, H.; Tanaka, T.; Asano, T.; Kaneko, M.K.; Kato, Y. Development of a Novel Anti-CD44 Variant 6 Monoclonal Antibody C44Mab-9 for Multiple Applications against Colorectal Carcinomas. *IJMS* **2023**, *24*, 4007. [CrossRef]
24. Robey, R.W.; Polgar, O.; Deeken, J.; To, K.W.; Bates, S.E. ABCG2: Determining Its Relevance in Clinical Drug Resistance. *Cancer Metastasis Rev.* **2007**, *26*, 39–57. [CrossRef]
25. Wang, X.; Xia, B.; Liang, Y.; Peng, L.; Wang, Z.; Zhuo, J.; Wang, W.; Jiang, B. Membranous ABCG2 Expression in Colorectal Cancer Independently Correlates with Shortened Patient Survival. *CBM* **2013**, *13*, 81–88. [CrossRef]
26. Cave, D.D.; Di Guida, M.; Costa, V.; Sevillano, M.; Ferrante, L.; Heeschen, C.; Corona, M.; Cucciardi, A.; Lonardo, E. TGF-B1 Secreted by Pancreatic Stellate Cells Promotes Stemness and Tumourigenicity in Pancreatic Cancer Cells through L1CAM Downregulation. *Oncogene* **2020**, *39*, 4271–4285. [CrossRef]
27. Cave, D.D.; Buonaiuto, S.; Sainz, B.; Fantuz, M.; Mangini, M.; Carrer, A.; Di Domenico, A.; Iavazzo, T.T.; Andolfi, G.; Cortina, C.; et al. LAMC2 Marks a Tumor-Initiating Cell Population with an Aggressive Signature in Pancreatic Cancer. *J. Exp. Clin. Cancer Res.* **2022**, *41*, 315. [CrossRef] [PubMed]
28. Sałagacka-Kubiak, A.; Zawada, D.; Saed, L.; Kordek, R.; Jeleń, A.; Balcerczak, E. ABCG2 Gene and ABCG2 Protein Expression in Colorectal Cancer—In Silico and Wet Analysis. *IJMS* **2023**, *24*, 10539. [CrossRef] [PubMed]

29. Kuol, N.; Godlewski, J.; Kmiec, Z.; Vogrin, S.; Fraser, S.; Apostolopoulos, V.; Nurgali, K. Cholinergic Signaling Influences the Expression of Immune Checkpoint Inhibitors, PD-L1 and PD-L2, and Tumor Hallmarks in Human Colorectal Cancer Tissues and Cell Lines. *BMC Cancer* **2023**, *23*, 971. [CrossRef] [PubMed]
30. Carroll, R.C. The M3 Muscarinic Acetylcholine Receptor Differentially Regulates Calcium Influx and Release through Modulation of Monovalent Cation Channels. *EMBO J.* **1998**, *17*, 3036–3044. [CrossRef] [PubMed]
31. Cheng, K.; Xie, G.; Khurana, S.; Heath, J.; Drachenberg, C.B.; Timmons, J.; Shah, N.; Raufman, J.-P. Divergent Effects of Muscarinic Receptor Subtype Gene Ablation on Murine Colon Tumorigenesis Reveals Association of M3R and Zinc Finger Protein 277 Expression in Colon Neoplasia. *Mol. Cancer* **2014**, *13*, 77. [CrossRef] [PubMed]
32. Lobbes, L.A.; Schütze, M.A.; Droeser, R.; Arndt, M.; Pozios, I.; Lauscher, J.C.; Hering, N.A.; Weixler, B. Muscarinic Acetylcholine Receptor M3 Expression and Survival in Human Colorectal Carcinoma—An Unexpected Correlation to Guide Future Treatment? *IJMS* **2023**, *24*, 8198. [CrossRef] [PubMed]
33. Pino, M.S.; Chung, D.C. The Chromosomal Instability Pathway in Colon Cancer. *Gastroenterology* **2010**, *138*, 2059–2072. [CrossRef] [PubMed]
34. Ferguson, L.R.; Chen, H.; Collins, A.R.; Connell, M.; Damia, G.; Dasgupta, S.; Malhotra, M.; Meeker, A.K.; Amedei, A.; Amin, A.; et al. Genomic Instability in Human Cancer: Molecular Insights and Opportunities for Therapeutic Attack and Prevention through Diet and Nutrition. *Semin. Cancer Biol.* **2015**, *35*, S5–S24. [CrossRef]
35. Martins, F.; Sofiya, L.; Sykiotis, G.P.; Lamine, F.; Maillard, M.; Fraga, M.; Shabafrouz, K.; Ribi, C.; Cairoli, A.; Guex-Crosier, Y.; et al. Adverse Effects of Immune-Checkpoint Inhibitors: Epidemiology, Management and Surveillance. *Nat. Rev. Clin. Oncol.* **2019**, *16*, 563–580. [CrossRef]
36. Wong, S.K.; Beckermann, K.E.; Johnson, D.B.; Das, S. Combining Anti-Cytotoxic T-Lymphocyte Antigen 4 (CTLA-4) and -Programmed Cell Death Protein 1 (PD-1) Agents for Cancer Immunotherapy. *Expert. Opin. Biol. Ther.* **2021**, *21*, 1623–1634. [CrossRef]
37. Yin, Q.; Wu, L.; Han, L.; Zheng, X.; Tong, R.; Li, L.; Bai, L.; Bian, Y. Immune-Related Adverse Events of Immune Checkpoint Inhibitors: A Review. *Front. Immunol.* **2023**, *14*, 1167975. [CrossRef]
38. Krekeler, C.; Wethmar, K.; Mikesch, J.-H.; Kerkhoff, A.; Menck, K.; Lenz, G.; Schildhaus, H.-U.; Wessolly, M.; Hoffmann, M.W.; Pascher, A.; et al. Complete Metabolic Response to Combined Immune Checkpoint Inhibition after Progression of Metastatic Colorectal Cancer on Pembrolizumab: A Case Report. *IJMS* **2023**, *24*, 12056. [CrossRef]

Disclaimer/Publisher's Note: The statements, opinions and data contained in all publications are solely those of the individual author(s) and contributor(s) and not of MDPI and/or the editor(s). MDPI and/or the editor(s) disclaim responsibility for any injury to people or property resulting from any ideas, methods, instructions or products referred to in the content.

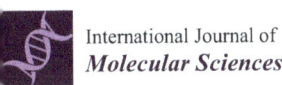

Article

Bafilomycin A1 Molecular Effect on ATPase Activity of Subcellular Fraction of Human Colorectal Cancer and Rat Liver

Solomiia Bychkova [1], Mykola Bychkov [2], Dani Dordevic [3], Monika Vítězová [4], Simon K.-M. R. Rittmann [5,*] and Ivan Kushkevych [4,*]

1. Department of Human and Animal Physiology, Faculty of Biology, Ivan Franko National University of Lviv, 79005 Lviv, Ukraine; solomiya.bychkova@lnu.edu.ua
2. Department of Therapy No. 1, Medical Diagnostic and Hematology and Transfusiology of Faculty of Postgraduate Education, Danylo Halytsky Lviv National Medical University, 79010 Lviv, Ukraine; mbychkov21@gmail.com
3. Department of Plant Origin Food Sciences, Faculty of Veterinary Hygiene and Ecology, University of Veterinary Sciences Brno, 612 42 Brno, Czech Republic; dordevicd@vfu.cz
4. Department of Experimental Biology, Faculty of Science, Masaryk University, 625 00 Brno, Czech Republic; vitezova@sci.muni.cz
5. Department of Functional and Evolutionary Ecology, Archaea Physiology & Biotechnology Group, Universität Wien, 1030 Wien, Austria
* Correspondence: simon.rittmann@univie.ac.at (S.K.-M.R.R.); kushkevych@mail.muni.cz (I.K.); Tel.: +420-549-49-5315 (I.K.)

Abstract: Bafilomycin A1 inhibits V-type H$^+$ ATPases on the molecular level, which acidifies endolysosomes. The main objective of the study was to assess the effect of bafilomycin A1 on Ca^{2+} content, NAADP-induced Ca^{2+} release, and ATPase activity in rat hepatocytes and human colon cancer samples. Chlortetracycline (CTC) was used for a quantitative measure of stored calcium in permeabilized rat hepatocytes. ATPase activity was determined by orthophosphate content released after ATP hydrolysis in subcellular post-mitochondrial fraction obtained from rat liver as well as from patients' samples of colon mucosa and colorectal cancer samples. In rat hepatocytes, bafilomycin A1 decreased stored Ca^{2+} and prevented the effect of NAADP on stored Ca^{2+}. This effect was dependent on EGTA–Ca^{2+} buffers in the medium. Bafilomycin A1 significantly increased the activity of Ca^{2+} ATPases of endoplasmic reticulum (EPR), but not plasma membrane (PM) Ca^{2+} ATPases in rat liver. Bafilomycin A1 also prevented the effect of NAADP on these pumps. In addition, bafilomycin A1 reduced Na$^+$/K$^+$ ATPase activity and increased basal Mg^{2+} ATPase activity in the subcellular fraction of rat liver. Concomitant administration of bafilomycin A1 and NAADP enhanced these effects. Bafilomycin A1 increased the activity of the Ca^{2+} ATPase of EPR in the subcellular fraction of normal human colon mucosa and also in colon cancer tissue samples. In contrast, it decreased Ca^{2+} ATPase PM activity in samples of normal human colon mucosa and caused no changes in colon cancer. Bafilomycin A1 decreased Na$^+$/K$^+$ ATPase activity and increased basal Mg^{2+} ATPase activity in normal colon mucosa samples and in human colon cancer samples. It can be concluded that bafilomycin A1 targets NAADP-sensitive acidic Ca^{2+} stores, effectively modulates ATPase activity, and assumes the link between acidic stores and EPR. Bafilomycin A1 may be useful for cancer therapy.

Keywords: molecular mechanisms; colon cancer; ATPase; autophagy; hepatocytes; liver; NAADP; biomarkers; bafilomycin A1; Ca^{2+} store

Citation: Bychkova, S.; Bychkov, M.; Dordevic, D.; Vítězová, M.; Rittmann, S.K.-M.R.; Kushkevych, I. Bafilomycin A1 Molecular Effect on ATPase Activity of Subcellular Fraction of Human Colorectal Cancer and Rat Liver. *Int. J. Mol. Sci.* **2024**, *25*, 1657. https://doi.org/10.3390/ijms25031657

Academic Editor: Donatella Delle Cave

Received: 10 January 2024
Revised: 24 January 2024
Accepted: 25 January 2024
Published: 29 January 2024

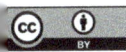

Copyright: © 2024 by the authors. Licensee MDPI, Basel, Switzerland. This article is an open access article distributed under the terms and conditions of the Creative Commons Attribution (CC BY) license (https://creativecommons.org/licenses/by/4.0/).

1. Introduction

A class of macrolide antibiotics known as bafilomycins is created from several different streptomycetes. These compounds' chemical structure is determined by a 16-membered lactone ring scaffold. A variety of biological activities, including anti-parasitic, anti-tumor, immunosuppressive, and anti-fungal action, are connected with bafilomycins [1].

Bafilomycin A1 is widely used as an autophagy inhibitor in various tissues [2–4]. In addition, bafilomycin A1 is also used as a specific inhibitor of V-type H$^+$ ATPase [5,6], which pumps protons into the lumen of organelles such as lysosomes [7]. It is well known that endosomes and lysosomes are important membrane-bound organelles that are essential for the normal functioning of the eukaryotic cell. Interaction disruption between endosomes and lysosomes may contribute to cancer development [8].

By preventing V-ATPase-dependent acidification and autophagosome-lysosome fusion, bafilomycin A1 has been demonstrated to interfere with autophagic flux [9]. Because autophagy involves the recycling of organelles and lysosomal breakdown, it is thought to be a crucial survival strategy for both cancerous and healthy cells. Research has demonstrated that bafilomycin A1-induced macroautophagy suppression reduces colon cancer cell proliferation and triggers apoptosis [10], suppresses the growth of HCC cells [11], inhibits autophagy flux in diffuse large B-cell lymphoma [12], and inhibits respiration in mitochondria of Nemeth-Kellner lymphoma [13]. Thus, bafilomycin A1 could be an effective therapeutic agent in cancer therapy [14]. Furthermore, bafilomycin A1 inhibited autophagosome–lysosome fusion and acidification, which resulted in a marked rise in cytosolic calcium concentration [9]. These acidic organelles are known to contain high amounts of Ca^{2+} [15]. Faris and others demonstrated that nicotinic acid adenine dinucleotide phosphate (NAADP) induces intracellular Ca^{2+} release in primary cultures of metastatic colorectal cancer Ca^{2+} imaging and molecular biology techniques [16]. The ATPase activity of the subcellular fraction of human colon cancer samples has recently been revealed to be impacted by NAADP, which helps to stimulate Ca^{2+} release from acidic organelles [17]. Bafilomycin A1 has been shown to inhibit NAADP-induced Ca^{2+} release from these organelles in rat hepatocytes [18], though it is unknown how bafilomycin A1 affects ATPase activity in cancer tissues.

Ca^{2+} ATPases are in charge of creating sharp Ca^{2+} gradients across intracellular membranes or the plasma membrane and preserving a low baseline Ca^{2+} level in the cytoplasm. [19], and remodeling Ca^{2+} signaling is an important step in cancer progression [19–21]. The growth of cancer is facilitated by changes in colon cancer cells' expression of the plasma Ca^{2+} pump (PMCA) and the corresponding modifications in the calcium released by the cell [21,22]. Differentiation of HT-29 colon cancer cells is associated with the upregulation of PMCA4, but no significant change in PMCA1 [22]. It was found that the simultaneous presence of bafilomycin A1 and NAADP completely inhibits PMCA activity in mouse NK/Ly cells [23], but the effect of bafilomycin A1 on PMCA activity in human colon cancer has not been studied.

Maintenance of high endoplasmic reticulum calcium concentration through the action of sarco/endoplasmic reticulum calcium ATPases (SERCAs) is critical for many cellular functions involved in intracellular signaling, control of proliferation, programmed cell death, or synthesis of mature proteins [24]. Increased expression of SERCA 2 was found in human colorectal cancer and was associated with advanced tumor stage and tumorigenesis [25]. Meanwhile, in several other cancers, SERCA3 expression is selectively downregulated [24]. We found that NAADP decreased the activity of SERCA and basal Mg^{2+} ATPase in the post-mitochondrial fraction of mouse lymphomas, and bafilomycin A1 prevented the effects of NAADP on the activity of these pumps [13]. This confirmed the function of these pumps in the context of bafilomycin-sensitive acid stores. Recently, it was found that NAADP causes a decrease in Ca^{2+} ATPase EPR activities and an increase in basal ATPase activity in human colon cancer samples [17], but the effect of bafilomycin A1 on the activity of these pumps has not been studied. It is known that Na$^+$/K$^+$ ATPases are crucial for cancer cell adhesion, motility, and migration [20,26]. Inhibitors of Na$^+$/K$^+$ ATPase (ouabain and digoxin) showed anti-tumor effects on multicellular tumor spheroids of hepatocellular carcinoma [27], and another inhibitor (gentiopicrin) exerted anticancer activity on human colon cancer [28]. Such glycosides as gentiopicrin are known to be used in traditional medicine for the treatment of heart disease, as they selectively inhibit Na$^+$/K$^+$ ATPase and increase intracellular Ca^{2+} concentration.

NAADP decreased Na$^+$/K$^+$ ATPase activity in mouse NK/Ly cells [13], and the simultaneous presence of bafilomycin A1 and NAADP caused a stronger inhibition of Na$^+$/K$^+$ ATPase activity and, at the same time, a strong decrease in molecular oxygen consumption in mitochondria and uncoupling of oxidative phosphorylation and respiration was observed in mouse NK/Ly cells [13]. Moreover, there was a dramatic decrease in Na$^+$/K$^+$ ATPase activity by application of NAADP, which could be explained by the release of Ca^{2+} from acid stores by NAADP in human colon cancer tissue samples [17]. Thus, attacking acid stores is an effective tool in cancer therapy. The effect of bafilomycin A1 on Na$^+$/K$^+$ ATPase activities in human colon cancer remains unexplored.

Therefore, the primary goal of the investigation was to determine the functional connections between acid Ca^{2+} storage (endo-lysosomes), extracellular phosphatase (EPR), and other active ion transport systems (ATPases) by examining the impact of bafilomycin A1 on Ca^{2+} content, NAADP-induced Ca^{2+} release, and ATPase activity in rat hepatocytes. The study also included an investigation into the impact of bafilomycin A1 on ATPase activity in human colon cancer samples to evaluate its potential use as a pharmacological agent in cancer therapy.

2. Results

2.1. Bafilomycin A1 Effect on ATPase Activity in Subcellular Fraction of Human Colon Mucosal Tissue Samples and Colorectal Cancer Tissue Samples

It was found that the average Na$^+$/K$^+$ ATPase activity in the human colon mucosa samples was 4.00 ± 0.61 μmol P$_i$/mg protein per h. After the addition of bafilomycin A1 (0.001 mM) to the incubation solution of the post-mitochondrial subcellular fraction, this index decreased to 2.43 ± 0.23 μmol P$_i$/mg protein per h. Consequently, 1.6 times less Na$^+$/K$^+$ ATPase activity was seen in the subcellular portion of human colon mucosal tissue when bafilomycin A1 (0.001 mM) was added ($n = 10$; $p \leq 0.05$) (Figure 1).

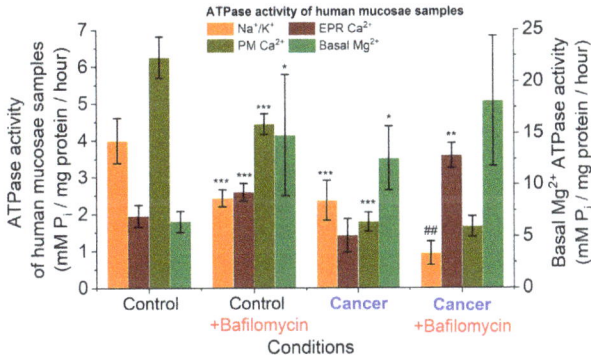

Figure 1. ATPase activity of subcellular fraction of colorectal cancer samples (cancer) and unchanged tissue (control): *** $p \leq 0.001$ vs. control; ** $p \leq 0.01$ vs. control; * $p \leq 0.05$ vs. control, ## $p \leq 0.05$ vs. cancer.

In the subcellular fraction of human colon cancer samples, the average Na$^+$/K$^+$ ATPase activity was 2.37 ± 0.34 μmol P$_i$/mg protein per h. Bafilomycin A1 (0.001 mM) caused the statistically significant ($n = 10$; $p \leq 0.05$) decrease in this index to 0.94 ± 0.32 μmol P$_i$/mg protein per h. Thus, bafilomycin A1 (0.001 mM) decreased Na$^+$/K$^+$ ATPase activity in the subcellular fraction of human colorectal cancer samples by 2.52 folds. This effect is more pronounced than in samples of healthy mucosa.

The median gene expression of Na$^+$/K$^+$-ATPase subunits (Figure 2) of colon tumor vs. normal samples for Na$^+$/K$^+$ ATPase (ATP1A1)—2.88-fold increase in cancer (535.19 cancer/186.04 normal); Na$^+$/K$^+$ ATPase (ATP1B1)—3.47-fold increase in cancer (235.35 cancer/67.88 normal); Na$^+$/K$^+$ ATPase (ATP1B3)—1.46-fold increase in cancer

(174.84 cancer/119.05 normal) according to Gepia (http://gepia.cancer-pku.cn/detail.php? gene, accessed on 9 January 2024).

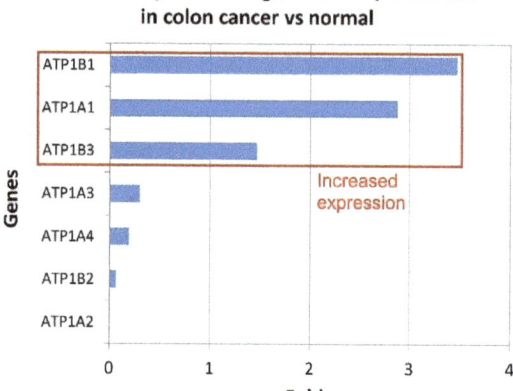

Figure 2. Increased expression of Na^+/K^+ ATPase' genes subunits in colon cancer vs. normal (according to Gepia (http://gepia.cancer-pku.cn/detail.php?gene, accessed on 9 January 2024).

In the human colon mucosa samples, the values of endoplasmic reticulum Ca^{2+} ATPase of EPR activity were 1.95 ± 0.30 µmol P_i/mg protein per h (Figure 1). After the addition of bafilomycin A1 (0.001 mM), the activity of EPR Ca^{2+} ATPase increased to 2.59 ± 0.24 µmol P_i/mg protein per h. Thus, bafilomycin A1 increased the activity of Ca^{2+} ATPase of EPR by 1.32-fold in the colon mucosa tissue samples ($n = 10$; $p \leq 0.05$). In human colon cancer samples, Ca^{2+} ATPase EPR activity was 1.42 ± 0.45 µM µmol P_i/mg protein per h (Figure 1). After the addition of bafilomycin A1 (0.001 mM) to the incubation medium of the cancer tissue samples, the average value of ATPase activity was 3.59 ± 0.34 µmol P_i/mg protein per h. Thus, bafilomycin A1 (0.001 mM) statistically ($n = 10$; $p \leq 0.05$) increased the activity of Ca^{2+} ATPase EPR in colon cancer tissue samples by 2.58-fold. In human colon mucosal tissue samples, plasmatic membrane (PM) Ca^{2+} ATPase activity was 6.25 ± 0.56 µmol P_i/mg protein per h. Under the influence of bafilomycin A1, the activity of the Ca^{2+} ATPase of the PM was 4.44 ± 0.28 µmol P_i/mg protein per h. Thus, bafilomycin A1 (0.001 mM) decreased PM Ca^{2+} ATPase activity 1.40-fold in human intestinal mucosal tissue samples ($n = 10$; $p \leq 0.05$). In human colon cancer samples, PM Ca^{2+} ATPase activity averaged 1.79 ± 0.26 µmol P_i/mg protein per h. After the addition of bafilomycin A1, the average Ca^{2+} ATPase activity of PM was 1.66 ± 0.28 µmol P_i/mg protein per h. Thus, bafilomycin A1 caused no changes in the Ca^{2+} ATPase activity of PM in the cancer tissue samples. In the colon mucosa tissue samples, the basal ATPase activity was 6.41 ± 1.03 µmol P_i/mg protein per h.

When bafilomycin (0.001 mM) was added, the basal ATPase activity increased to 14.78 ± 6.21 µM µmol P_i/mg protein per h. Thus, bafilomycin A1 increased basal ATPase activity 2.30-fold in human intestinal mucosal tissue samples ($n = 10$; $p \leq 0.05$). In colon cancer tissue samples, the indicators of basal ATPase activity varied from 2.10 to 25.63 and averaged 12.56 ± 3.11 µmol P_i/mg protein per h (see Figure 1). When bafilomycin A1 (0.001 mM) was added to the cancer samples, the indicators of ATPase activity ranged from 3.34 to 35.72, with an average value of 18.60 ± 6.29 µmol P_i/mg protein per h. Thus, the results are underlying the statistically 1.48-fold increase in basal ATPase activity of human colon cancer tissue samples by bafilomycin A1 ($n = 10$; $p \leq 0.05$).

2.2. Modulation of ATPase Activity by Bafilomycin A1 and Its Impact on NAADP-Induced Effects in Subcellular Rat Liver Fractions

To investigate the effect of bafilomycin A1 (0.001 mM) on ATPase activity, the post-mitochondrial subcellular fraction of rat liver obtained by the differential centrifugation method was used. The results indicate that the mean activity of Na^+/K^+ ATPase of the post-mitochondrial fraction in rat liver was 3.20 ± 0.24 µmol P_i/mg protein per h ($n = 6$) in the control (Figure 3).

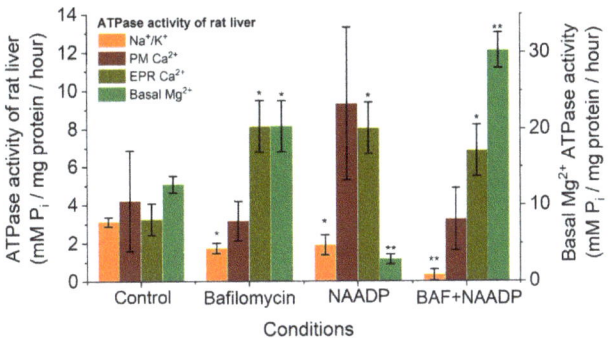

Figure 3. Simultaneous effect of bafilomycin A1 (0.001 mM) and NAADP (7 µM) on ATPase activity of rat liver post mitochondrial fraction: * $p \leq 0.05$ vs. control; ** $p \leq 0.01$ vs. control.

Bafilomycin A 1 (0.001 mM) addition to the incubation medium of the post-mitochondrial fraction of rat liver resulted in a decrease in the mean activity of Na^+/K^+ ATPase to 1.95 ± 0.98 µmol P_i/mg protein per h ($n = 6$). Thus, bafilomycin A 1 (0.001 mM) reduced Na^+/K^+ ATPase activity by 41.67% ($p > 0.05$) in the post-mitochondrial fraction of rat liver. Bafilomycin A1 (0.001 mM) significantly increased the activity of Ca^{2+} ATPases of EPR in the subcellular fraction of rat liver from 3.03 ± 0.93 to 8.09 ± 4.47 µmol P_i/mg protein per h. This was an approximately three-fold increase in Ca^{2+} pump activity of EPR ($p \leq 0.05$, $n = 6$). In contrast, bafilomycin A1 (0.001 mM) did not statistically alter PM Ca^{2+} ATPase activity of the post-mitochondrial fraction in rat liver, but it increased basal Mg^{2+} ATPase activity more than two-fold from 12.26 ± 1.29 to 20.33 ± 2.50 µmol P_i/mg protein per h ($p \leq 0.05$, $n = 6$) (Figure 3).

Simultaneous addition of bafilomycin A1 (0.001 mM) and NAADP (7 µM) to the incubation medium caused a greater decrease in the activity of Na^+/K^+ pumps of the rat liver subcellular fraction compared with the control (0.33 ± 0.29 µmol Pi/mg protein per h) ($p \leq 0.05$, $n = 6$). NAADP and bafilomycin A1 caused a greater increase in basal ATPase activity to 30.24 ± 2.32 µmol P_i/mg protein per h, statistically significant compared with both the medium containing NAADP alone and bafilomycin A1 alone. The activity of Ca^{2+} ATPases of PM in the simultaneous presence of bafilomycin A1 and NAADP in the incubation medium was 3.25 ± 1.63 µmol P_i/mg protein per h. This was statistically significant ($p \leq 0.05$) compared with the medium containing bafilomycin A1 alone and much lower compared with the medium containing NAADP. The activity of the Ca^{2+} ATPases EPR of the rat liver subcellular fraction was 6.85 ± 2.57 µmol P_i/mg protein per h when bafilomycin A1 and NAADP were added simultaneously to the incubation medium (see Figure 3). This was not statistically authentic to the medium with NAADP or to the medium with bafilomycin A1 alone. Thus, bafilomycin A1 also prevented the effect of NAADP on the activity of the Ca^{2+} ATPases of EPR in rat liver.

2.3. Bafilomycin Affected Stored Calcium Content and Prevented NAADP-Induced Changes of Stored Calcium in Rat Hepatocytes

In the first phase of our investigation, we assessed the effects of bafilomycin in a medium without EGTA–Ca^{2+} buffer on the calcium content in permeabilized rat hepatocytes as well as the simultaneous effects of bafilomycin (20, 0.001 mM) and NAADP on the calcium content in the permeabilized rat (Figure 4).

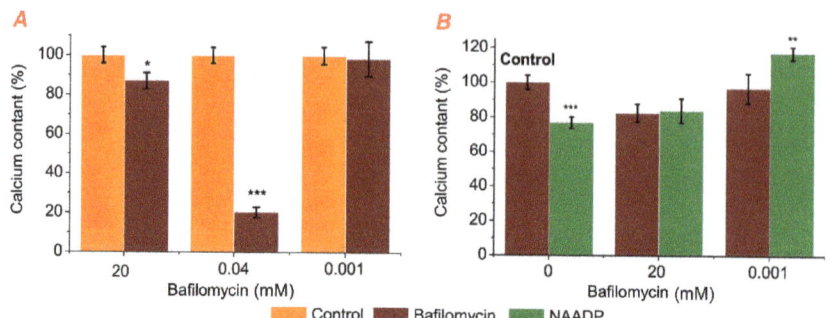

Figure 4. Bafilomycin (20; 0.04; 0.001 mM) addition effect in the medium without EGTA–Ca^{2+} buffers on calcium content in permeabilized rat hepatocytes (**A**) and simultaneous effect of bafilomycin (20, 0.001 mM) and NAADP (7 µM) on calcium content in permeabilized rat hepatocytes (**B**): * $p \leq 0.05$ vs. control, ** $p \leq 0.01$ vs. NAADP, *** $p \leq 0.001$ vs. control.

To find out the effect of bafilomycin A1 on endo-lysosomal stores, its effect on Ca^{2+} content in permeabilized rat hepatocytes was investigated. Bafilomycin A1 at different concentrations (20; 0.04; 0.001 mM) was used to study its effect on stored calcium in permeabilized rat hepatocytes incubated in a medium without EGTA–Ca^{2+} buffer. We observed that bafilomycin A1 significantly decreased CTC–Ca^{2+} chemiluminescence in the millimolar concentration range (20 and 0.04 mM), corresponding to the decrease in the content of Ca^{2+} in intracellular organelles of permeabilized rat hepatocytes. The amount of calcium that was stored remained unchanged despite the reduced bafilomycin A1 concentration (0.001 mM) (Figure 4A).

To investigate the relationships between NAADP-sensitive stores and bafilomycin-sensitive ones, we used these two drugs in the incubation medium. No changes in stored calcium were observed in permeabilized hepatocytes incubated in the medium with simultaneous presence of bafilomycin A1 (20 mM) and NAADP (7 µM) compared with the medium with only bafilomycin A1 (Figure 4B). The simultaneous effect of a lower concentration of Bafilomycin A1 (0.001 mM) and NAADP (7 µM) resulted in a statistically significant increase in stored calcium by 40.23 ± 3.47% ($p \geq 0.001$) compared to the medium with bafilomycin A1 (0.001 mM) alone. These series of experiments were performed in an incubation solution without chelating agents. Previously, we found that NAADP releases Ca^{2+} in permeabilized rat hepatocytes and that the NAADP-induced changes in Ca^{2+} storage in these cells depend on the concentration of EGTA–Ca^{2+} buffer in the cell incubation medium.

A series of experiments were conducted using EGTA–Ca^{2+} buffers to change the concentration of free calcium in the incubation medium in order to control the amount of calcium present better (Figure 5).

Ca^{2+} salts (0.050 mM) and EGTA (0.100 mM) were present in high amounts in medium A, while EGTA (0.05 mM) and Ca^{2+} salts (0.025 mM) were present in lower concentrations in medium B. The EGTA–Ca^{2+} buffer solution kept the concentration of free calcium constant in both situations at 240 nM, which is the hepatocytes' physiological resting state.

In any solution containing Ca^{2+} chelators, bafilomycin A1 (0.001 mM) did not affect the amount of calcium that was stored in rat hepatocytes (see Figure 4). The impact of NAADP was influenced by the concentration of EGTA, as we have found in our previous work [18]. In medium B with low EGTA content as well as in medium without chelators, NAADP (7 µM) led to a reduction in calcium that was stored. When bafilomycin A1 (0.001 mM) and NAADP (7 µM) were mixed, we discovered that the calcium content increased by 41.36 ± 3.92% ($p \geq 0.001$) compared to NAADP alone (Figure 5B). However, this effect was not statistically significant against either the control or bafilomycin A1. Consequently, it was found that bafilomycin A1 (0.001 mM) blocked NAADP's effects across all medium types.

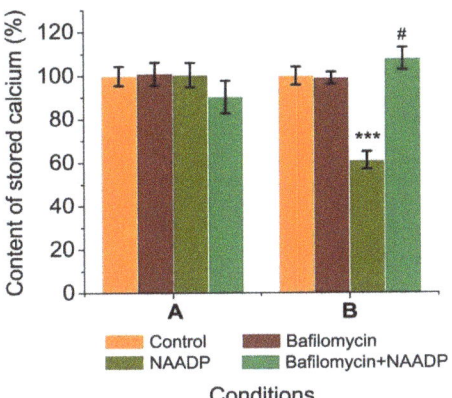

Figure 5. Simultaneous effect of bafilomycin (0.001 mM) and NAADP (7 µM) on calcium content (%) in permeabilized rat hepatocytes in the medium with different EGTA–Ca^{2+} buffers: [Ca^{2+}]$_{cyt.}$ = 243 nM (EGTA: 100 µM, CaCl$_2$: 50 µM) (A); [Ca^{2+}]$_{cyt.}$ = 240 nM (EGTA: 50 µM, CaCl$_2$: 25 µM) (B). *** $p \leq 0.001$ vs. control; # $p \leq 0.01$ vs. NAADP.

3. Discussion

Previously, we found that NAADP affects ATPase activity in cancer samples, probably due to Ca^{2+} release from acidic stores, as we had suspected [17]. In this article, we investigated the effect of bafilomycin A1 on the ATPase activity of human colon cancer tissue samples. It is well known that differentiation of colorectal cancer cells is associated with altered Ca^{2+} homeostasis and expression of specific sarcoplasmic/endoplasmic reticulum calcium ATPase (ERCA) isoforms [21]. Changes in SERCA expression and activity cause cellular cancer, induce ER stress, and trigger apoptosis linked to ER stress. [29]. In addition to the Ca^{2+} ATPase of the EPR (SERCA), the important role of the Ca^{2+} ATPase of the PM (PMCA) has also been demonstrated, playing an important role in remodeling Ca^{2+} homeostasis in human colon cancer cells [22].

We observed a three-fold higher activity of Ca^{2+} ATPase of PM compared with the activity of Ca^{2+} ATPase of EPR in normal human colon mucosa (6.25 ± 0.56 vs. 1.95 ± 0.30 µmol P$_i$/mg protein per h) (Figure 1). However, in colon cancer tissue samples, the activity of these two pumps was low (1.79 ± 0.26 µmol P$_i$/mg protein per h for PMCA). At the same time, the activity of the Ca^{2+} ATPase of EPR (SERCA) only tended to decrease and remained low in colon cancer tissues (1.42 ± 0.45 µmol P$_i$/mg protein per h). It is important to note that the activity of PMCA was reduced more than 3.5-fold in cancer tissue compared to healthy mucosa (Figure 1). Our results are consistent with other studies on colorectal cancer that have shown lower PMCA4 expression in tumors compared to normal tissues [21,30,31], and loss of SERCA3 expression was an early event during colon carcinogenesis [24,32]. Additionally, it has been shown that the expression of the SERCA3 protein is down-regulated in gastric and colorectal cancer cell lines, indicating that cell differentiation in vitro enhances its expression [33]. Moreover, the expression of Ca^{2+} pumps was shown to be highly regulated in breast cancer cells in a subtype-specific manner [34]. Thus, we observed decreased activity of both Ca^{2+} ATPase of EPR and PM in cancer tissues compared to normal human mucosa, which is consistent with protein expression data obtained by other research groups. It was found here that bafilomycin A1 (Figure 1) effectively increased EPR Ca^{2+} ATPase activity in both normal human mucosa and colon cancer tissue samples by 1.32-fold in colon mucosa tissue samples ($n = 10$; $p \leq 0.05$) and by 2.58-fold ($n = 10$; $p \leq 0.05$) in colon cancer tissue samples. We hypothesize that this is due to the release of Ca^{2+} from endo-lysosomal stores due to inhibition of the H^+ pump by bafilomycin A1, resulting in locally high Ca^{2+} concentrations that activate the Ca^{2+} ATPase of the EPR. This is further confirmation of a very close and strong contact site between these different Ca^{2+} pools (lysosomes and EPR), which are still present even in the subcellular fraction under these experimental conditions. A clearly visible membrane contact sites between lysosomes and ER membranes in human cardiac mesenchymal stromal cells were recently confirmed by transmission electron microscopy [16,35], and early similar nanojunctions between lysosomes and sarcoplasmic reticulum were shown in pulmonary artery smooth muscle cells [36]. Therefore, bafilomycin A1 increases the activity of the EPR Ca^{2+} pump due to tight colocalization of EPR membranes with lysosomes. Based on our experimental data, we hypothesized that there are similar contact sites between bafilomycin-sensitive acidic stores and EPR in the subcellular fraction of normal human intestinal mucosa as in colorectal cancer. This assumption is consistent with the observations of other research groups [35–37].

We also observed that bafilomycin A1 decreased the activity of Ca^{2+} ATPase of PM by 1.40-fold in human colon mucosa tissue samples ($n = 10$; $p \leq 0.05$). This may be due to the fact that bafilomycin A1 induces a significantly lower cytosolic pH due to the inhibition of the H^+ pump of the acidic store. It is known that cytosolic acidification can inhibit PMCA [38], just as PMCA simultaneously affects intracellular Ca^{2+} regulation and pH [39].

It was also shown that in the subcellular fraction of human colorectal tissue samples bafilomycin A1 did not alter the activity of Ca^{2+} ATPase of PM (Figure 1). We hypothesized that the Ca^{2+} ATPase of PM in cancer cells is not in close colocalization with the endo lysosomal system, possibly as a consequence of a disturbance in membrane circulation. It was found that the activity of basal Mg^{2+} ATPase was two-fold higher in the subcellular fraction of human colorectal cancer tissue samples than in normal mucosa tissue.

It was observed that bafilomycin A1 increased basal ATPase activity in normal human intestinal mucosal tissue samples as well as in human colon cancer tissue samples. This effect could not be related to the release of Ca^{2+} from acidic stores because basal Mg^{2+} ATPase activity was estimated in solution with EGTA. The effect of bafilomycin A1 on basal Mg^{2+} ATPase activity is realized by a change in pH due to inhibition of the H^+ pump. It was shown that the pH dependence of the enzymatic activity of basal Mg^{2+} ATPase was not bell-shaped [40] but was characterized by the linearity in the range of values of hydrogen index 6.0–8.0 [41].

It was found that the activity of Na^+/K^+ ATPase of the subcellular fraction was higher in the human colon mucosa samples than in the colon cancer samples (4.00 ± 0.61 vs 2.37 ± 0.34 µmol P_i/mg protein per h). Apparently, this is related to the type of isoform of Na^+/K^+ ATPase. It was shown that the alpha-3 isoform of Na^+/K^+ ATPase was upregulated in human colon cancer (Figure 2), but the alpha-1 isoform was downregulated [42]. The activity of Na^+/K^+ ATPase can lead to the invasion of endocrine-resistant breast cancer cells [43]. High expression of the alpha-1 subunit of Na^+/K^+ ATPase has been associated with tumor development and clinical outcomes in gastric cancer [44]. We also observed that bafilomycin A1 decreased Na^+/K^+ ATPase activity in human colon mucosal tissue samples and in human colon cancer samples. Importantly, the inhibitory effect of bafilomycin A1 on Na^+/K^+ pump activity was more pronounced in cancer tissue than in healthy tissue (see Figure 1). Previously, we observed a similar effect of NAADP on the activity of this protein in colon cancer tissue samples [17]. The simultaneous presence of bafilomycin A1 and NAADP resulted in a stronger inhibition of Na^+/K^+ ATPase activity in mouse NK/Ly cells [13]. There is a favorable correlation between the expression levels of the sodium pump-α3 subunit and metastasis in colorectal cancer [45]. Thus, inhibition of Na^+/K^+ ATPase could significantly inhibit the migration of colorectal cancer cells. Our results imply that endo-lysosomal agents bafilomycin A1 or NAADP [17] or both [13] are effective in inhibiting Na^+/K^+ ATPase activity in various cancers.

The ATPase activity of the rat subcellular fraction under the combined action of bafilomycin A1 was also examined (Figure 3). We found that bafilomycin A1 significantly increased the activity of the Ca^{2+} ATPases of the EPR in the subcellular fraction of rat liver but not that of the Ca^{2+} ATPases of the PM. This observation fully confirmed our assumption about the activation of the Ca^{2+} ATPase of the EPR by bafilomycin A1, as we had suspected above on the basis of experiments on its effect on Ca^{2+} content in rat hepatocytes. Furthermore, because bafilomycin A1 increases the activity of the Ca^{2+} ATPase in the EPR but not the PM, it was postulated that the bafilomycin-responsive acid storage is tightly associated with the EPR but not the PM. This observation is consistent with Ronco V. (2015) [37] that there is a functional Ca^{2+}-mediated cross-talk between endolysosomal and endoplasmic reticulum Ca^{2+} pools during NAADP-induced Ca^{2+} signaling.

It was also observed that bafilomycin A1 reduced Na^+/K^+ ATPase activity in the post-mitochondrial fraction of rat liver (Figure 3). It is important to note that the subcellular fraction is a heterogeneous mixture of membrane vesicles formed from different membranes: endosomes, lysosomes, EPR, and PM. In addition to Na^+/K^+ ATPase in the PM, it is also possible that it is present in the membranes of the endo-lysosomal store [36] as a result of PM invagination. Most likely, the effect of bafilomycin A1 on Na^+/K^+ ATPase is realized by a change in pH or/and released Ca^{2+}. It is likely that the Ca^{2+} that bafilomycin A1 releases from acidic storage inhibits the function of Na^+/K^+ ATPase. Higher intracellular Ca^{2+} has been shown to have this inhibitory impact on the sodium pump in human red blood cells, for instance [46]. Another explanation could be that bafilomycin A1 decreases Na^+/K^+ ATPase activity due to a change in pH. It has been shown that acidification to pH values below 6.0 inhibits this protein [41]. In lysosomal membranes of the liver, in addition to the bafilomycin A1-sensitive H^+ ATPase, the bafilomycin A1-insensitive Mg^{2+} ATPase has also been identified [47]. Bafilomycin A1 was also found to increase the activity of basal Mg^{2+} ATPase by more than two-fold. It is explained that the effect of bafilomycin A1 on the activity of basal Mg^{2+} ATPase is more likely due to a change in pH. The combined action of bafilomycin A1 and NAADP causes an even greater inhibition of Na^+/K^+ pump activity and results in an even greater increase in basal ATPase activity. It has already been established that NAADP decreases the activity of basal Mg^{2+} ATPase and the activity of Na^+/K^+ ATPase [48].

Therefore, bafilomycin enhances the effect of NAADP on inhibiting the activity of Na^+/K^+ pumps. We hypothesize that Na^+/K^+ ATPase may be active in endosomal organelles, i.e., bafilomycin and NAADP may reduce pump activity by increasing acidification. It is also possible that there is a NAADP-sensitive but bafilomycin-insensitive store in this intracellular fraction. The basal activity of Mg^{2+} ATPase is determined in the presence of Mg^{2+} and ATP ions at millimolar concentrations and with the addition of EGTA. Thus, the effect of bafilomycin A1 on basal Mg^{2+} ATPase is not associated with an increase in Ca^{2+} concentration due to the presence of high EGTA in the incubation medium of the subcellular fraction. The effect is most likely due to the pH change caused by bafilomycin. It is known that basal Mg^{2+} ATPase activity has a distinct optimum at physiological pH values (7.5–8.5) in the membrane of various tissues and significantly inhibits higher and lower pH values [49–51]. Therefore, NAADP, like bafilomycin A1, exerts a unidirectional effect on these systems of active ion transport. Therefore, our assumption above was correct: the effect of bafilomycin A1 on the activity of the Na^+/K^+ pump and basal Mg^{2+} ATPase is achieved by a change in pH or Ca^{2+}. NAADP was previously found to cause a significant increase in Ca^{2+} ATPase activity of the subcellular fraction of rat liver [48] due to the increase in Ca^{2+} ATPase of EPR and PM. NAADP has been found to release Ca^{2+} from lysosomal organelles through TPCs, and this, in turn, causes the release of Ca^{2+} from the ER store, which has possible morphological and functional links with acidic cell compartments in rat hepatocytes [18]. In the present article, we have shown that the combined influence of bafilomycin A1 and NAADP prevents the effect of NAADP on the activity of Ca^{2+} ATPases EPR in the subcellular fraction of rat liver (Figure 3). This demonstrates the relationship between acid storage and EPR in rat liver cells. Bafilomycin A1 most likely inhibited the H^+ gradient at the acid store's membranes, which is what drives the transit of Ca^{2+} ions, by blocking the acid store's H^+ pump. As a result, NAADP did not release calcium, which in turn did not alter the Ca^{2+} activity of the EPR pump. This confirms that NAADP-responsive receptors are localized in the endo-lysosomal store closely associated with the EPR. Apparently, there is some morphological contact between the EPR and the endo-lysosomal store [36,37], persisting even after obtaining the subcellular fraction by centrifugation. The combined effect of bafilomycin A1 and NAADP prevented the effect of NAADP on the activity of Ca^{2+} ATPases of PM; bafilomycin alone caused no change in the activity of this pump but prevented the effect of NAADP. This implies that the NAADP-induced increase in the activity of the Ca^{2+} ATPases of the PM is also dependent on a bafilomycin-sensitive store. Thus, our experiments in rat hepatocytes demonstrate that bafilomycin A1, targeting the endo-lysosomal system, that is, the NAADP-sensitive Ca^{2+} store, effectively modulates ATPase activity in membranes that are in close co-localization with the acidic store.

Initially, the experiments were performed on rat hepatocytes to investigate the effect of bafilomycin A1 on Ca^{2+} stores. We found that Ca^{2+} stores in rat hepatocytes decreased with the application of bafilomycin A1 (20 and 0.04 mM). Since it is known [52] that CTC is utilized to monitor Ca^{2+} signal from the EPR (pH 7.2) as well as from weakly acidic organelles presented by endosomes with pH between 6 and 6.4, it is likely that this drop (Figure 4A) represents a change in Ca^{2+} concentration primarily in the EPR and/or endosomes. Lysosomes have substantially lower pH values, typically between 4.5 and 5 [53]. This decrease in the stored calcium in rat hepatocytes by bafilomycin (20 and 0.04 µM) can be explained as follows (Figure 6): the direct binding of bafilomycin A1 to the H$^+$ pump of the acid store membranes prevents the filling of these organelles with calcium because the driving force for its transport—the proton gradient—is disrupted, releasing calcium from the lysosomes, as shown for epithelial cell lines [54], which should create local areas of increased calcium concentration like "hot spots" [55–57], activating the EPR Ca^{2+} pump to fill the EPR, with possible subsequent release of Ca^{2+} from the EPR due to overload, and/or activating the EPR Ca^{2+} channels, possibly via Ca^{2+} induced Ca^{2+} release (CIRC). The interaction between various calcium stores, attributed to the Calcium-Induced Calcium Release (CIRC) mechanism, has also been documented by other researchers [37,58]. The lysosomal Ca^{2+} release, which was caused by bafilomycin A1, may also be amplified by the release of Ca^{2+} from EPR through the CICR. Thus, applying bafilomycin A1 (20 and 0.04 mM) caused decreased calcium content in EPR after calcium release from acidic stores (autophagosomes, late endosomes, and lysosomes). The effect of bafilomycin A1 (0.04 mM) is stronger than that of bafilomycin A1 (20 mM) because, at higher concentrations, bafilomycin A1 likely inhibits SERCA to pump Ca^{2+} into the ER, so no subsequent CICR occurs (Figure 4).

The absence of changes in stored Ca^{2+} under the action of bafilomycin A1 (0.001 mM) (see Figure 4A) could be explained by the fact that its action at this concentration is restricted only to lysosomes and does not affect other Ca^{2+} stores, such as EPR and therefore does not alter the fluorescence intensity of the Ca^{2+}–CTC complex therein. Next, the effect of bafilomycin A1 (0.001 mM) on NAADP-induced calcium release in permeabilized rat hepatocytes was examined (Figure 4B) to determine the role of acidic stores (autophagosomes, late endosomes, and lysosomes) in this process. It is known that NAADP is able to release Ca^{2+} from acidic stores [28,59], which has been confirmed for various tissues [16,35], including rat hepatocyte microsomes [60], liver lysosomes [28], and rat hepatocytes [18]. Previously, it was shown that the effects of NAADP on stored Ca^{2+} depend on the concentration of buffers in the cell incubation medium of rat hepatocytes [18].

Thus, two different types of solutions were performed with the addition of an EGTA buffer (Figure 4) or without an EGTA buffer (Figure 4B). It was observed that the fluorescence intensity of the Ca^{2+}–CTC complex in permeabilized hepatocytes did not change with simultaneous exposure to bafilomycin A1 (20 or 0.04 mM) and NAADP (7 µM) compared with the medium with bafilomycin A1 alone in a medium without EGTA–Ca^{2+} buffer (Figure 4B). This indicates that bafilomycin A1 (20 µM) effectively inhibits the effect of NAADP. In contrast, the simultaneous action of NAADP (7 µM) and a lower concentration of bafilomycin (0.001 mM) resulted in an increase in stored calcium, which we assume is due to its accumulation in the EPR. This is possible because, in the series described above, the incubation medium was used without EGTA–Ca^{2+} buffer. When used in different combinations to maintain free calcium at physiological levels, bafilomycin A1 (0.001 µM) did not alter the stored calcium content of rat hepatocytes (Figure 4), but it prevented the effects of NAADP. This is confirmation that the bafilomycin-sensitive Ca^{2+} store is also NAADP-sensitive, corresponding to the endo-lysosomal organelle of the cell. In addition, the effect of bafilomycin A1 on NAADP-induced changes in Ca^{2+} content in rat hepatocytes was found to be dependent on the presence of EGTA–Ca^{2+} buffer in the cell incubation medium. This may indirectly confirm that Ca^{2+} "hotspots" and/or CICR play an important role in the interplay between the lysosome and EPR in bafilomycin A1-induced Ca^{2+} release in rat hepatocytes, as hypothesized above.

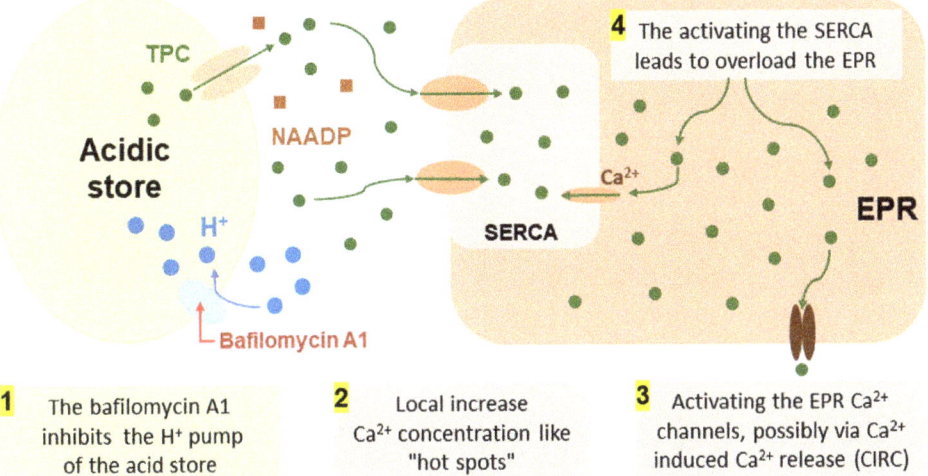

Figure 6. The hypothetical scheme of the molecular mechanisms of bafilomycin A1 effect on acid Ca^{2+} store and EPR: the bafilomycin A1 inhibits the H^+ pumps of acid store (1), this creates a local areas of increased calcium concentration like "hot spots" close to membranes of EPR (2), Activating the SERCA to fill the EPR by Ca^{2+} (3), this leads to overload the EPR and next activating the EPR Ca^{2+} channels (4), possibly via Ca^{2+} induced Ca^{2+} release (CIRC). Explanation: green dots and arrows—movement of Ca^{2+} ion; blue dots and arrows—movement of H^+ protons; the red arrow indicates the inhibition of the H^+-pump by bafilomycin A1; brown squares are NAADP molecules.

Thus, the obtained results show promise for modulating ion transport across the membrane of cancer cells by affecting the "acid stores" (autophagosomes, late endosomes, and lysosomes), which could be used as a potential new approach for the treatment of colorectal cancer. Moreover, with the results, potential therapeutic targets for the treatment of cancer could be identified and contribute to the understanding of the mechanisms behind carcinogenesis and the function of NAADP-sensitive acid storage in these processes.

4. Materials and Methods

4.1. Ethical Standards and Characteristics of Patients

Under the authorization of the Bioethics Committee of the Biological Faculty of the National Ivan Franko University of Lviv, Protocol No. 11/10, 2022, all procedures involving animals were carried out in compliance with the "International Convention for Working with Animals". The Institutional Review Board (Ethics Committee) of the Department of Therapy No. 1, Medical Diagnostics and Haematology and Transfusiology of the Faculty of Postgraduate Education, Danylo Halytsky Lviv National Medical University, approved the study using human samples on 2 September 2022, in accordance with the Declaration of Helsinki's guidelines. A total of 20 patients with colorectal cancer (mean age 54.3 ± 1.7 years) were complexly studied, all of whom agreed to give colonic mucosa samples during endoscopy.

We analyzed cancer samples from 12 women and 8 men. Six women had colorectal cancer type I, and 6 had type II (Table 1). Among men, 5 patients had cancer of type I and 3 had type II. Neoplasms without nodes and metastases, when the cancer affected the submucosa, were included in the It type of cancer. The type II tumor invades through the muscularis propria into the subserosa with no nodes and no metastases.

Table 1. The characteristics of patients, types, and stages of colorectal cancer.

Number of pts.	Age of pts.	Sex	Stage	Definition
1	53	female	I	The tumor invades the submucosa—no nodes, no metastases
2	52	female	I	The tumor invades the submucosa—no nodes, no metastases
3	76	female	II	The tumor invades through the muscularis propria into the subserosa—no nodes, no metastases
4	53	female	II	The tumor invades through the muscularis propria into the subserosa—no nodes, no metastases
5	52	female	I	The tumor invades the submucosa—no nodes, no metastases
6	50	female	II	The tumor invades through the muscularis propria into the subserosa—no nodes, no metastases
7	74	female	I	The tumor invades the submucosa—no nodes, no metastases
8	51	female	I	The tumor invades the submucosa—no nodes, no metastases
9	51	female	I	The tumor invades the submucosa—no nodes, no metastases
10	48	female	II	The tumor invades through the muscularis propria into the subserosa—no nodes, no metastases
11	45	female	II	The tumor invades through the muscularis propria into the subserosa—no nodes, no metastases
12	56	female	II	The tumor invades through the muscularis propria into the subserosa—no nodes, no metastases
13	55	male	I	The tumor invades the submucosa—no nodes, no metastases
14	45	male	I	The tumor invades the submucosa—no nodes, no metastases
15	56	male	I	The tumor invades the submucosa—no nodes, no metastases
16	55	male	II	The tumor invades through the muscularis propria into the subserosa—no nodes, no metastases
17	50	male	II	The tumor invades through the muscularis propria into the subserosa—no nodes, no metastases
18	54	male	II	The tumor invades through the muscularis propria into the subserosa—no nodes, no metastases
19	50	male	I	The tumor invades the submucosa—no nodes, no metastases
20	60	male	I	The tumor invades the submucosa—no nodes, no metastases
M	54.3			
m	1.7			

Samples of the patients' colonic mucosa were taken during endoscopy from both the cancer-affected and healthy (control) regions of their mucosa. Two samples—one of malignant tissue and the other of unaltered tissue—were taken from a single patient (control). The vehicle control of the study had the same parameters as "control" because we added to the control the same volume of solution without reagents. Before being a part of the initiative, every patient signed an informed permission form for diagnosis and tissue sample research.

4.2. Rat Hepatocytes Isolation

The "two-step" collagenase II type (Sigma, Burlington, MA, USA) perfusion method was used to generate hepatocytes, as previously mentioned [18]. Briefly, male wild-type rats (180–200 g) were anesthetized by inhalation of chloroform and then decapitated. The liver was isolated and digested using the "two-step" collagenase perfusion method as recommended for the preparation of isolated hepatocytes [61]. The liver is nonrecirculatingly perfused with Hank's Balanced Salt Solution (HBSS), which is free of Ca^{2+} and Mg^{2+} and contains EGTA (0.1 mM) for 10 min. The liver is then briefly washed with EGTA-free HEPES-containing (10 mM) buffer at 37 °C for 2 min. After that, the blanched liver was perfused for ten to fifteen minutes with 0.01% collagenase in 1 mM HBSS that contained Ca^{2+}. Following the collagenase treatment, the liver was removed, chopped, and mixed with HBSS and Ca^{2+}. The resulting cell suspension was filtered using successive nylon mesh filters and centrifuged at 50× g for a duration of two minutes. Cells were resuspended in Ca^{2+}-containing HBSS supplemented with 10% fetal bovine serum after the supernatant was removed. Trypan blue exclusion was used to determine the vitality of hepatocytes, and each experiment's preparation contained about 90% viable cells. HBSS contained (mM): 137 NaCl, 5.4 KCl, 0.2 Na_2HPO_4, 0.4 KH_2PO_4, 0.4 $MgSO_4$, 1.3 $CaCl_2$, 4.1 Na_2CO_3, and 5.6 glucose. For Ca^{2+} and Mg^{2+} free HBSS, $CaCl_2$ and $MgSO_4$ were omitted from the medium.

4.3. Chlortetracycline Chemiluminescent Imaging as a Quantitative Measure of Stored Calcium in Rat Hepatocytes

Stored calcium was measured by chemiluminescence of the Ca^{2+} chlortetracycline complex (CTC). This Ca^{2+}-sensitive indicator is used to monitor the stored Ca^{2+} concentration [52,53] in the lumen of the organelle. Prior to Ca^{2+} imaging, isolated hepatocytes were permeabilized in suspension with saponin (0.1 mg/mL) for 10 min in an intracellular solution. Following an intracellular solution wash, the cells were treated with the suitable drug for ten minutes. Permeabilized hepatocyte suspensions were treated for 10 min in intracellular solutions containing the necessary reagents prior to being loaded with chlortetracycline (CTC). After that, an intracellular solution was used to wash the permeabilized cell suspensions. 20 NaCl, 120 KCl, 1.13 $MgCl_2$, 1.3 $CaCl_2$, 10 HEPES, 5 µg/mL oligomycin, 1 µg/mL rotenone, and 2 ATP (pH 7.0) were the contents of the intracellular solution (mM). Every step of the experiment was carried out at 37 °C. To adjust the amount of free calcium present in the permeabilized rat hepatocytes' incubation medium, we used EGTA–Ca^{2+} buffer with the following Ca^{2+} concentrations (maxchelator.stanford.edu/CaEGTA–TS.htm): $[Ca^{2+}]_{cyt.}$ = 2.47 nM (EGTA 100 µM, $CaCl_2$ 1 µM); $[Ca^{2+}]_{cyt.}$ = 243 nM (EGTA 100 µM, $CaCl_2$ 50 µM); $[Ca^{2+}]_{cyt.}$ = 240 nM (EGTA 50 µM, $CaCl_2$ 25 µM). Hepatocytes were loaded with 100 µM CTC and allowed to sit at room temperature for 20 min without light in order to measure the changes in internal Ca^{2+} concentrations. This Ca^{2+} sensitive chemiluminescent probe is widely used in biological systems [52,53] to monitor the free internal Ca^{2+} concentration in the lumen of organelles by the following mechanism: CTC permeates in neutral, uncomplexed form and internal and external CTC concentrations are equal at equilibrium. A tiny rise in chemiluminescence occurs within the lumen as a result of Ca^{2+} complexing with CTC. Additionally, this complex attaches itself to the membrane's inner surface, greatly enhancing chemiluminescence. As a result, it is believed that CTC-Ca^{2+} chemiluminescent signals the Ca^{2+} concentration in intracellular organelles following depolarization of the mitochondria.

As a selective inhibitor of H^+ pumps V-type, bafilomycin A1 (Sigma, USA) was introduced in concentrations of 20, 0.04, and 0.001 mM, and NAADP (Sigma, USA) in concentrations of 7 µM. Cells were plated on glass slides for Ca^{2+} measurements, and a LUMAM-I-1 luminous microscopy system (40× objective, NA 0.7) was used to examine individual cells. A light-emitting diode was used to stimulate the CTC at 380 nm, and emission fluorescence was measured between 505 and 520 nm. Each subset of studies involved the examination of a set of thirty cells within the field of view. The relative variations in Ca^{2+} in CTC chemiluminescence were standardized to a 100% control value.

4.4. Assay of ATPase Activity in Subcellular Post-Mitochondrial Fraction of Rat Liver and Human Samples of Colon Mucosa

Isolation of the subcellular post-mitochondrial fraction was performed as previously described for rat liver [23,48,62] and for human colon mucosa and human colorectal samples [17], the determination of ATPase activity was based on the determination of the content of inorganic phosphorus by the spectrophotometric method. ATPase activity was estimated in the post-mitochondrial subcellular fraction obtained by differential centrifugation. In summary, tissue samples were homogenized at 0 °C to 2 °C for 10 min at 300 rpm using a glass-glass homogenizer. Supernatant 1 included mitochondria, whereas the homogenate was centrifuged at $3000\times g$ for 10 min using a Jouan MR 1812 centrifuge (Saint-Herblain, France) to precipitate nuclei, large cell fragments, and undisturbed cells. Following another centrifugation of this supernatant for 10 min at $8500\times g$ (0–2 °C), the mitochondrial fraction was sedimented. Supernatant 2, or the subcellular post-mitochondrial fraction, was separated after the mitochondria were sedimented, and it was utilized for the ATPase activity test. It was separated at $14,000\times g$ for 20 min.

Using the Fiske-Subbarow method, which estimates the quantity of inorganic phosphorus (Pi) released during the ATP hydrolase reaction and expresses it in μmol Pi/mg protein per h, ATPase activity was evaluated spectrophotomically. The goal was to transfer the post-mitochondrial subcellular fraction, which was obtained using differential centrifugation, to an internal standard solution that contained the following components (in milligrams) at 37 °C: NaCl 50.0, KCl 100, Tris–NCl 20, $MgCl_2$ 3, $CaCl_2$ 0.01, and pн 7.0. The addition of 3 mM ATP (Sigma, Burlington, MA, USA) initiated the process. To measure their impact on ATPase activity, bafilomycin A1 (Sigma, USA) and NAADP (Sigma, USA) were added to the incubation suspension. The difference in Pi between the medium containing and excluding ouabain was used to indicate the activity of Na^+/K^+ ATPase (Sigma, USA). Instead, equivalent volumes of incubation media were present in the samples (devoid of ouabain). Baseline Mg^{2+} ATPase activity was assessed in an incubation medium with ouabain and EGTA but no $CaCl_2$. It was decided to add thapsigargin (Sigma, USA) in order to suppress the Ca^{2+} ATP-dependent EPR. Additionally, the difference in Pi between the medium containing inhibitors (thapsigargin and ouabain) and the one without these substances was used to quantify the activity of Ca^{2+} ATP of EPR. The incubation medium was present in identical amounts in the samples (which did not contain thapsigargin or ouabain). Prior to being introduced to the incubation medium at a concentration of 1 μmol, thapsigargin and ouabain were dissolved in DMSO in a separate aliquot and then dissolved in an internal solution in another aliquot. Other samples (apart from thapsigargin and ouabain) had the same quantity of an incubation medium present. Micromoles of inorganic phosphorus, or 1 mg of protein every hour (μmol Pi/mg protein per hour), were used to express ATPase activity.

4.5. Specific ATPase Activity Calculation

The difference of inorganic phosphorus in the media with varying compositions was used to calculate the total ATPase activity of the post-mitochondrial fraction: (a) specific Na^+/K^+ ATPase activity was calculated as the difference of inorganic phosphorus content in the medium with or without ouabain (1 mM); (b) the difference between total Ca^{2+}/Mg^{2+} and Na^+/K^+ ATPase activity was quantified; (c) the amount of SERCA (sarcoendoplasmic reticulum Ca^{2+} ATPase) that contributes to the overall Ca^{2+}/Mg^{2+} ATPase activity was calculated using thapsigargin (d) in an incubation medium without ouabain and containing 1 mM EGTA. The incubation medium served as a control for the enzymatic hydrolysis of ATP in each experiment.

4.6. Statistical Analysis

The data in the text are expressed as mean ± SEM [63]. ANOVA test to estimate the significance of differences between experimental groups: $p < 0.05$ was conducted with the statistical software using Origin Pro 2018 (www.originlab.com).

5. Conclusions

Bafilomycin A1 significantly raised the basal ATPase activity in both the normal mucosa and the subcellular portion of colon cancer tissue in patient colon samples. It also successfully boosted the Ca^{2+} ATPase of EPR activity. It was shown that bafilomycin A1 decreased the activity of Ca^{2+} ATPase of PM in human colon mucosal tissue samples and caused no changes in the activity of Ca^{2+} ATPase of PM in the subcellular fraction of human colon cancer tissue. It was shown that bafilomycin A1 decreased the activity of Na^+/K^+ ATPase in human colon mucosa tissue samples as well as in cancer samples. In rat hepatocytes, bafilomycin A1 effectively reduced calcium stores and blocked NAADP's impact on them. In the subcellular fraction of rat liver, bafilomycin A1 decreased Na^+/K^+ ATPase activity and elevated baseline Mg^{2+} and EPR Ca^{2+} ATPase activities. When compared to the medium containing NAADP, the combination action of bafilomycin A1 and NAADP fully inhibits any change in Ca^{2+} ATPase and basal Mg^{2+} ATPase activities. The obtained results support the following statement: the EPR Ca^{2+} ATPases and the bafilomycin-sensitive storage are in close functional and physical contact. We explained the effect of bafilomycin A1 on these ATPase activities by acidification. Thus, the obtained results show promising targets for modulating ion transport across the membrane of cancer cells by affecting the "acidic stores" (autophagosomes, late endosomes, and lysosomes) as a possible new approach for the treatment of colorectal cancer.

Author Contributions: Conceptualization, S.B. and M.B.; methodology, S.B., M.B., D.D., M.V. and I.K.; software, I.K.; formal analysis, D.D., M.V., S.K.-M.R.R. and I.K.; investigation, S.B. and M.B.; writing—original draft preparation, S.B., M.B., D.D., M.V., S.K.-M.R.R. and I.K.; writing—review and editing, D.D., M.V., S.K.-M.R.R. and I.K.; visualization, I.K.; supervision, S.B. and M.B.; project administration, S.B. All authors have read and agreed to the published version of the manuscript.

Funding: This research was supported by the Grant Agency of Masaryk University (MUNI/A/1280/2022). Open access funding by the University of Vienna.

Institutional Review Board Statement: The study was conducted according to the guidelines of the Declaration of Helsinki and approved by the Institutional Review Board (Ethics Committee) of the Department of Therapy No. 1, Medical Diagnostic and Hematology and Transfusiology of Faculty of Postgraduate Education, Danylo Halytsky Lviv National Medical University (protocol code: No. 5, 2 September 2021).

Informed Consent Statement: All participants received information about this research and their participation and signed a digital informed consent form.

Data Availability Statement: The datasets generated and/or analyzed during the current study are not publicly available due to privacy but are available from the corresponding author upon reasonable request.

Conflicts of Interest: The authors declare no conflict of interest.

References

1. Dröse, S.; Altendorf, K. Bafilomycins and concanamycins as inhibitors of V-ATPases and P-ATPases. *J. Exp. Biol.* **1997**, *200*, 1–8. [CrossRef]
2. Sun, J.; Li, Y.; Yang, X.; Dong, W.; Yang, J.; Hu, Q.; Zhang, C.; Fang, H.; Liu, A. Growth differentiation factor 11 accelerates liver senescence through the inhibition of autophagy. *Aging Cell* **2022**, *21*, e13532. [CrossRef] [PubMed]
3. Park, H.-S.; Song, J.-W.; Park, J.-H.; Lim, B.-K.; Moon, O.-S.; Son, H.-Y.; Lee, J.-H.; Gao, B.; Won, Y.-S.; Kwon, H.-J. TXNIP/VDUP1 attenuates steatohepatitis via autophagy and fatty acid oxidation. *Autophagy* **2021**, *17*, 2549–2564. [CrossRef]
4. Lee, D.H.; Park, J.S.; Lee, Y.S.; Han, J.; Lee, D.-K.; Kwon, S.W.; Han, D.H.; Lee, Y.-H.; Bae, S.H. SQSTM1/p62 activates NFE2L2/NRF2 via ULK1-mediated autophagic KEAP1 degradation and protects mouse liver from lipotoxicity. *Autophagy* **2020**, *16*, 1949–1973. [CrossRef]

5. Lu, X.; Chen, L.; Chen, Y.; Shao, Q.; Qin, W. Bafilomycin A1 inhibits the growth and metastatic potential of the BEL-7402 liver cancer and HO-8910 ovarian cancer cell lines and induces alterations in their microRNA expression. *Exp. Ther. Med.* **2015**, *10*, 1829–1834. [CrossRef]
6. Wang, R.; Wang, J.; Hassan, A.; Lee, C.-H.; Xie, X.-S.; Li, X. Molecular basis of V-ATPase inhibition by bafilomycin A1. *Nat. Commun.* **2021**, *12*, 1782. [CrossRef] [PubMed]
7. Futai, M.; Sun-Wada, G.-H.; Wada, Y.; Matsumoto, N.; Nakanishi-Matsui, M. Vacuolar-type ATPase: A proton pump to lysosomal trafficking. *Proc. Jpn. Acad. Ser. B* **2019**, *95*, 261–277. [CrossRef] [PubMed]
8. Jeger, J.L. Endosomes, lysosomes, and the role of endosomal and lysosomal biogenesis in cancer development. *Mol. Biol. Rep.* **2020**, *47*, 9801–9810. [CrossRef]
9. Mauvezin, C.; Neufeld, T.P. Bafilomycin A1 disrupts autophagic flux by inhibiting both V-ATPase-dependent acidification and Ca-P60A/SERCA-dependent autophagosome-lysosome fusion. *Autophagy* **2015**, *11*, 1437–1438. [CrossRef]
10. Wu, Y.C.; Wu, W.K.K.; Li, Y.; Yu, L.; Li, Z.J.; Wong, C.C.M.; Li, H.T.; Sung, J.J.Y.; Cho, C.H. Inhibition of macroautophagy by bafilomycin A1 lowers proliferation and induces apoptosis in colon cancer cells. *Biochem. Biophys. Res. Commun.* **2009**, *382*, 451–456. [CrossRef]
11. Yan, Y.; Jiang, K.; Liu, P.; Zhang, X.; Dong, X.; Gao, J.; Liu, Q.; Barr, M.P.; Zhang, Q.; Hou, X.; et al. Bafilomycin A1 induces caspase-independent cell death in hepatocellular carcinoma cells via targeting of autophagy and MAPK pathways. *Sci. Rep.* **2016**, *6*, 37052. [CrossRef]
12. Li, F.; Hu, Y.; Hu, Y.; Zhou, R.; Mao, Z. Bafilomycin A1 Induces Caspase-Dependent Apoptosis and Inhibits Autophagy Flux in Diffuse Large B Cell Lymphoma. *Med. Pharmacol.* **2021**, 2021070520. [CrossRef]
13. Hreniukh, V.; Bychkova, S.; Kulachkovsky, O.; Babsky, A. Effect of bafilomycin and NAADP on membrane-associated ATPases and respiration of isolated mitochondria of the murine Nemeth-Kellner lymphoma: Mitochondria and ATPase activities in lymphoma. *Cell Biochem. Funct.* **2016**, *34*, 579–587. [CrossRef] [PubMed]
14. Bychkova, S.V.; Stasyshyn, A.R.; Bychkov, M.A. The role of bafilomycin as a therapeutic agent in the modulation of endo-lysosomal store of rat hepatocytes. *Med. Perspekt.* **2022**, *27*, 22–26. [CrossRef]
15. Morgan, A.J. Ca^{2+} dialogue between acidic vesicles and ER. *Biochem. Soc. Trans.* **2016**, *44*, 546–553. [CrossRef]
16. Faris, P.; Pellavio, G.; Ferulli, F.; Di Nezza, F.; Shekha, M.; Lim, D.; Maestri, M.; Guerra, G.; Ambrosone, L.; Pedrazzoli, P.; et al. Nicotinic Acid Adenine Dinucleotide Phosphate (NAADP) Induces Intracellular Ca^{2+} Release through the Two-Pore Channel TPC1 in Metastatic Colorectal Cancer Cells. *Cancers* **2019**, *11*, 542. [CrossRef]
17. Kushkevych, I.; Bychkov, M.; Bychkova, S.; Gajdács, M.; Merza, R.; Vítězová, M. ATPase Activity of the Subcellular Fractions of Colorectal Cancer Samples under the Action of Nicotinic Acid Adenine Dinucleotide Phosphate. *Biomedicines* **2021**, *9*, 1805. [CrossRef]
18. Bychkova, S.V.; Chorna, T.I. NAADP-sensitive Ca^{2+} stores in permeabilized rat hepatocytes. *Ukr. Biochem. J.* **2014**, *86*, 65–73. [CrossRef] [PubMed]
19. Chen, J.; Sitsel, A.; Benoy, V.; Sepúlveda, M.R.; Vangheluwe, P. Primary Active Ca^{2+} Transport Systems in Health and Disease. *Cold Spring Harb. Perspect. Biol.* **2020**, *12*, a035113. [CrossRef] [PubMed]
20. Peters, A.A.; Milevskiy, M.J.G.; Lee, W.C.; Curry, M.C.; Smart, C.E.; Saunus, J.M.; Reid, L.; da Silva, L.; Marcial, D.L.; Dray, E.; et al. The calcium pump plasma membrane Ca^{2+}-ATPase 2 (PMCA2) regulates breast cancer cell proliferation and sensitivity to doxorubicin. *Sci. Rep.* **2016**, *6*, 25505. [CrossRef] [PubMed]
21. Aung, C.S.; Ye, W.; Plowman, G.; Peters, A.A.; Monteith, G.R.; Roberts-Thomson, S.J. Plasma membrane calcium ATPase 4 and the remodeling of calcium homeostasis in human colon cancer cells. *Carcinogenesis* **2009**, *30*, 1962–1969. [CrossRef]
22. Aung, C.S.; Kruger, W.A.; Poronnik, P.; Roberts-Thomson, S.J.; Monteith, G.R. Plasma membrane Ca^{2+}-ATPase expression during colon cancer cell line differentiation. *Biochem. Biophys. Res. Commun.* **2007**, *355*, 932–936. [CrossRef] [PubMed]
23. Bychkova, S.; Hreniuh, V. Activity of ATPases in postmitichondtial fraction of lymphoma NK/Ly cells under bafilomicine and NAADP presence. *Biol. Stud.* **2015**, *9*, 31–38. [CrossRef]
24. Papp, B.; Launay, S.; Gélébart, P.; Arbabian, A.; Enyedi, A.; Brouland, J.-P.; Carosella, E.D.; Adle-Biassette, H. Endoplasmic Reticulum Calcium Pumps and Tumor Cell Differentiation. *Int. J. Mol. Sci.* **2020**, *21*, 3351. [CrossRef] [PubMed]
25. Chung, F.-Y.; Lin, S.-R.; Lu, C.-Y.; Yeh, C.-S.; Chen, F.-M.; Hsieh, J.-S.; Huang, T.-J.; Wang, J.-Y. Sarco/Endoplasmic Reticulum Calcium-ATPase 2 Expression as a Tumor Marker in Colorectal Cancer. *Am. J. Surg. Pathol.* **2006**, *30*, 969–974. [CrossRef] [PubMed]
26. Da Silva, C.I.; Gonçalves-de-Albuquerque, C.F.; de Moraes, B.P.T.; Garcia, D.G.; Burth, P. Na/K-ATPase: Their role in cell adhesion and migration in cancer. *Biochimie* **2021**, *185*, 1–8. [CrossRef] [PubMed]
27. Song, Y.; Lee, S.-Y.; Kim, S.; Choi, I.; Kim, S.-H.; Shum, D.; Heo, J.; Kim, A.-R.; Kim, K.M.; Seo, H.R. Inhibitors of Na^+/K^+ ATPase exhibit antitumor effects on multicellular tumor spheroids of hepatocellular carcinoma. *Sci. Rep.* **2020**, *10*, 5318. [CrossRef]
28. Zhang, F.; Xia, M.; Li, P.-L. Lysosome-dependent Ca^{2+} release response to Fas activation in coronary arterial myocytes through NAADP: Evidence from CD38 gene knockouts. *Am. J. Physiol. Cell Physiol.* **2010**, *298*, C1209–C1216. [CrossRef]
29. Chemaly, E.R.; Troncone, L.; Lebeche, D. SERCA control of cell death and survival. *Cell Calcium* **2018**, *69*, 46–61. [CrossRef]
30. Rüschoff, J.H.; Brandenburger, T.; Strehler, E.E.; Filoteo, A.G.; Heinmöller, E.; Aumüller, G.; Wilhelm, B. Plasma Membrane Calcium ATPase Expression in Human Colon Multistep Carcinogenesis. *Cancer Investig.* **2012**, *30*, 251–257. [CrossRef]

31. Rüschoff, J.; Hanna, W.; Bilous, M.; Hofmann, M.; Osamura, R.Y.; Penault-Llorca, F.; van de Vijver, M.; Viale, G. HER2 testing in gastric cancer: A practical approach. *Mod. Pathol.* **2012**, *25*, 637–650. [CrossRef]
32. Brouland, J.-P.; Gélébart, P.; Kovàcs, T.; Enouf, J.; Grossmann, J.; Papp, B. The Loss of Sarco/Endoplasmic Reticulum Calcium Transport ATPase 3 Expression Is an Early Event during the Multistep Process of Colon Carcinogenesis. *Am. J. Pathol.* **2005**, *167*, 233–242. [CrossRef] [PubMed]
33. Ribiczey, P.; Tordai, A.; Andrikovics, H.; Filoteo, A.G.; Penniston, J.T.; Enouf, J.; Enyedi, Á.; Papp, B.; Kovács, T. Isoform-specific up-regulation of plasma membrane Ca^{2+} ATPase expression during colon and gastric cancer cell differentiation. *Cell Calcium* **2007**, *42*, 590–605. [CrossRef]
34. Varga, K.; Hollósi, A.; Pászty, K.; Hegedűs, L.; Szakács, G.; Tímár, J.; Papp, B.; Enyedi, Á.; Padányi, R. Expression of calcium pumps is differentially regulated by histone deacetylase inhibitors and estrogen receptor alpha in breast cancer cells. *BMC Cancer* **2018**, *18*, 1029. [CrossRef]
35. Faris, P.; Casali, C.; Negri, S.; Iengo, L.; Biggiogera, M.; Maione, A.S.; Moccia, F. Nicotinic Acid Adenine Dinucleotide Phosphate Induces Intracellular Ca^{2+} Signalling and Stimulates Proliferation in Human Cardiac Mesenchymal Stromal Cells. *Front. Cell Dev. Biol.* **2022**, *10*, 874043. [CrossRef]
36. Fameli, N.; Ogunbayo, O.A.; van Breemen, C.; Evans, A.M. Cytoplasmic nanojunctions between lysosomes and sarcoplasmic reticulum are required for specific calcium signaling. *F1000Research* **2014**, *3*, 93. [CrossRef]
37. Ronco, V.; Potenza, D.M.; Denti, F.; Vullo, S.; Gagliano, G.; Tognolina, M.; Guerra, G.; Pinton, P.; Genazzani, A.A.; Mapelli, L.; et al. A novel Ca^{2+}-mediated cross-talk between endoplasmic reticulum and acidic organelles: Implications for NAADP-dependent Ca^{2+} signalling. *Cell Calcium* **2015**, *57*, 89–100. [CrossRef] [PubMed]
38. Yoshida, H.; Shimamoto, C.; Ito, S.; Daikoku, E.; Nakahari, T. HCO_3^--dependent transient acidification induced by ionomycin in rat submandibular acinar cells. *J. Physiol. Sci.* **2010**, *60*, 273–282. [CrossRef] [PubMed]
39. Hwang, S.-M.; Lee, J.Y.; Park, C.-K.; Kim, Y.H. The Role of TRP Channels and PMCA in Brain Disorders: Intracellular Calcium and pH Homeostasis. *Front. Cell Dev. Biol.* **2021**, *9*, 584388. [CrossRef]
40. Kushkevych, I.; Fafula, R.; Parák, T.; Bartoš, M. Activity of Na^+/K^+-activated Mg^{2+}-dependent ATP-hydrolase in the cell-free extracts of the sulfate-reducing bacteria *Desulfovibrio piger* Vib-7 and *Desulfomicrobium* sp. Rod-9. *Acta Vet. Brno* **2015**, *84*, 3–12. [CrossRef]
41. Kosterin, S.O.; Veklich, T.O.; Pryluts′kyĭ, I.I.; Borysko, P.O. Kinetic interpretation of the original pH-dependence of enzymatic activity of "basal" Mg(2+)-ATPase of the smooth muscle sarcolemma. *Ukr. Biokhim. Zh. (1999)* **2005**, *77*, 37–45. [PubMed]
42. Sakai, H.; Suzuki, T.; Maeda, M.; Takahashi, Y.; Horikawa, N.; Minamimura, T.; Tsukada, K.; Takeguchi, N. Up-regulation of Na^+, K^+-ATPase α3-isoform and down-regulation of the α1-isoform in human colorectal cancer. *FEBS Lett.* **2004**, *563*, 151–154. [CrossRef] [PubMed]
43. Khajah, M.A.; Mathew, P.M.; Luqmani, Y.A. Na^+/K^+ ATPase activity promotes invasion of endocrine resistant breast cancer cells. *PLoS ONE* **2018**, *13*, e0193779. [CrossRef] [PubMed]
44. Nakamura, K.; Shiozaki, A.; Kosuga, T.; Shimizu, H.; Kudou, M.; Ohashi, T.; Arita, T.; Konishi, H.; Komatsu, S.; Kubota, T.; et al. The expression of the alpha1 subunit of Na+/K+-ATPase is related to tumor development and clinical outcomes in gastric cancer. *Gastric Cancer* **2021**, *24*, 1278–1292. [CrossRef] [PubMed]
45. Wu, D.; Yu, H.-Q.; Xiong, H.-J.; Zhang, Y.-J.; Lin, X.-T.; Zhang, J.; Wu, W.; Wang, T.; Liu, X.-Y.; Xie, C.-M. Elevated Sodium Pump α3 Subunit Expression Promotes Colorectal Liver Metastasis via the p53-PTEN/IGFBP3-AKT-mTOR Axis. *Front. Oncol.* **2021**, *11*, 743824. [CrossRef] [PubMed]
46. Brown, A.M.; Lew, V.L. The effect of intracellular calcium on the sodium pump of human red cells. *J. Physiol.* **1983**, *343*, 455–493. [CrossRef] [PubMed]
47. Arai, K.; Shimaya, A.; Hiratani, N.; Ohkuma, S. Purification and characterization of lysosomal H(+)-ATPase. An anion-sensitive v-type H(+)-ATPase from rat liver lysosomes. *J. Biol. Chem.* **1993**, *268*, 5649–5660. [CrossRef] [PubMed]
48. Bychkova, S. Influence of NAADP and bafilomycine A1 on activity of ATPase in liver postmitochondrial fraction. *Biol. Stud.* **2015**, *9*, 31–40. [CrossRef]
49. Hohmann, J.; Kowalewski, H.; Vogel, M.; Zimmerman, H. Isolation of a Ca^{2+} or Mg^{2+}-activated ATPase (ecto-ATPase) from bovine brain synaptic membranes. *Biochim. Biophys. Acta BBA Biomembr.* **1993**, *1152*, 146–154. [CrossRef]
50. Konno, Y.; Kato, K.; Dairaku, N.; Koike, T.; Iijima, K.; Imatani, A.; Sekine, H.; Ohara, S.; Shimosegawa, T. Expression of Mg^{2+}-dependent, HCO_3^--stimulated adenine triphosphatase in the human duodenum. *J. Gastroenterol. Hepatol.* **2004**, *19*, 18–23. [CrossRef]
51. Wang, H.; Gilles-Baillien, M. Ca^{2+}-ATPase and Mg^{2+}-ATPase activities distinct from alkaline phosphatase in rat jejunal brush-border membranes. *Arch. Int. Physiol. Biochim. Biophys.* **1993**, *101*, 387–393. [CrossRef]
52. Jacob, J.; Chandran, D.; Sasidharan, R.; Kuruvila, L.; Madhusudan, U.K.; Rao, N.L.; Banerjee, D. Chlortetracycline, a fluorescent probe for pH of calcium stores in cells. *Curr. Sci.* **2003**, *2003*, 671–674.
53. Colacurcio, D.J.; Nixon, R.A. Disorders of lysosomal acidification—The emerging role of v-ATPase in aging and neurodegenerative disease. *Ageing Res. Rev.* **2016**, *32*, 75–88. [CrossRef]
54. Kim, H.-K.; Lee, G.-H.; Bhattarai, K.R.; Lee, M.-S.; Back, S.H.; Kim, H.-R.; Chae, H.-J. TMBIM6 (transmembrane BAX inhibitor motif containing 6) enhances autophagy through regulation of lysosomal calcium. *Autophagy* **2021**, *17*, 761–778. [CrossRef] [PubMed]

55. Fitzpatrick, J.S.; Hagenston, A.M.; Hertle, D.N.; Gipson, K.E.; Bertetto-D'Angelo, L.; Yeckel, M.F. Inositol-1,4,5-trisphosphate receptor-mediated Ca^{2+} waves in pyramidal neuron dendrites propagate through hot spots and cold spots: Ca^{2+} waves propagate through hot and cold spots. *J. Physiol.* **2009**, *587*, 1439–1459. [CrossRef]
56. Giacomello, M.; Drago, I.; Bortolozzi, M.; Scorzeto, M.; Gianelle, A.; Pizzo, P.; Pozzan, T. Ca^{2+} Hot Spots on the Mitochondrial Surface Are Generated by Ca^{2+} Mobilization from Stores, but Not by Activation of Store-Operated Ca^{2+} Channels. *Mol. Cell* **2010**, *38*, 280–290. [CrossRef]
57. Tepikin, A.V. Mitochondrial junctions with cellular organelles: Ca^{2+} signalling perspective. *Pflügers Arch. Eur. J. Physiol.* **2018**, *470*, 1181–1192. [CrossRef] [PubMed]
58. Hulsurkar, M.M.; Lahiri, S.K.; Karch, J.; Wang, M.C.; Wehrens, X.H.T. Targeting calcium-mediated inter-organellar crosstalk in cardiac diseases. *Expert Opin. Ther. Targets* **2022**, *26*, 303–317. [CrossRef]
59. Calcraft, P.J.; Ruas, M.; Pan, Z.; Cheng, X.; Arredouani, A.; Hao, X.; Tang, J.; Rietdorf, K.; Teboul, L.; Chuang, K.-T.; et al. NAADP mobilizes calcium from acidic organelles through two-pore channels. *Nature* **2009**, *459*, 596–600. [CrossRef]
60. Mándi, M.; Tóth, B.; Timár, G.; Bak, J. Ca^{2+} release triggered by NAADP in hepatocyte microsomes. *Biochem. J.* **2006**, *395*, 233–238. [CrossRef]
61. Blaauboer, B.J.; Boobis, A.R.; Castell, J.V.; Coecke, S.; Groothuis, G.M.M.; Guillouzo, A.; Hall, T.J.; Hawksworth, G.M.; Lorenzon, G.; Miltenburger, H.G.; et al. The Practical Applicability of Hepatocyte Cultures in Routine Testing: The Report and Recommendations of ECVAM Workshop 1. *Altern. Lab. Anim.* **1994**, *22*, 231–241. [CrossRef]
62. Ferents, I.M.; Bychkova, S.V.; Bychkov, M.A. Peculiarities of the effects of bile acids on atpase activity of the colon mucosa in patients with overweight and irritable bowel syndrome. *Wiad. Lek.* **2020**, *73*, 574–577. [CrossRef] [PubMed]
63. Bailey, N.T.J. *Statistical Methods in Biology*, 3rd ed.; Cambridge University Press: Cambridge, UK, 1995; Volume 75, p. 515. 255p.

Disclaimer/Publisher's Note: The statements, opinions and data contained in all publications are solely those of the individual author(s) and contributor(s) and not of MDPI and/or the editor(s). MDPI and/or the editor(s) disclaim responsibility for any injury to people or property resulting from any ideas, methods, instructions or products referred to in the content.

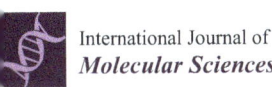

Article

Pictilisib-Induced Resistance Is Mediated through FOXO1-Dependent Activation of Receptor Tyrosine Kinases in Mucinous Colorectal Adenocarcinoma Cells

Murali R. Kuracha [1,*], Venkatesh Govindarajan [2], Brian W. Loggie [3], Martin Tobi [4] and Benita L. McVicker [1,5,*]

1. Department of Internal Medicine, University of Nebraska Medicine, Omaha, NE 68198, USA
2. Department of Medical Education, Creighton University School of Medicine, Omaha, NE 68178, USA
3. Department of Surgery, Creighton University School of Medicine, Omaha, NE 68124, USA
4. Research and Development Service, Detroit VAMC, Detroit, MI 48201, USA
5. Research Service, Nebraska-Western Iowa Health Care System, Omaha, NE 68105, USA
* Correspondence: murali.kuracha@siriusmindshare.com (M.R.K.); bmcvicker@unmc.edu (B.L.M.); Tel.: +1-402-995-3369 (B.L.M.)

Abstract: The phosphatidylinositol (PI3K)/AKT/mTOR axis represents an important therapeutic target to treat human cancers. A well-described downstream target of the PI3K pathway is the forkhead box O (FOXO) transcription factor family. FOXOs have been implicated in many cellular responses, including drug-induced resistance in cancer cells. However, FOXO-dependent acute phase resistance mediated by pictilisib, a potent small molecule PI3K inhibitor (PI3Ki), has not been studied. Here, we report that pictilisib-induced adaptive resistance is regulated by the FOXO-dependent rebound activity of receptor tyrosine kinases (RTKs) in mucinous colorectal adenocarcinoma (MCA) cells. The resistance mediated by PI3K inhibition involves the nuclear localization of FOXO and the altered expression of RTKs, including *ErbB2*, *ErbB3*, *EphA7*, *EphA10*, *IR*, and *IGF-R1* in MCA cells. Further, in the presence of FOXO siRNA, the pictilisib-induced feedback activation of RTK regulators (pERK and pAKT) was altered in MCA cells. Interestingly, the combinational treatment of pictilisib (Pi3Ki) and FOXO1i (AS1842856) synergistically reduced MCA cell viability and increased apoptosis. These results demonstrate that pictilisib used as a single agent induces acute resistance, partly through FOXO1 inhibition. Therefore, overcoming PI3Ki single-agent adaptive resistance by rational design of FOXO1 and PI3K inhibitor combinations could significantly enhance the therapeutic efficacy of PI3K-targeting drugs in MCA cells.

Keywords: FOXO; pictilisib; mucinous colorectal adenocarcinomas

1. Introduction

Phosphatidylinositol 3-kinase (PI3K)-targeting drugs are creating great interest as therapeutics for human cancers [1]. PI3Ks belong to the lipid kinase family that is divided into three classes. Class I is further subdivided into classes IA and IB, with class IA PI3Ks implicated in human cancers [2]. Class IA PI3Ks are heterodimeric, comprised of a regulatory subunit (p85α, p55α, p50α, p85β, and p55γ) and a catalytic subunit (p110α, p110β, and p110γ) encoded by the gene PI3KCA [3]. Commonly, PI3KCA gene mutations occur in the kinase domain (e.g., H1047R) or in the regulatory domain (e.g., E542K and E545K). These mutations diminish inhibitory interactions leading to constitutive activation of PI3K and downstream effectors (e.g., AKT, mTOR, and S6 kinase) [4]. The hyperactivation of these signaling nodes regulates the PI3K/AKT axis towards the growth and survival of the cancer cell [2]. However, several small molecule inhibitors that target the key nodes of the PI3K pathway have been developed and are currently in various preclinical and clinical trials [5]. Effective PI3K-inhibiting drugs are especially desired for hard-to-treat aggressive tumors. Mucinous colorectal adenocarcinomas (MCA) tend to be very aggressive and comprise a significant portion (10–20%) of colorectal cancers (CRC). MCAs are a highly disseminated heterogeneous group of tumors with a propensity to metastasize to the liver and peritoneal cavity [6–11]. Clinically, higher mutational rates for *KRAS*, *BRAF*, and PI3KCA have been reported in MCA rather than non-mucinous CRCs [12]. Pictilisib is a small molecule inhibitor of PI3K that has been used in chemotherapeutic regimens for a variety of human cancers, including MCA [13,14]. However, the effectiveness of pictilisib as a single-agent therapy is limited due to the potential development of drug-induced resistance.

Forkhead (FOXO) family transcription factors, FOXO1, FOXO3a, and FOXO4, are direct downstream targets of the PI3K/AKT pathway [15,16]. Importantly, FOXO proteins are involved in several post-translational modifications, including cell cycle inhibition [17], apoptosis [18,19], defense against oxidative stress, and DNA repair [20,21]. Moreover, FOXOs can act as critical modulators in cellular processes, including drug-induced resistance in many cell types [18,22]. In particular, FOXO1 is known to modulate paclitaxel-mediated cytotoxic resistance in ovarian cancers [23,24]. Such drug-induced resistance in cancer cells could be a result of FOXO1 nuclear migration and subsequent transcriptional activity. Currently, there is limited information concerning mechanisms and transcriptional changes mediated by drugs that induce resistance in cancer cells.

In the present study, we examined the consequence of FOXO1 nuclear localization in mucinous colorectal cancer cell lines associated with PI3K inhibition and pictilisib-induced resistance.

2. Results

2.1. Nuclear Localization of FOXO Transcription Factors after Pi3K Inhibition in MCA Cells

FOXO protein localization in response to PI3K inhibition in mucinous colorectal cancer cells (LS174T and RW7213) was examined using immunocytochemistry. Interestingly, FOXO1 was strongly stained in the nuclear compartment in MCA cells treated with pictilisib for 96 h compared to DMSO-treated control cells. In both MCA cell lines, the staining intensity of FOXO1 was significantly elevated in response to pictilisib single-agent treatment (Figure 1A–D'). Quantification of nuclear stain intensity showed a significant increase in the number of FOXO1 nuclear-stained positive cells in pictilisib-treated compared to DMSO-treated LS174T and RW7213 cells (Figure 1E,F). It was also determined that the FOXO3 protein was nuclear-localized following PI3K inhibition in the MCA cells.

2.2. Characterization of FOXO Nuclear Migration following Pictilisib Treatment in LS174T Cells

Western blot was performed to characterize the translocation of FOXO1, FOXO3, and FOXO4 protein localization in MCA cells. The majority of the FOXO proteins were nuclear-localized following PI3K inhibition in LS174T cells (Figure 2). In DMSO-treated control cells, the nuclear fraction of FOXOs was decreased (Figure 2A,B). Surprisingly, FOXO4 proteins were totally restricted to the nucleus after 72 or 96 h of pictilisib and DMSO vehicle treatment (Figure 2C). Overall, of the FOXO family proteins, FOXO1 and FOXO3 were found to migrate into the nucleus as a result of PI3Ki treatment. Therefore, these results suggest that the nuclear fraction of FOXO1 proteins was comparable in PI3Ki-treated cells and are available for transcriptional enhancement of RTK activity and cell resistance associated with PI3K inhibition by pictilisib.

2.3. FOXO Knockdown in MCA Cells Mitigates PI3K and MAP Kinase Signaling Induced by Pictilisib Treatment

To understand the functional role of the FOXO protein in PI3K-inhibited MCA cells, we performed targeted gene knockdown in LS174T cells. FOXO siRNA (short-interference RNA) or non-silencing siRNAs were transfected into LS174T cells, and FOXO protein expression was assessed by Western blot analysis. Results indicate that FOXO protein was remarkably attenuated in LS174T cells following siRNA-mediated knockdown (Figure 3). Interestingly, FOXO1 and FOXO3 siRNAs efficiently knocked down target genes at lower concentrations compared to the FOXO4 siRNA gene attenuation that was achieved at higher siRNA concentrations (Figure 3C). Specificity was shown with the non-silencing siRNA having no effect on FOXO expression levels. Overall, FOXO target genes were efficiently knocked down using FOXO siRNAs, revealing the relevance of investigating FOXO factors in PI3K drug-induced resistance in MCA cells.

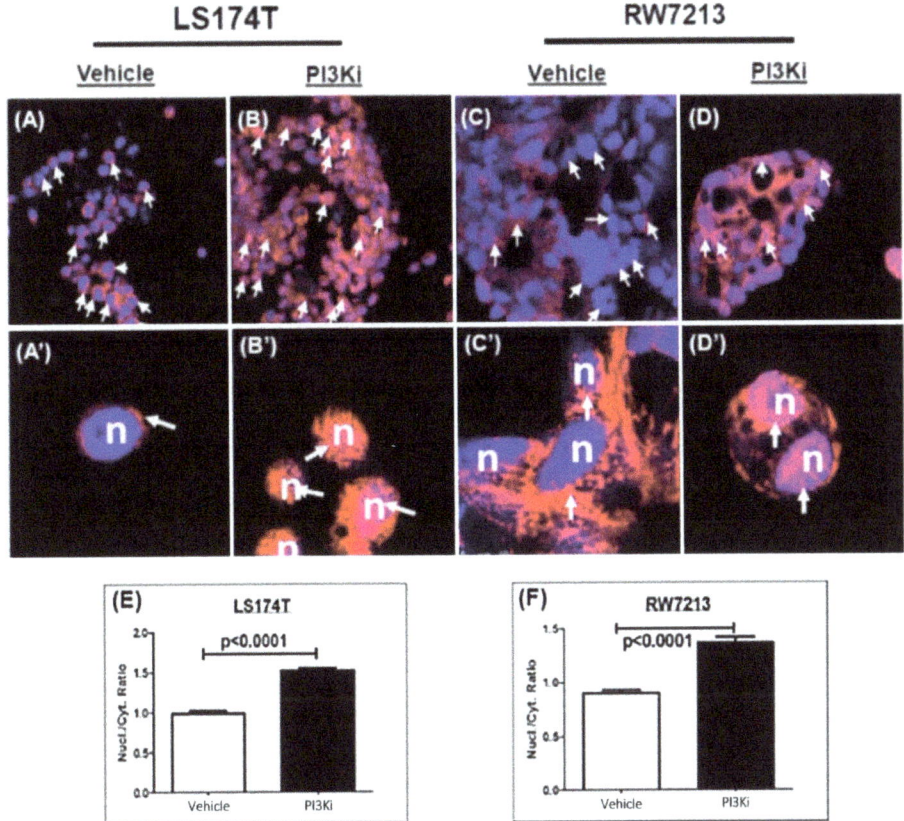

Figure 1. Nuclear enrichment of FOXOs in PI3Ki-treated MCA cells. (**A**,**A'**,**C**,**C'**): DMSO vehicle-treated LS174T and RW7213 cells expressed FOXO1 after 96 h. (**B**,**B'**,**D**,**D'**): LS174T and RW7213 cells exhibit FOXO1 staining in the nuclear compartment after 96 h of pictilisib treatment. Nuclei were assigned with pseudo-colored blue and FOXO1 with red. Nuclear enrichment of FOXO1 was seen at 96 h in both MCA cell lines (nuclei appear pink due to the red–blue overlap (white arrows). Cytoplasmic FOXO1 peri nuclear red-stained in (**A'**,**C'**) (white arrows). Scale bar: (**A**–**D**): 25 µm; (**A'**,**B'**,**D'**): 7.5 µm; (**C'**):10 µm. Statistical significance of nuclear FOXO1 staining intensity was measured in both MCA cell lines using a two-tail *t*-test (**E**,**F**): LS174T (vehicle, n = 230 cells; PI3Ki, n = 249 cells), RW7213 (vehicle = DMSO control, n = 236 cells; PI3Ki, n = 114 cells). *p*-value significance $p < 0.001$; error bars: standard error mean values were plotted.

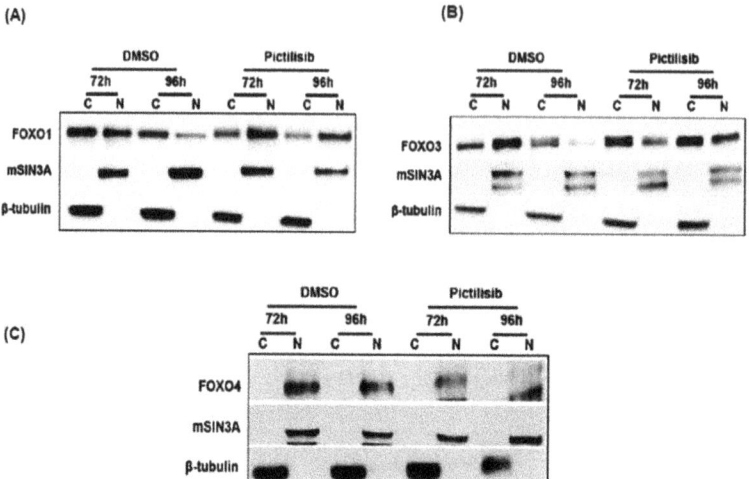

Figure 2. Enrichment of FOXO proteins in nuclear fractions after PI3Ki treatment. FOXO1 (**A**), FOXO3 (**B**), and FOXO4 (**C**) proteins from nuclear and cytoplasmic fractions of the vehicle or PI3Ki-treated (for 72 or 96 h) LS17T cells were resolved, blotted, and probed with respective antibodies: FOXO1, FOXO3, FOXO4, mSIN3A, and β-tubulin. Nuclear FOXOs were normalized to mSIN3A, and cytoplasmic FOXOs were normalized to β-tubulin. Notably, the nuclear fraction of FOXO1 at 72–96 h was elevated in the PI3Ki-treated cells (**A**), while FOXO4 proteins were restricted only to the nucleus with or without PI3K inhibition (1C). C = cytoplasmic; N = nuclear; vehicle = DMSO control.

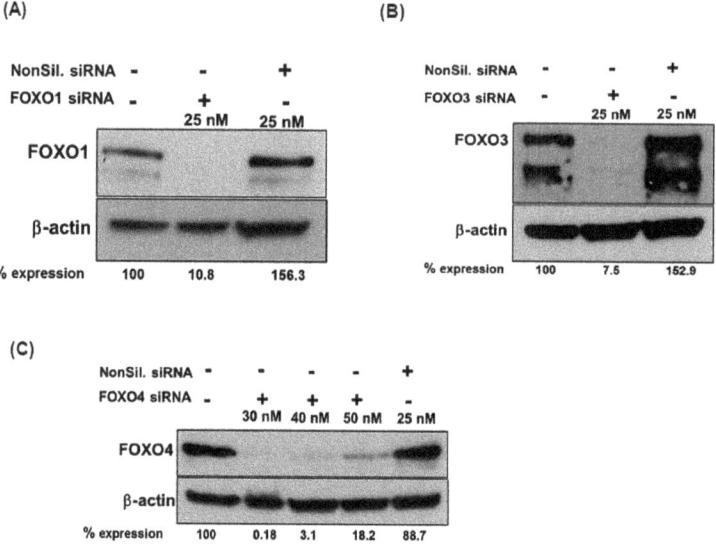

Figure 3. FOXO1, FOXO3, and FOXO4 were deleted in MCA cells by siRNA-mediated knockdown. (**A–C**): LS174T cells were transfected with siRNA smart pools (Dharmacon), targeting FOXO1, FOXO3, FOXO4, and non-silencing RNA as off-target transfection control. Western blot analysis showed effective knockdown of FOXO1, 3, and 4 in LS17T cells. Expression levels of proteins on Western blots were quantified by densitometry, and the percentages of FOXO protein expression relative to untreated (−) controls are shown below the blots. All values were normalized to β-actin as a loading control.

To determine the significance of FOXO protein attenuation during PI3K inhibition and resistance in MCA cells, we next examined the effect of FOXO knockdown in pictilisib-treated LS174T cells. The activity of downstream effector molecules (PI3K and MAP kinase signaling pathways) was evaluated in response to FOXO protein knockdown. In previous studies, we showed that ERK and AKT phosphorylation is initially reduced after short-term (24–48 h) pictilisib treatment but later increased after longer treatment periods (72–96 h) [13]. Here, FOXO1 siRNA transfection followed by pictilisib treatment for 96 h resulted in reduced pERK1/2 and pAKT activity compared to non-silencing or other FOXO siRNAs alone or in combination (Figure 4A,B). In contrast, phosphorylated-ERK activity remained elevated in non-silencing siRNA and pictilisib-treated MCA cells. Moreover, phosphorylation of AKT, a downstream factor of the PI3K survival pathway, was altered by FOXO siRNA in PI3Ki-induced LS174T-resistant cells (Figure 4B). FOXO1, FOXO3 alone, and FOXO4 siRNA showed markedly reduced AKT phosphorylation in PI3Ki-resistant LS174T cells (Figure 4B). FOXO1 alone knockdown resulted in the complete inhibition of pAKT, whereas other forms of FOXO siRNAs, including non-target siRNA, alone or in combination, led to less of a reduction in AKT phosphorylation in the PI3Ki-resistant cells. Thus, the resistance of MCA cells to pictilisib single-agent treatment was mitigated by FOXO1 functional gene attenuation and could be correlated to rebound activation of MAPK and AKT survival pathways. Thus, pictilisib single-agent induction of survival and growth in resistant cells depends on FOXO1-dependent pERK and pAKT activation.

2.4. FOXO1 Mediates the Redirection of Receptor Tyrosine Kinase mRNA Expression in PI3Ki-Induced LS174T-Resistant Cells

The contribution of RTK mRNA expression in MCA cell resistance was evaluated by RT-PCR to determine the possible correlation between pictilisib drug-induced resistance and FOXO1 attenuation in LS174T cells. The RTKs evaluated included the insulin receptor (*IR*), insulin growth factor receptor 1 (*IGF-R1*), *ErbB2*, *ErbB3*, and ephrin receptor A10 (*EphA10*). The results indicate that the rebound activity of FOXO1-mediated RTKs is seen with PI3K inhibition that is associated with pictilisib treatment of MCA cells (Figure 5). The statistical analysis revealed that remarkably elevated levels of RTK mRNA expression were seen with PI3K inhibition at 96 h. In contrast, FOXO1 knockdown rescued pictilisib-induced rebound activity of RTK mRNA overexpression in the LS174T cells (Figure 5A). Further, we confirmed that RTK mRNA expression positively correlated with FOXO transcription factors using the Cignal Reporter GFP (green fluorescent protein) expression assay. As shown in Figure 5B, DMSO-treated MCA cells displayed cytoplasmic GFP expression. However, functional FOXO/TRE/GFP plasmid transfection followed by pictilisib treatment resulted in reporter GFP expression that was localized in the nucleus of LS174T cells (Figure 5C). This indicates that the nuclear fraction of FOXO1 promoter activity is required for the rebound activation of RTKs in pictilisib-treated MCA cells. Taken together, these data suggest that FOXO1-dependent RTK mRNA expression is elevated during pictilisib single-agent treatment.

2.5. FOXO1 Knockdown Sensitizes the Rebound Activity of RTKs during PI3K Inhibition in Drug-Induced Resistant MCA Cells

The potential of FOXO1 as a regulator of the PI3K pathway led us to investigate the loss of the FOXO1 functional gene during pictilisib-induced rebound activity of RTKs and upstream elements of these signaling pathways. The RTK proteome profile array was analyzed in cells transfected with FOXO1 and non-silencing siRNA along with pictilisib treatment. Results indicate that FOXO siRNA followed by pictilisib treatment exhibited less phosphorylation of IGF-R1, IR, EphA10, EphA7, ERbB2, and ErbB3 at 96 h, whereas transfection with non-silencing siRNA led to significantly elevated RTK phosphorylation (Figure 6). Our previous reports demonstrated that pictilisib has a synergistic effect. For instance, linsitinib (IR and IGFR1 inhibitor) vs. pictilisib and lapatinib and EGFR and ErbB2 inhibitor vs. pictilisib. This combinational synergism resulted in a loss of viability in MCA cell lines [13]. However, ephrin receptors have been identified as key modulators to regulate RAS/MAPK and PI3K/AKT pathways in tumor progression [25]. At present, there are no inhibitors available to target EphA7 or EphA10. Taken together, the results show that FOXOs, especially FOXO1, are sensitizing pictilisib drug-induced rebound activity by attenuating RTKs in MCA cells.

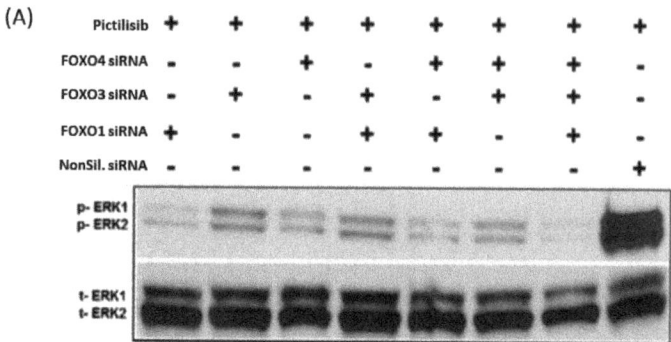

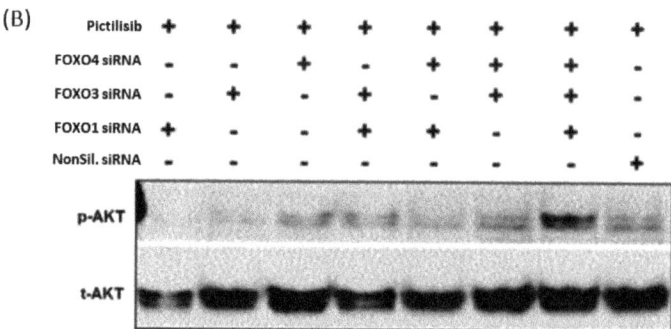

Figure 4. Rebound activation of pERK1/2 and pAKT seen in response to PI3K inhibition and FOXO knockdown. LS174T cells were transfected with FOXO1, FOXO3, or FOXO4 siRNA alone or in combination, grown for 24 h, and treated with PI3Ki for 96 h. (**A**) Western blots were performed using anti-pERK (pERK1 and ERK2), and (**B**) anti-pAKT and anti-total-ERK (tERK1 and ERK2), and total-AKT antibodies. The blot signals were quantified using densitometry and were normalized to non-silencing controls. Phospho-ERK1/2 levels were reduced in all PI3Ki-treated cells with FOXO knockdown compared to non-silencing controls (**A**). A more pronounced reduction in FOXO1 (**A**) and FOXO4 (**A**) siRNA-treated cells was seen than in FOXO3 siRNA-treated cells (**A**). Phospho-ERK1/2 levels were reduced when all three FOXO genes were knocked down, but this reduction was comparable to FOXO1 single knockdown, suggesting that FOXO1 may be the most critical FOXO protein for mediating rebound activation of pERK levels in response to PI3Ki-treatment. Similarly, phospho-AKT levels were reduced in FOXO1 (**B**), FOXO3 (**B**), and FOXO1 + FOXO4 siRNA-treated PI3Ki-resistant cells compared to FOXO3, non-silencing siRNA treated cells. Phospho-AKT levels were reduced with FOXO1 gene knockdown (**B**). Compared to all other FOXOs alone or together, knockdown indicates that the FOXO1 protein could be a critical modulator to influence PI3K inhibitor-treated resistant cell survival through AKT phosphorylation.

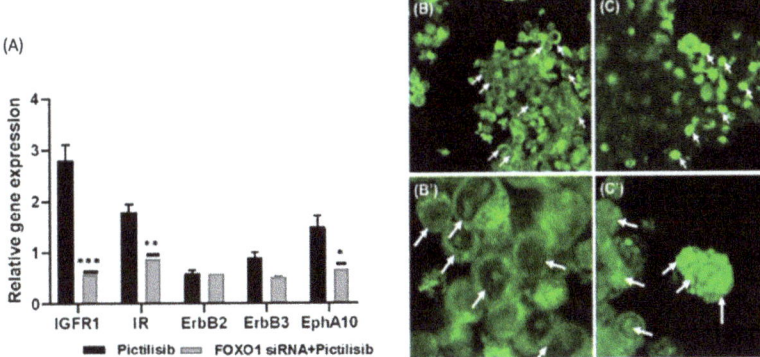

Figure 5. FOXO1-mediated differential expression of receptor tyrosine kinases (RTKs) in PI3Ki-induced resistant MCA cells. (**A**). Quantitative RT-PCR results show a reduction in *IGFR1*, *IR*, *ErbB2*, *ErbB3*, and *EphA10* mRNA relative gene expression levels in LS174T cells transfected with FOXO1 siRNA subjected to PI3Ki treatment. *ErbB2* and *ErbB3* mRNA relative gene expression was not significantly reduced. Error bars indicate the standard error of the mean of relative gene expression levels (n = 4). *p*-value significance (* $p < 0.01$, ** $p < 0.001$, and *** $p < 0.0001$). Error bars: standard error mean values were plotted. (**B–C′**): FOXO transcriptional activity monitored in PI3Ki-treated LS174T cells and DMSO vehicle control cells. (**B,B′**): FOXO1 transcriptional promoter element contained GFP reporter construct transfected 24 h, upon DMSO vehicle treatment for 96 h. Cytoplasmic GFP expression (white arrows) was seen in LS174T control cells. (**C,C′**): FOXO1 responsive promoter element contained GFP reporter construct transfected 24 h followed by PI3Ki treatment. After 96 h, nuclear GFP expression (white arrows) was seen in PI3Ki-resistant LS174T cells. Scale bar: (**B–C′**) 20 µm.

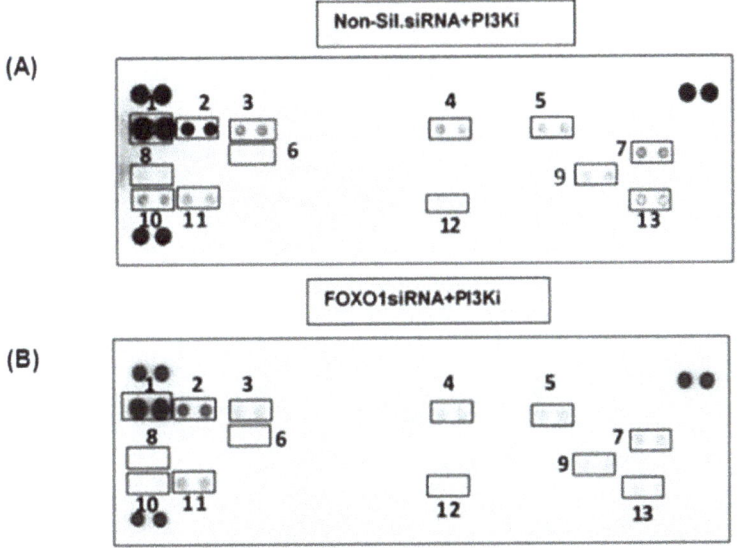

Figure 6. *Cont.*

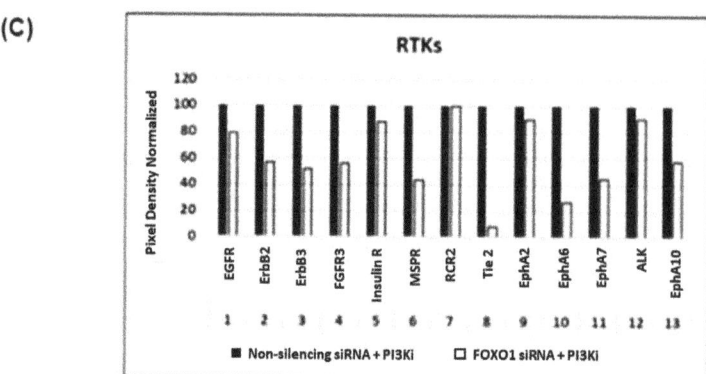

Figure 6. RTK phosphorylation in response to FOXO1 knockdown and prolonged exposure to PI3K inhibitor. (**A,B**): After 96 h, FOXO1 and non-silencing siRNA followed by PI3Ki treated LS174T cell lysates were incubated with RTK profiler antibody array containing 49 RTKs (R&D Biosystems), followed by the anti-phospho-tyrosine antibody. The RTKs that were elevated and downregulated in the boxes indicate RTK expression. (**C**): Pixel densities were quantified using ImageJ analysis software 1.44. The numbers on the *x*-axis correspond to RTKs and fold elevation relative to non-silencing siRNA + PI3Ki controls. The *x*-axis number 1 to 13 corresponds to EGFR, ErbB2, ErbB3, FGFR3, Insulin R, MSPR, RCR2, Tie 2, Eph A2, Eph A7, ALK, and Eph A10. These RTKs activity was normalized with non-silencing siRNA + PI3Ki.

2.6. PI3Ki and FOXO1i Synergy in MCA Cell Lines

A major pathway targeted by therapeutic drugs in human cancers is the PI3K/AKT/mTOR signaling pathway. Several small-molecule inhibitors have been developed to target PI3K; however, the development of PI3K-dependent resistance mechanisms has limited their success in the clinical spectrum [1]. In our previous studies, we evaluated IC50 values and initial sensitivity to pictilisib [13]. However, resistance occurred within 72 h of pictilisib treatment. Here, we investigated the hypothesis that combined inhibition of PI3K and FOXO1 would diminish drug-induced resistance. To test this hypothesis, MCA cell lines (LS174T and RW7213) were treated with increasing concentrations of pictilisib and the FOXO1 inhibitor (AS1842856). Our results demonstrate that both MCA cell lines are sensitized after individual treatments for 96 h (Supplementary Figure S1A,B). A four-parameter logistic/sigmoidal dose–response model was used to assess the sensitivity of both MCA lines to FOXO1i (IC50: 0.28 μM (LS174T) and 0.17 μM (RW7213)). Subsequently, synergistic responsive experiments were performed with AS1842856 and pictilisib in the MCA cells. Importantly, the combinational treatment of pictilisib and AS1842856 synergistically increased cell cytotoxicity in both MCA cell lines (Supplementary Figure S1C,D). A combination index (CI) value of <1 [26] was seen in both MCA cell lines (CI = 0.54 for LS174T and CI = 0.47 for RW7213), suggesting synergy between the two drugs in reducing MCA viability in vitro. Thus, these results demonstrate that the drug-induced resistance to pictilisib single-agent inhibition in MCA cells could be bypassed using FOXO1i and PI3Ki combination therapy.

3. Discussion

Although the PI3K/AKT/mTOR axis is a target for cancers, the current use of small molecule inhibitors against this axis is limited by the development of drug resistance in patients [23,27,28]. We confirmed that similar resistance occurs with MCA cells in vitro and that pictilisib-induced drug-resistance can lead to cancer cell survival and aggressiveness in MCA cells. Additionally, studies have reported that FOXO proteins are putative markers for poor chemotherapeutic response in various cancer models [24,29]. However, the molecular mechanism of drug-induced phase resistance in MCA is still uncertain.

In the present study, we explored the possible underlying mechanism of FOXO protein involvement in MCA cell drug-induced resistance that is mediated by pictilisib administered as a single agent. The results revealed that pictilisib treatment led to an increased accumulation of nuclear FOXO1 compared to vehicle-treated LS174T cells. FOXO transcription factors are highly competitive transcriptional binders involved in determining the fate of target cells [30]. Nuclear FOXO1 is most likely to be involved in cell fate decisions with the influence of RTK gene transcription in resistant cells. MCA cells are sensitized during pictilisib treatment by FOXO1 proteins migrating from the cytoplasm to the nucleus and their involvement in the process of drug-induced resistance. It could be possible that acute phase resistance to pictilisib leads to FOXO1-dependent RTK gene transcription and reduction in pro-apoptotic gene (e.g., BIM) activity that results in MCA cell survival following the drug treatment. For instance, a recent study showed that FOXO1 influences AKT phosphorylation in hepatocytes by suppressing the expression of Tribble 3 (Trb3), a pseudokinase capable of binding to AKT to block phosphorylation [31]. However, the rebound activation of RTK receptors, the phosphorylation of ERK and AKT, and the nuclear accumulation of FOXO1 were clearly observed in response to pictilisib treatment at 96 h in MCA cells. It appears there is clear evidence that the FOXO1-dependent positive feedback loop to the MAPK and PI3K/AKT pathways could support the development of drug-induced resistance and survival in MCA cells. Indeed, several studies have reported that inhibition of the PI3K/AKT axis leads to enhanced phosphorylation of ERK and AKT in several cancer models, including breast, prostate, and lung cancers [32–34]. However, Serra et al. reported that acquired ERK activity is a major cause of resistance to PI3K inhibitors in cancer treatment [34]. Similarly, our results show that pictilisib-treated LS174T cells have elevated ERK1/2 phosphorylation. However, FOXO siRNA followed by pictilisib treatment of LS174T cells leads to a reduction in IR, IGF-R1, ErbB2, ErbB3, EphA7, and EphA10 receptor activity and phosphorylation of AKT and ERK. These results suggest that FOXO-based promoter activity is essential to synthesize target gene receptors which are involved in cell survival and growth in resistant cancer cells [23,27,31,35]. In addition, earlier studies demonstrated that the inhibition of the PI3K/AKT axis inhibition leads to the nuclear localization of FOXO proteins and promotes transcriptional activation of RTK receptors through ERK signaling in breast cancer cells [33,34]. Here, we observed that targeting FOXO proteins by blocking functional activity with siRNAs resulted in decreased AKT and ERK phosphorylation in MCA cells. Thus, the FOXO1-mediated attenuation of RTKs (MAPK and PI3K signaling pathways) represents a more proximal mechanism that controls pictilisib drug-induced phosphorylation of ERK (Supplementary Figure S2). We suggest that FOXO1 acts as a pleiotropic effector on multiple signaling pathways, targeting drug-induced resistance by interfering with RTK signaling and the apoptotic pathway. In addition, the utilization of a small-molecule inhibitor against FOXO1 could effectively target PI3Ki-induced resistance and reduce ERK and AKT activity.

FOXO1i (AS1842856) is emerging as a selective chemotherapeutic drug against FOXO1 which is currently used for the treatment of Type II diabetic mullites (T2DM) [36,37]. Despite the recognition of FOXO1 nuclear localization in the development of pictilisib drug-induced resistance, how effectively FOXO1i treatment with a combination of PI3Ki causes ERK activation remains elusive. Based on previous studies, inhibition of the PI3K/AKT axis induces nuclear accumulation of FOXO proteins [33,34,38,39]. Our results suggest that pictilisib single-agent treatment increases RTK expression and that ERK1/2 phosphorylation is mediated by the nuclear localization of FOXO1. Importantly, we show that this effect is completely abolished by FOXO siRNA-mediated knockdown or FOXO1 inhibitor administered as a co-treatment with pictilisib. Our findings propose that pictilisib single-agent treatment induces nuclear localization of FOXO1 transcriptional activity, which is rescued by FOXO1 siRNA or the combinational inhibition of pictilisib with a FOXO1 inhibitor. FOXO1i (AS1842856) and pictilisib synergy represent a key mechanism responsible for RTK rebound activity and drug resistance in MCA cells. Therefore, this study suggests that FOXO1 involvement is a critical event in PI3K/AKT axis inhibition that mediates resistance in MCA cells. Thus, our results suggest that (a) drug-induced resistance by pictilisib is mediated by FOXO1 transcription factors in MCA cells; (b) FOXO siRNA attenuates RTK rebound activity and diminishes ERK and AKT phosphorylation; (c) FOXO1i and PI3Ki combinational synergy are more effective in reducing MCA cell viability and increasing apoptosis.

In summary, we demonstrated that FOXO1 nuclear accumulation correlates with the acute resistance created in MCA cells following pictilisib treatment. We provide evidence that FOXO1 regulates RTK rebound activity in pictilisib drug-induced resistant cells. Further, FOXO siRNA attenuates phospho-ERK1/2 and phospho-AKT levels in pictilisib given as a single agent to MCA cells. Most importantly, FOXO1i (AS1842856) and pictilisib combinational synergy increase efficacy through cell toxicity and apoptosis. Although these data were generated from in vitro studies, it is likely that in vivo analyses will confirm the findings and the potential therapeutic value of FOXO1i/PI3Ki treatment in MCA cells. We speculate that FOXO1 might be a co-target to rescue PI3Ki single-agent resistance in MCA therapy.

4. Materials and Methods

4.1. Cell Lines

Mucinous colorectal adenocarcinoma cell lines (LS174T and RW7213) were cultured as described in our previous studies [13]. Briefly, LS174T (American Type Culture Collection; Manassas, VA, USA) and RW7213 (gifted from John Mariadason; Ludwig Cancer Institute, Melbourne, Australia) cell lines were grown as monolayer cultures in RPMI1640 (Hyclone Laboratories, Logan, UT, USA) supplemented with 4.5 g/L glucose (Invitrogen, Carlsbad, CA, USA), 10% FBS (Invitrogen, Carlsbad, CA, USA), 2 mM L-glutamine, 20 mM HEPES, 1X MEAA, 100 IU/mL penicillin, and streptomycin in a humidified atmosphere of 5% CO_2 at 37 °C. The cell lines were tested for interspecies cross-contamination and mycoplasma infection and authenticated by short tandem repeat [10] analysis using 16 STR markers (IDEXX Bio-Analytics, Columbia, MO, USA).

4.2. Immunocytochemistry

LS174T or RW7213 cells were grown on chamber slides and treated for 72 and 96 h with pictilisib or Dimethyl sulfoxide (DMSO) vehicle control. Subsequently, the cells were washed with 1X cold PBS and fixed in 4% PFA. Following incubation with blocking solution (0.1% TritonX-100 at RT for 1 h), the cells were incubated with rabbit-anti FOXO1 (1:50 dilution; Cell Signaling Technology, Boston, MA, USA) in a humid chamber overnight at 4 °C. For the visualization of FOXO1, Alexa594 conjugated anti-rabbit secondary antibody (Invitrogen, Carlsbad, CA, USA) was applied to the cells for 1 hour at RT and DAPI-containing anti-fade mounting media was used for nuclear counterstaining. The positive cytoplasmic and nuclear-stained cells were counted in both PI3Ki and DMSO vehicle control cells.

4.3. Fluorescence Microscopy

Images of pictilisib and DMSO-treated LS174T and RW7213 cells were obtained using multiphoton confocal microscopy (Leica TCS SP8 MP Microsystems Inc., Buffalo Grove, IL, USA). Images were captured using AxioVision software version 4.8 and quantified using meta soft analysis.

4.4. FOXO Signal Reporter Assays

LS174T cells were transfected using a Cignal FOXO reporter kit (cat # CCS-6022G Qiagen, Germantown, MD, USA) according to the manufacturer's protocol. In brief, LS174T cells were transfected with FOXO/TRE/GFP construct for 24 h, followed by PI3Ki treatment for 96 h. GFP fluorescence identification of transfected cells was performed using ImageXpress Ultra microscope and MetaXpress software version 2.6.

4.5. siRNA Knockdown Studies

Three pairs of siRNA Smart pool reagents (cat # M-003006-03-0010; cat # M-003007-02-0010; cat # M-003016-02-0010 Dharmacon, Lafayette, CO, USA) were used against FOXO1, FOXO3, and FOXO4 gene targets. The siRNA transfection protocol was performed according to the manufacturer's instructions with FOXO siRNAs introduced with DharmaFECT transfecting reagent (cat # 8T-2001-01). As a transfection control, on-target and off-targeting siRNA pools were used (cat # D-001810-10-20). Seventy-two hours after transfection, 12.5–30 nM siRNA-treated cell proteins were harvested, and total protein concentration was measured using the BCA method.

4.6. Western Blots

Total cell proteins were lysed in radioimmunoprecipitation (RIPA) lysis buffer containing protease phosphatase cocktail inhibitor (Cell Signaling; Danvers, MA, USA). After centrifugation (2000× g at 4 °C), the supernatant was mixed with an equal volume of Laemmli sample buffer and boiled. The denatured proteins were resolved by precast SDS-PAGE (sodium dodecyl sulphate–polyacrylamide gel electrophoresis) 4–15% gradient gels followed by electrotransfer to polyvinylidene fluoride or polyvinylidene difluoride (PVDF) membranes (Millipore; St. Louis, MO, USA). The blots were blocked with 5% skim milk for 1 h at RT and probed with the following antibodies overnight at 4 °C: anti-FOXO1 (cat # 8H0003845), anti-FOXO3 (cat # 550485), FOXO4 (cat # 550982), phosphorylated ERK (pERK) (cat # 4376), total ERK (tERK) (cat # 4695), phosphorylated AKT (pAKT) (cat # 4060), and total AKT (tAKT) (cat # 4691), all from Cell Signaling, and anti-β-actin (cat # A5441, Sigma Aldrich; Saint Louis, MO, USA). The blots were then washed three times with 1X TBST (Tris-buffered saline with 0.1% Tween® 20) detergent and incubated with the appropriate secondary antibody for 1 h at RT. The antigen–antibody complex was detected by enhanced chemiluminescence according to the manufacturer's instructions (ThermoFisher; Denver, CO, USA). Signals on the blots were quantified by densitometry software (Quantity one 4.6.5, Bio-Rad, Hercules, CA, USA). All the Western blots were performed in triplicate.

4.7. RTK Arrays

The RTK (Receptor Tyrosine Kinase) Proteome Profile Array Kit (cat # 8ARY001B, R&D systems, Minneapolis, MN, USA) was used to measure alterations in RTK phosphorylation in response to FOXO1 siRNA, non-silencing siRNA, or following PI3Ki treatment in LS174T cells as previously described [13]. Following treatments, the cells were washed with cold PBS (phosphate-buffered saline), lysed in NP40 lysis buffer, and 300 μg of cell lysates were incubated with blocked membranes overnight. Membranes were subsequently washed and incubated with an HRP (horseradish peroxidase)-conjugated anti-phosphotyrosine antibody (supplied with the kit) for 1 h at RT, washed, and ultimately incubated with a chemiluminescent substrate according to the manufacturer's protocol. The membrane was then exposed to X-ray film, and the results (image spot intensity and pixel density) were quantified by Image J analysis software 1.44.

4.8. Quantitative Real-Time PCR

Pictilisib-induced, FOXO-dependent RTK target gene expression in MCA cells was assessed by quantitative real-time PCR (qRT-PCR). Total RNA was extracted from FOXO1 and non-silencing siRNA expressing pictilisib (PI3Ki)-treated LS174T cells using the ToTally RNA kit (cat # AM1910, Ambion, Austin, TX, USA). RNA was treated with RNase-free DNase (Invitrogen) for 30 min at RT, and the first-strand cDNA was synthesized from 1 μg of DNase-treated RNA by MMLV reverse transcriptase (cat # New England Biolabs, Ipswich, MA). For qRT-PCR, 1μL of cDNA was mixed with 10 μL of 2X Fast SYBR green mix (cat # Applied Biosystems, Foster, CA, USA), oligonucleotides, and RT-PCR run using ABI 7500 machine (Applied Biosystems). Supplementary Table S1 lists the oligonucleotides used for the amplification of IGF-1R, IR, ErbB2, ErbB3, EphA10, and GAPDH as a reference control. In order to rule out probable contamination of genomic DNA, negative controls were performed in parallel by directly using RNA as a template for PCR. For data analysis, target gene Ct (cycle threshold) values were normalized to the GAPDH housekeeping gene and 2ddct values were reported as fold change relative to the control.

4.9. Cell Viability Assays

Cells were treated for 96 h with pictilisib (PI3Ki) (16 nM to 1 mM) or AS1842856 (FOXO1i) (1 nM to 1 mM), and cell viability was measured using the WST-1 cell viability assay (cat # 2198 Bio-Vision; Milpitas, CA, USA). The concentration of the drug resulting in 50% of maximal inhibition (IC50) was calculated from a four-parameter sigmoidal dose–response model (XLfit, IDBS). In vitro synergy studies were performed by the addition of PI3K and FOXO1 inhibitors in a fixed ratio ranging from 0.0039X to 4X IC50 of each drug, either alone or in combination. The synergy between drugs was followed based on our previously described studies [13] using the Compusyn program described by Chou and Talalay [26].

4.10. Statistical Analyses

Statistical analysis of all data was presented as mean ± SEM using Graph Pad Prism 8. A comparison between groups was carried out by a two-tail t-test, and values of $p < 0.05$ were considered statistically significant.

Supplementary Materials: The supporting information can be downloaded at: https://www.mdpi.com/article/10.3390/ijms241512331/s1.

Author Contributions: M.R.K., V.G., B.W.L., B.L.M. and M.T.; methodology, M.R.K., V.G. and B.W.L.; validation, M.R.K., V.G., B.W.L., B.L.M. and M.T.; formal analysis, M.R.K., B.L.M. and M.T.; resources, M.R.K., V.G., B.W.L. and B.L.M.; data curation, M.R.K.; writing—original draft preparation, M.R.K., V.G. and B.W.L.; writing—review and editing, M.R.K., V.G., B.W.L., B.L.M. and M.T.; funding acquisition, B.L.M. and M.T. All authors have read and agreed to the published version of the manuscript.

Funding: This research was funded in part by Biomedical Laboratory Research and Development, VA Office of Research and Development, Grant #BX004127 (B.L.M and M.T.).

Institutional Review Board Statement: Not applicable.

Informed Consent Statement: Not applicable.

Data Availability Statement: Once the database is finalized, it can be made available for data-sharing.

Acknowledgments: The study is dedicated to the memory of Peter Thomas, Creighton University, Omaha, NE. Peter was our mentor, colleague, and dear friend who departed this world earlier this year. He was a gifted scientist who pioneered major discoveries in the metabolism and role of carcinoembryonic antigen during primary colorectal cancers and CRC metastasis to the peritoneum and liver. Peter oversaw much of the research presented here, and we are forever grateful for his contributions to the field. The authors also thank John Mariadason (Ludwig Cancer Institute, Melbourne, Australia) for providing the RW7213 cell line and Genentech (San Francisco, CA, USA) for providing pictilisib.

Conflicts of Interest: The authors declare no conflict of interest.

Abbreviations

AKT	AKT kinase (Protein Kinase B or PKB)
AS1842856	FOXO1 inhibitor
BCA	Bicinchoninic Acid
BRAF	Murine sarcoma viral oncogene homolog B
DAPI	4,6-diamidino-2-phenylindole
DMSO	Dimethyl sulfoxide
EphA7	EPH Receptor A7
EphA10	EPH Receptor A10
ErbB2	Erb-B2 Receptor Tyrosine Kinase 2

ErbB3	Erb-B2 Receptor Tyrosine Kinase 3
FGFR 3	Fibroblast Growth Factor Receptor 3
GFP	Green Fluorescent Protein
IGF-R1	Insulin Growth Factor Receptor 1
INSR	Insulin Receptor pERK: phosphor-ERK1&2
KRAS	Kirsten rat sarcoma virus
MAP Kinase	Mitogen-activated protein kinase
MSP R	Macrophage Stimulating 1 Receptor
mTOR	Mechanistic Target Of Rapamycin Kinase
pAKT	Phosphor-AKT
PBS	Phosphate-buffered saline
PFA	Paraformaldehyde
PI3K	Phosphatidylinositol Kinase 3
pictilisib	PI3K inhibitor
ROR2	Receptor Tyrosine Kinase-Like Orphan Receptor 2
S6 Kinase	Ribosomal Protein S6 Kinase
siRNA	Small interfering RNA
Tie-2	Tyrosine Kinase with Immunoglobulin-Like and EGF-Like Domains 2
TRE	Tetracycline response element (TRE)

References

1. Tan, J.; Yu, Q. Molecular mechanisms of tumor resistance to PI3K-mTOR-targeted therapy. *Chin. J. Cancer* **2013**, *32*, 376–379. [CrossRef]
2. Vivanco, I.; Sawyers, C.L. The phosphatidylinositol 3-Kinase–AKT pathway in human cancer. *Nat. Rev. Cancer* **2002**, *2*, 489–501. [CrossRef]
3. Engelman, J.A.; Luo, J.; Cantley, L.C. The evolution of phosphatidylinositol 3-kinases as regulators of growth and metabolism. *Nat. Rev. Genet.* **2006**, *7*, 606–619. [CrossRef]
4. Chou, T.C.; Talalay, P. Quantitative analysis of dose-effect relationships: The combined effects of multiple drugs or enzyme in-hibitors. *Adv. Enzym. Regul.* **1984**, *22*, 27–55. [CrossRef]
5. Josephs, D.H.; Sarker, D. Pharmacodynamic Biomarker Development for PI3K Pathway Therapeutics. *Transl. Oncogenomics* **2015**, *7*, 33–49. [CrossRef]
6. Debunne, H.; Ceelen, W. Mucinous Differentiation in Colorectal Cancer: Molecular, Histological and Clinical Aspects. *Acta Chir. Belg.* **2013**, *113*, 385–390. [CrossRef] [PubMed]
7. Symonds, D.A.; Vickery, A.L. Mucinous carcinoma of the colon and rectum. *Cancer* **1976**, *37*, 1891–1900. [CrossRef] [PubMed]
8. Catalano, V.; Loupakis, F.; Graziano, F.; Torresi, U.; Bisonni, R.; Mari, D.; Fedeli, S.L. Mucinous histology predicts for poor response rate and overall survival of patients with colorectal cancer and treated with first-line oxaliplatin- and/or irinotecan-based chemotherapy. *Br. J. Cancer* **2009**, *100*, 881–887. [CrossRef] [PubMed]
9. Hugen, N.; van de Velde, C.J.H.; de Wilt, J.H.W.; Nagtegaal, I.D. Metastatic pattern in colorectal cancer is strongly influenced by histological subtype. *Ann. Oncol. Off. J. Eur. Soc. Med. Oncol.* **2014**, *25*, 651–657. [CrossRef]
10. Mekenkamp, L.J.; Heesterbeek, K.J.; Koopman, M.; Tol, J.; Teerenstra, S.; Venderbosch, S.; Punt, C.J.; Nagtegaal, I.D. Mucinous adenocarcinomas: Poor prognosis in metastatic colorectal cancer. *Eur. J. Cancer* **2012**, *48*, 501–509. [CrossRef]
11. Luo, C.; Cen, S.; Ding, G.; Wu, W. Mucinous colorectal adenocarcinoma: Clinical pathology and treatment options. *Cancer Commun.* **2019**, *39*, 13. [CrossRef] [PubMed]
12. Hugen, N.; Simons, M.; Halilović, A.; van der Post, R.S.; Bogers, A.J.; Marijnissen-van Zanten, M.A.; Nagtegaal, I. The molecular background of mucinous carcinoma beyond MUC2. *J. Pathol. Clin. Res.* **2015**, *1*, 3–17. [CrossRef] [PubMed]
13. Kuracha, M.R.; Thomas, P.; Loggie, B.W.; Govindarajan, V. Bilateral blockade of MEK- and PI3K-mediated pathways downstream of mutant KRAS as a treatment approach for peritoneal mucinous malignancies. *PLoS ONE* **2017**, *12*, e0179510. [CrossRef]
14. Schöffski, P.; Cresta, S.; Mayer, I.A.; Wildiers, H.; Damian, S.; Gendreau, S.; Rooney, I.; Morrissey, K.M.; Spoerke, J.M.; Ng, V.W.; et al. A phase Ib study of pictilisib (GDC-0941) in combination with paclitaxel, with and without bevacizumab or trastuzumab, and with letrozole in advanced breast cancer. *Breast Cancer Res.* **2018**, *20*, 109. [CrossRef]
15. Brunet, A.; Bonni, A.; Zigmond, M.J.; Lin, M.Z.; Juo, P.; Hu, L.S.; Anderson, M.J.; Arden, K.C.; Blenis, J.; Greenberg, M.E. Akt Promotes Cell Survival by Phosphorylating and Inhibiting a Forkhead Transcription Factor. *Cell* **1999**, *96*, 857–868. [CrossRef] [PubMed]
16. Kops, G.P.L.; De Ruiter, N.D.; De Vries-Smits, A.M.M.; Powell, D.R.; Bos, J.L.; Burgering, B.M. Direct control of the Forkhead transcription factor AFX by protein kinase B. *Nature* **1999**, *398*, 630–634. [CrossRef]
17. Dijkers, P.F.; Medema, R.H.; Pals, C.; Banerji, L.; Thomas, N.S.B.; Lam, E.W.-F.; Burgering, B.M.T.; Raaijmakers, J.A.M.; Lammers, J.-W.J.; Koenderman, L.; et al. Forkhead Transcription Factor FKHR-L1 Modulates Cytokine-Dependent Transcriptional Regulation of p27^{KIP1}. *Mol. Cell. Biol.* **2000**, *20*, 9138–9148. [CrossRef]

18. Sunters, A.; de Mattos, S.F.; Stahl, M.; Brosens, J.J.; Zoumpoulidou, G.; Saunders, C.A.; Coffer, P.J.; Medema, R.H.; Coombes, R.C.; Lam, E.W.-F. FoxO3a Transcriptional Regulation of Bim Controls Apoptosis in Paclitaxel-treated Breast Cancer Cell Lines. *J. Biol. Chem.* **2003**, *278*, 49795–49805. [CrossRef]
19. Fitzwalter, B.E.; Towers, C.G.; Sullivan, K.D.; Andrysik, Z.; Hoh, M.; Ludwig, M.; O'Prey, J.; Ryan, K.M.; Espinosa, J.M.; Morgan, M.J.; et al. Autophagy Inhibition Mediates Apoptosis Sensitization in Cancer Therapy by Relieving FOXO3a Turnover. *Dev. Cell* **2018**, *44*, 555–565.e3. [CrossRef]
20. Kops, G.J.; Dansen, T.B.; Polderman, P.E.; Saarloos, I.; Wirtz, K.W.A.; Coffer, P.J.; Huang, T.-T.; Bos, J.L.; Medema, R.H.; Burgering, B.M. Forkhead transcription factor FOXO3a protects quiescent cells from oxidative stress. *Nature* **2002**, *419*, 316–321. [CrossRef]
21. Nemoto, S.; Fergusson, M.M.; Finkel, T. Nutrient availability regulates SIRT1 through a forkhead-dependent pathway. *Science* **2004**, *306*, 2105–2108. [CrossRef] [PubMed]
22. Kajihara, T.; Jones, M.; Fusi, L.; Takano, M.; Feroze-Zaidi, F.; Pirianov, G.; Mehmet, H.; Ishihara, O.; Higham, J.M.; Lam, E.W.-F.; et al. Differential Expression of FOXO1 and FOXO3a Confers Resistance to Oxidative Cell Death upon Endometrial Decidualization. *Mol. Endocrinol.* **2006**, *20*, 2444–2455. [CrossRef] [PubMed]
23. Goto, T.; Takano, M.; Albergaria, A.; Briese, J.; Pomeranz, K.M.; Cloke, B.; Fusi, L.; Feroze-Zaidi, F.; Maywald, N.; Sajin, M.; et al. Mechanism and functional consequences of loss of FOXO1 expression in endometrioid endometrial cancer cells. *Oncogene* **2007**, *27*, 9–19. [CrossRef]
24. Han, C.-Y.; Cho, K.-B.; Choi, H.-S.; Han, H.-K.; Kang, K.-W. Role of FoxO1 activation in MDR1 expression in adriamycin-resistant breast cancer cells. *Carcinogenesis* **2008**, *29*, 1837–1844. [CrossRef]
25. Nievergall, E.; Lackmann, M.; Janes, P.W. Eph-dependent cell-cell adhesion and segregation in development and cancer. *Cell. Mol. Life Sci.* **2011**, *69*, 1813–1842. [CrossRef]
26. Chou, T.-C. Drug combination studies and their synergy quantification using the Chou-Talalay method. *Cancer Res.* **2010**, *70*, 440–446. [CrossRef]
27. Vaziri-Gohar, A.; Zheng, Y.; Houston, K.D. IGF-1 Receptor Modulates FoxO1-Mediated Tamoxifen Response in Breast Cancer Cells. *Mol. Cancer Res.* **2017**, *15*, 489–497. [CrossRef]
28. Murugan, A.K. mTOR: Role in cancer, metastasis and drug resistance. *Semin. Cancer Biol.* **2019**, *59*, 92–111. [CrossRef]
29. Hui, R.C.-Y.; Francis, R.E.; Guest, S.K.; Costa, J.R.; Gomes, A.R.; Myatt, S.S.; Brosens, J.J.; Lam, E.W.-F. Doxorubicin activates FOXO3a to induce the expression of multidrug resistance gene *ABCB1* (*MDR1*) in K562 leukemic cells. *Mol. Cancer Ther.* **2008**, *7*, 670–678. [CrossRef] [PubMed]
30. Rao, P.; Pang, M.; Qiao, X.; Yu, H.; Wang, H.; Yang, Y.; Ren, X.; Hu, M.; Chen, T.; Cao, Q.; et al. Promotion of β-catenin/Foxo1 signaling ameliorates renal interstitial fibrosis. *Lab. Investig.* **2019**, *99*, 1689–1701. [CrossRef]
31. Matsumoto, M.; Han, S.; Kitamura, T.; Accili, D. Dual role of transcription factor FoxO1 in controlling hepatic insulin sensitivity and lipid metabolism. *J. Clin. Investig.* **2006**, *116*, 2464–2472. [CrossRef] [PubMed]
32. Robertson, B.W.; Bonsal, L.; Chellaiah, M.A. Regulation of Erk1/2 activation by osteopontin in PC3 human prostate cancer cells. *Mol. Cancer* **2010**, *9*, 260. [CrossRef]
33. Chandarlapaty, S.; Sawai, A.; Scaltriti, M.; Rodrik-Outmezguine, V.; Grbovic-Huezo, O.; Serra, V.; Majumder, P.K.; Baselga, J.; Rosen, N. AKT Inhibition Relieves Feedback Suppression of Receptor Tyrosine Kinase Expression and Activity. *Cancer Cell* **2011**, *19*, 58–71. [CrossRef] [PubMed]
34. Serra, V.; Scaltriti, M.; Prudkin, L.; Eichhorn, P.J.A.; Ibrahim, Y.H.; Chandarlapaty, S.; Markman, B.; Rodriguez, O.; Guzman, M.; Rodriguez, S.; et al. PI3K inhibition results in enhanced HER signaling and acquired ERK dependency in HER2-overexpressing breast cancer. *Oncogene* **2011**, *30*, 2547–2557. [CrossRef] [PubMed]
35. Pan, C.; Jin, X.; Zhao, Y.; Pan, Y.; Yang, J.; Karnes, R.J.; Zhang, J.; Wang, L.; Huang, H. AKT-phosphorylated FOXO1 suppresses ERK activation and chemoresistance by disrupting IQGAP1-MAPK interaction. *EMBO J.* **2017**, *36*, 995–1010. [CrossRef] [PubMed]
36. Xia, P.; Chen, J.; Liu, Y.; Fletcher, M.; Jensen, B.C.; Cheng, Z. Doxorubicin induces cardiomyocyte apoptosis and atrophy through cyclin-dependent kinase 2–mediated activation of forkhead box O1. *J. Biol. Chem.* **2020**, *295*, 4265–4276. [CrossRef]
37. Nagashima, T.; Shigematsu, N.; Maruki, R.; Urano, Y.; Tanaka, H.; Shimaya, A.; Shimokawa, T.; Shibasaki, M. Discovery of Novel Forkhead Box O1 Inhibitors for Treating Type 2 Diabetes: Improvement of Fasting Glycemia in Diabetic *db/db* Mice. *Mol. Pharmacol.* **2010**, *78*, 961–970. [CrossRef]
38. Sunters, A.; Madureira, P.A.; Pomeranz, K.M.; Aubert, M.; Brosens, J.J.; Cook, S.J.; Burgering, B.M.; Coombes, R.C.; Lam, E.W. Paclitaxel-Induced Nuclear Translocation of FOXO3a in Breast Cancer Cells Is Mediated by c-Jun NH2-Terminal Kinase and Akt. *Cancer Res.* **2006**, *66*, 212–220. [CrossRef]
39. Gan, L.; Chen, S.; Wang, Y.; Watahiki, A.; Bohrer, L.; Sun, Z.; Huang, H. Inhibition of the androgen receptor as a novel mechanism of taxol chemotherapy in prostate cancer. *Cancer Res.* **2009**, *69*, 8386–8394. [CrossRef]

Disclaimer/Publisher's Note: The statements, opinions and data contained in all publications are solely those of the individual author(s) and contributor(s) and not of MDPI and/or the editor(s). MDPI and/or the editor(s) disclaim responsibility for any injury to people or property resulting from any ideas, methods, instructions or products referred to in the content.

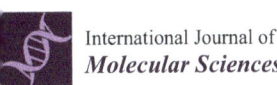

Article

ABCG2 Gene and ABCG2 Protein Expression in Colorectal Cancer—In Silico and Wet Analysis

Aleksandra Sałagacka-Kubiak [1,*], Dawid Zawada [1], Lias Saed [1], Radzisław Kordek [2], Agnieszka Jeleń [1] and Ewa Balcerczak [1]

1. Department of Pharmaceutical Biochemistry and Molecular Diagnostics, Medical University of Lodz, 92-213 Lodz, Poland; dawid.zawada2@gmail.com (D.Z.); lias.saed@stud.umed.lodz.pl (L.S.); agnieszka.jelen@umed.lodz.pl (A.J.)
2. Department of Pathology, Medical University of Lodz, 92-213 Lodz, Poland; radzislaw.kordek@umed.lodz.pl
* Correspondence: aleksandra.salagacka@umed.lodz.pl

Abstract: ABCG2 (ATP-binding cassette superfamily G member 2) is a cell membrane pump encoded by the *ABCG2* gene. ABCG2 can protect cells against compounds initiating and/or intensifying neoplasia and is considered a marker of stem cells responsible for cancer growth, drug resistance and recurrence. Expression of the *ABCG2* gene or its protein has been shown to be a negative prognostic factor in various malignancies. However, its prognostic significance in colorectal cancer remains unclear. Using publicly available data, *ABCG2* was shown to be underexpressed in colon and rectum adenocarcinomas, with lower expression compared to both the adjacent nonmalignant lung tissues and non-tumour lung tissues of healthy individuals. This downregulation could result from the methylation level of some sites of the *ABCG2* gene. This was connected with microsatellite instability, weight and age among patients with colon adenocarcinoma, and with tumour localization, population type and age of patients for rectum adenocarcinoma. No association was found between *ABCG2* expression level and survival of colorectal cancer patients. In wet analysis of colorectal cancer samples, neither *ABCG2* gene expression, analysed by RT-PCR, nor ABCG2 protein level, assessed by immunohistochemistry, was associated with any clinicopathological factors or overall survival. An ABCG2-centered protein–protein interaction network build by STRING showed proteins were found to be involved in leukotriene, organic anion and xenobiotic transport, endodermal cell fate specification, and histone methylation and ubiquitination. Hence, ABCG2 underexpression could be an indicator of the activity of certain signalling pathways or protein interactors essential for colorectal carcinogenesis.

Keywords: ABCG2; prognosis; survival; protein–protein interaction network; immunohistochemistry; qPCR

1. Introduction

Despite the existence of effective screening techniques and the unquestionable advancement in treatment options, colorectal cancer remains the third most common cancer type worldwide. According to GLOBOCAN, the condition was responsible for almost one million deaths in 2020, with nearly two million new cases that year [1]. It also predicted that the number of new cases and the number of deaths will increase by about 70% of today's values by 2040 [2]. Currently, the major obstacles to the successful management of colorectal cancer are difficulties in accurate prediction of the further course of colorectal cancer and choosing the optimal treatment schedule, as well as predicting the response to applied therapy. Thus, the research efforts focused on new biological markers related to the neoplastic process that can be transferable to clinical practice.

ABCG2 (ATP-binding cassette superfamily G member 2), encoded by the *ABCG2* gene, is an ATP-dependent transporter belonging to the ATP-binding cassette (ABC) protein superfamily. The ABCG2 localized in the cell membrane pumps the drug molecules

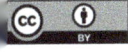

from the cytoplasm out of the cells (Figure 1). This diminishes access of the drug to the cellular target, and thus reduces the effectiveness of the applied therapy. As ABCG2 is characterized by low substrate specificity, and its substrates include drugs from various therapeutic groups and their metabolites, it may provide resistance to a wide variety of anticancer drugs—a phenomenon termed multidrug resistance (MDR) [3]. Some studies have suggested that the *ABCG2* gene and its protein may act as indicators for the prediction of irinotecan-based therapy outcomes in colorectal cancer patients (reviewed in [4]).

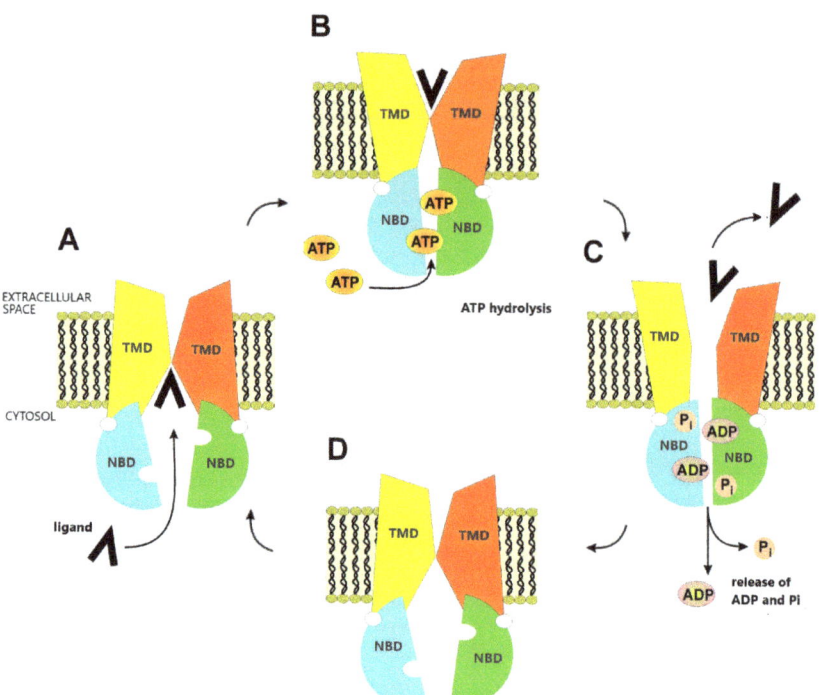

Figure 1. Scheme of the structure and the process of transport across the membrane with the participation of ABCG2. The transport takes place in four closely related stages. (**A**) Transmembrane domains (TMDs) adopt an inward-facing conformation with high affinity to the exported compound, which attaches itself to a special pocket formed by two TMD domains. This induces conformational changes in nucleotide-binding domains (NBDs) so that they increase their affinity for ATP. (**B**) Two ATP molecules are attached, resulting in NBFs approaching each other. This causes the TMDs to adopt an outward-facing conformation. (**C**) Transfer and release of the exported ligand across the membrane. ATP hydrolysis, phosphate and ADP release occur in parallel. (**D**) Relaxation of NBDs, return of TMDs to inward-facing conformation. The transporter is ready to accept the next ligand molecule, and the whole cycle can be repeated [5–8].

However, the role of ABCG2 in creating the MDR phenomenon is a manifestation of its physiological properties. ABCG2 is present in placental syncytiotrophoblast cells, epithelium of the intestine, liver tubules, ducts and lobes of the breast, renal proximal tubule cells, adrenal glands, stem cells and endothelium of capillaries and veins. It controls the absorption and excretion of endogenous and exogenous substances, creates tissue barriers and maintains the homeostasis of the physiological compartments of the body. These activities suggest that it may have an important role in the carcinogenesis of, inter alia, the colon and rectum. First, ABCG2 protects cells against compounds initiating and/or intensifying neoplasia. Dietrich et al. [9] identified elevated concentrations of 2-amino-1-methyl-6-phenylimidazo[4,5-b] pyridine (PhIP), a food-derived colon carcinogen and substrate of

ABCG2, in adenomas of ApcMin mice. Downregulation of ABCG2/Abcg2 was found to impair the barrier function of the intestine, thus leading to higher carcinogen concentrations in colorectal adenomas in mice and humans and promoting the adenoma–carcinoma sequence via DNA-bound accumulation of carcinogenic xenobiotics. Moreover, ABCG2 can affect the oral availability and tissue distribution of flavonoids, reducing their beneficial anticancer effect [10].

It is still not fully understood if the downregulation of *ABCG2* expression in colorectal cancer is a cause or a consequence of carcinogenesis. Previously, it was demonstrated that inflammation, a part of colorectal carcinogenesis, decreased the expression of ABC transporters in the intestines in animals. Significantly lower *Abcg2* mRNA levels were noted in the small intestines of adjuvant-induced arthritis rats compared with controls [11]. Englund et al. [12] demonstrated lower *ABCG2* expression in patients with active ulcerative colitis compared with controls, and the level negatively correlated with the *IL-6* mRNA level. Lower ABCG2 staining of the colonic epithelium was noted in inflamed tissues compared to healthy mucosa, and this was associated with disruption of the epithelial F-actin structure. It was also found that inflammation is needed to reduce *ABCG2* mRNA expression because it did not differ between patients in remission and healthy controls. Mossafa et al. [13] demonstrated that proinflammatory cytokines, such as IL-1β, IL-6 and TNF-α, were able to modulate the expression of ABCG2 at transcriptional and post-transcriptional levels in human cervix and gastric cancer cells. Moreover, ABCG2, along with other membrane transporters, is an important component of the intestinal barrier against xenobiotics such as drugs, bacterial toxins or carcinogens such as benzo[a]pyrene conjugates, 17 aflatoxin B1, 25 and PhIP18. Deuring et al. [14] showed that in patients with active inflammatory bowel disease, various inflammatory mediators can block the detoxification function of ABCG2 in intestine mucosa as a consequence of an unfolded protein response. The expression of ABCG2 in the intestine is directly influenced by the expression of the pregnane X receptor PXR, a key regulator in drug metabolism and efflux [15]. Hence, it can be suggested that the downregulation of *ABCG2* expression observed in colorectal cancer can result from inflammation in the bowel mucosa, and that this may represent a preliminary step in reducing its protective potential against cancer-promoting xenobiotics.

The human *ABCG2* gene harbours a variety of polymorphisms and mutations, which may significantly change its expression as well as its substrate binding and transporter activity through improper protein folding or cellular trafficking (reviewed in [16]). To et al. [17] found *ABCG2* mRNA variants that differ in the 3'UTR sequence, and the shorter forms of this sequence do not have a possible binding site for the corresponding microRNA, hsa-miR-519c, thus preventing mRNA degradation and/or repression on protein translation, resulting in transporter overexpression; this is observed in resistant S1MI80 colon cancer cells. Importantly, some studies indicate that *ABCG2* sequence variants may be involved in modulating colorectal cancer risk, as the expression and activity of the transporter in the bowels can differ between individuals, due at least in part to genetic polymorphisms of the *ABCG2* gene. Campa et al. [18] reported an association between colorectal cancer and rs2622621 and rs1481012 *ABCG2*. In addition, Kopp et al. [19] indicated that *ABCB1* rs1045642, *ABCG2* rs2231137 and *IL10* rs3024505 interacting with fibre intake significantly influenced colorectal cancer risk; however, this was contradicted by Andersen [20].

Additionally, ABCG2 is also considered a marker of cancer stem cells (CSCs), a subpopulation of tumour cells with stem cell characteristics; these are believed to be responsible for cancer growth, drug resistance and recurrence. Significantly increased expression of ABCG2 was observed in so-called side population (SP) cells isolated from various human gastrointestinal system cancer cell lines resembling stem cells [21]. Xie et al. [22] found that a fraction of SP cells obtained from colon cancer samples exhibited enhanced *ACBG2* expression compared to non-SP cells.

CSCs are often characterized by the presence of the CD133 cell surface marker. Ma et al. [23] found ABCG2 to be expressed in CD133-positive cancer stem cells from human colorectal tumours. siRNA-mediated knock-down of *ABCG2* expression lowered the self-renewal capacity of the cells and increased the efficiency of chemotherapy-induced apoptosis in colon adenocarcinoma cells and CD133-positive colorectal carcinoma cells. In addition, in SW480 cells, knockdown of *ABCG2* by lentivirus construct inhibits CD133 expression, sphere formation in vitro and tumour formation in vivo [24]. In CSCs, ABGC2 is able to transport compounds important for the growth, division and differentiation of the cells and pump out any harmful endo- and exogenous substances. Krishnamurthy et al. [25] demonstrated ABCG2 maintains CSC survival under hypoxic conditions by reducing the accumulation of protoporphyrins, i.e., toxic heme metabolites.

In addition, Gupta et al. [26] showed that *ABCG2* mRNA and protein levels are decreased several-fold in human colorectal cancer and liver tissue with metastasis from a colonic primary. They postulate that downregulation of ABCG2 may enhance the accumulation of protoporphyrins in the tumour cell, resulting in increased generation of heme, a cofactor for isoform I of nitric oxide synthases, and sustainable production of precancerous nitric oxide during malignancy. It appears that low activity of NOS may be cytostatic or cytotoxic for tumour cells, whereas high activity can have the opposite effect and promote tumour growth.

Some studies have reported the presence of ABCG2 in the nucleus in head and neck squamous cell carcinoma cells [27] and glioblastoma multiforme cells [28]. In lung cancer cells, Liang SC et al. [29] found ABCG2 protein to bind to the E-box of *CDH1* (E-cadherin) promoter inside the nucleus, where it regulates its transcription. Increased expression of ABCG2 causes an increase in E-cadherin and attenuates cell migration in vitro. In contrast, an increased level of ABCG2, and corresponding increase in E-cadherin, may induce circulating cancer cells to colonize at a distant site and form a metastatic tumour. Wang et al. [30] reported strong membranous staining of ABCG2 to be significantly linked with lymph node and distant metastasis, and that cytoplasmatic expression was connected with tumour stage. The researchers postulated that high ABCG2 expression can reduce ROS production and thus confer better OS and DFS, and that the protective role of ABCG2 was specific to the site.

Both the ABCG2 gene and protein expression have aroused considerable interest as potential prognostic factors in various cancers. Both have been shown to be negative prognostic factors associated with a more aggressive phenotype of haematological malignancies such as acute myeloid leukaemia [31] and adult acute lymphoblastic leukaemia [32], and solid tumours such as non-small-cell lung cancer [33], small-cell lung cancer [34], oesophageal squamous cell carcinoma [35–37], pancreatic cancer [38], pancreatic ductal adenocarcinoma [39], head and neck squamous cell carcinoma [40] and breast cancer [41]. The expression of ABCG2 protein is correlated with the expression of HER2 in breast cancer, suggesting that ABCG2 is not only a drug-resistance-related transporter but also a potential biomarker predicting the biological behaviour, clinical progression and prognosis of breast cancer [42]. In contrast, loss of ABCG2 protein was related to a worse prognosis and was an independent prognostic factor in patients with moderately or poorly differentiated intrahepatic cholangiocarcinoma [43]. Several studies on the prognostic significance of ABCG2 expression in colorectal cancer have been conducted; however, they have yielded inconsistent results [26,30,44–46] due to heterogeneity in the numbers of analysed samples and patient enrolment, stratification schemes, applied treatments and measurement of *ABCG2* gene and ABCG2 protein expression.

Therefore, the present study integrates data regarding *ABCG2* gene and protein expression from publicly available databases. Multiple bioinformatical and biostatistical analyses were conducted, including screening of *ABCG2* expression in a collection of various malignancies, comparing *ABCG2* expression in normal and malignant colon and rectum tissues, evaluating the relationship between the *ABCG2* expression level and clinical features of CRC and prognosis in colorectal cancer, and constructing the functional network of the ABCG2 protein. Furthermore, to validate findings from the in silico analysis, *ABCG2* gene and protein expression was measured in a cohort of colorectal cancer patients to determine their prognostic significance. The study also discusses the significance of the findings from the in silico and wet analysis with regard to those of previous studies.

2. Results

2.1. In Silico Analysis of OMICS Data Regarding ABCG2 Gene and ABCG2 Protein Expression in Colorectal Cancer

2.1.1. A Decrease in *ABCG2* mRNA Expression Level Is Common in Multiple Carcinomas

First, differences in *ABCG2* expression between cancers of various origins and comparable noncancerous tissue from healthy individuals were assessed via the Oncomine platform. Decreased *ABCG2* mRNA expression (blue) was observed in all except one analysed cancer, i.e., including various breast, ovarian, lung and liver tumours (Figure 2A). In 7 of 12 datasets collected in Oncomine, 17 out of 34 analyses found *ABCG2* to be among 10% of the top underexpressed genes in colorectal tumours (Figure 2B).

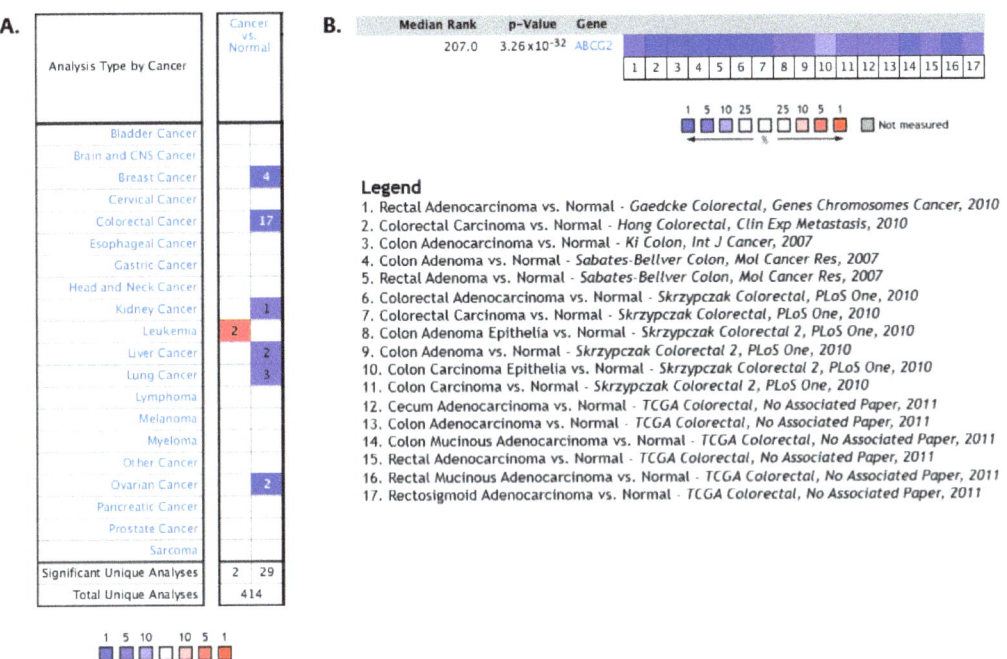

Figure 2. (**A**) The relative *ABCG2* mRNA levels in different types of cancer compared to matched normal tissue in Oncomine. Significantly ($p < 0.05$) increased and decreased levels of *ABCG2* are indicated in red and blue, respectively. The intensity of cell colour is determined by the best gene rank percentile for the analyses within the cell. The number in each cell represents the number of analyses that meet the given thresholds within the analysis and cancer types. (**B**) Comparison of *ABCG2* mRNA expression in colorectal cancer across 17 analyses. The rank given for the gene is the median rank for the gene across each of the analyses. The *p*-value for the gene is its *p*-value for the median-ranked analysis.

Comparable results were obtained from the TNMplot and TIMER 2.0 databases, where the majority of cancer types showed significantly decreased *ABCG2* expression (Figure 3A,B), e.g., bladder cancer, breast cancer, lung adenocarcinoma and squamous carcinoma, colon and rectum adenocarcinoma or uterine endometrial cancer. One exception was renal clear cell carcinoma, where significant overexpression of *ABCG2* was confirmed in both datasets.

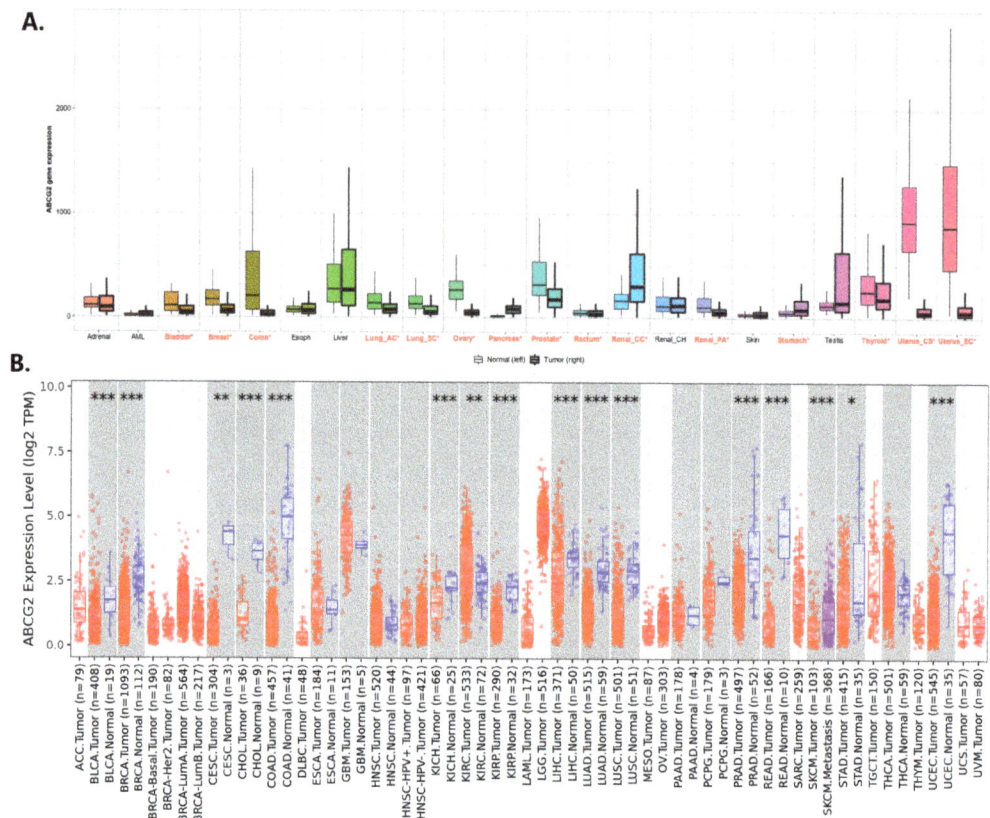

Figure 3. The level of *ABCG2* expression in different cancer types compared to the corresponding normal tissue: (**A**) TNMplot; cancer names where differences with $p < 0.01$ (Mann–Whitney U-test) were detected are typed in red and indicated by asterix. (**B**) TIMER2.0; the statistical significance (p-value) computed by the Wilcoxon test is annotated by the number of stars: * < 0.05; ** < 0.01; *** < 0.001; box plots in grey columns indicate cancer types where data for matched normal tissue were available; red and blue box plots indicate tumour and normal samples, respectively.

2.1.2. *ABCG2* Is Underexpressed in Colorectal Cancer in Comparison to Both Adjacent and Unpaired Normal Colorectal Tissue

To confirm whether *ABCG2* expression changes during carcinogenesis in the colon and rectum, paired colon or rectum cancer tumours and adjacent normal tissue collected from the same patients were compared using the TNMplot platform. As shown in Figure 4, *ABCG2* expression was significantly lower in colon cancer samples than in paired non-cancerous tissues ($p = 3.91 \times 10^{-25}$) indicated by DNA chip data, and significantly lower in both colon and rectum adenocarcinoma samples compared to paired normal tissues, assessed by RNA-seq ($p = 8.71 \times 10^{-8}$ and $p = 9.15 \times 10^{-3}$, respectively). Similar differences were noted between tumours and nonadjacent healthy tissue samples (Figure 5). *ABCG2* expression was substantially decreased in cancerous tissue samples compared to non-transformed tissue obtained from the separate subject cohort. Similar results were observed in the case of colon cancer, measured by DNA chip ($p = 9.62 \times 10^{-167}$), as for colon and rectum adenocarcinomas based on RNA-seq data ($p = 3.15 \times 10^{-65}$ and $p = 8.74 \times 10^{-3}$).

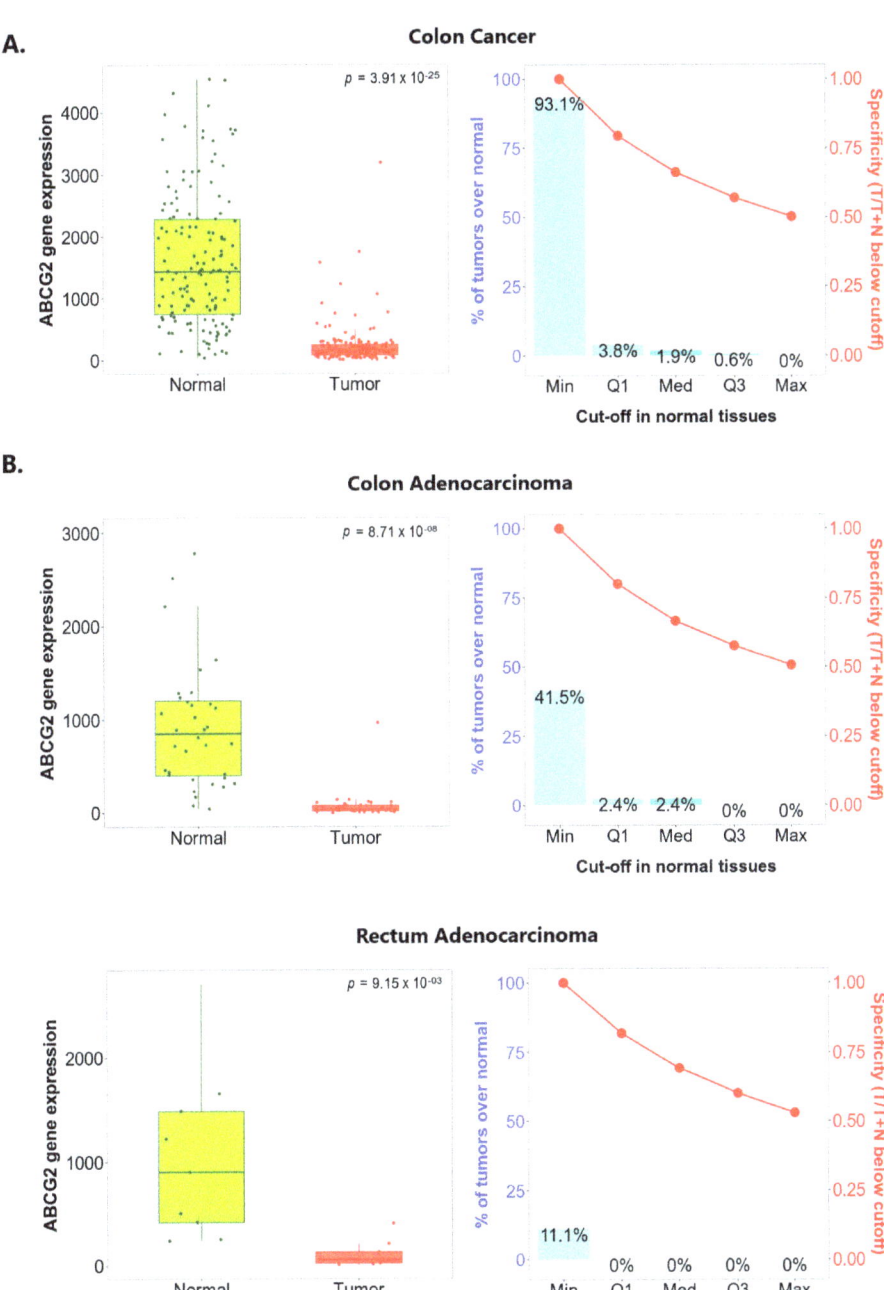

Figure 4. *ABCG2* expression level in paired tumour and adjacent normal tissue according to TNM-plot. (**A**) Gene chip data for colon cancer (**B**) RNA-Seq data for colon adenocarcinoma and rectum adenocarcinoma.

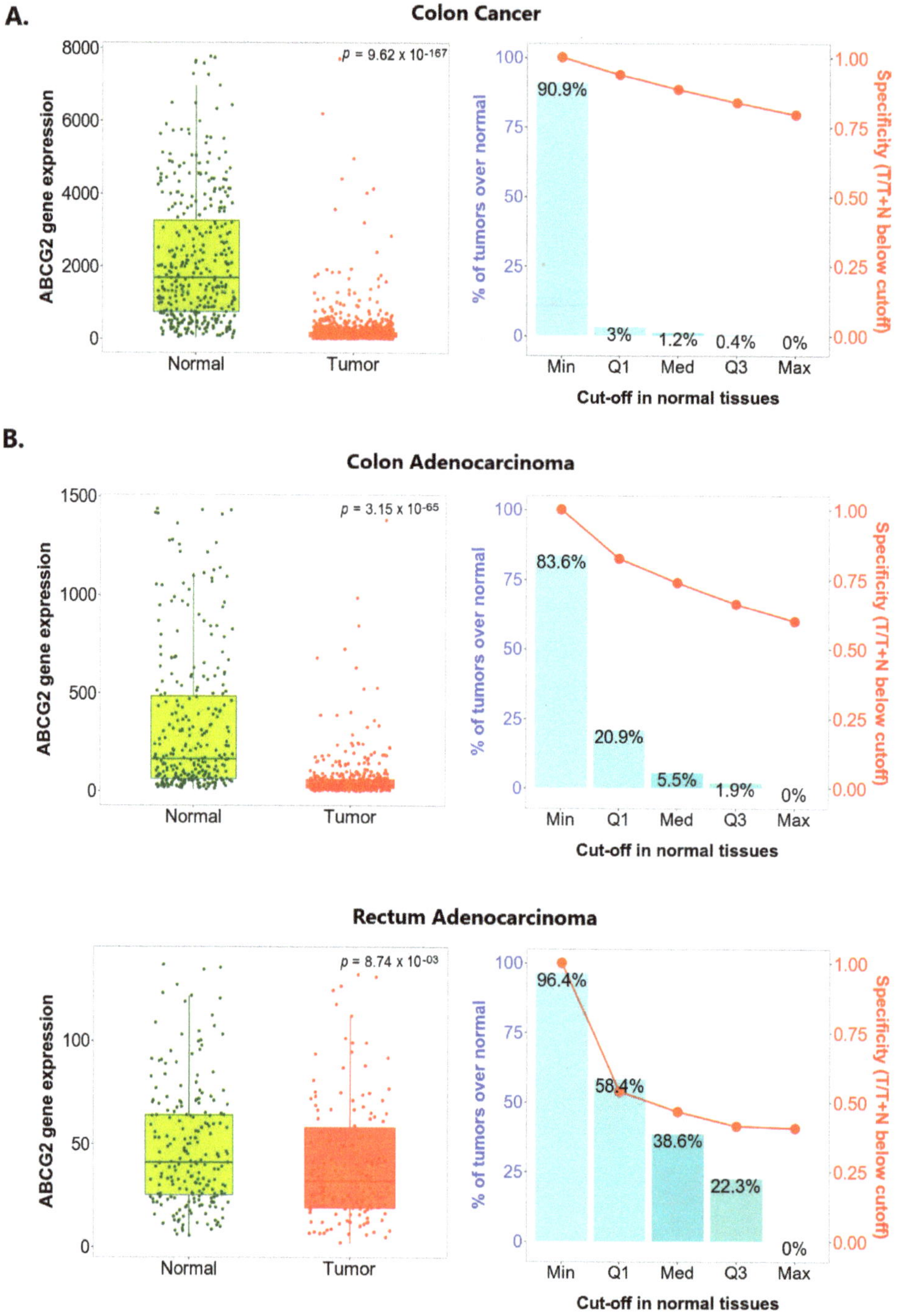

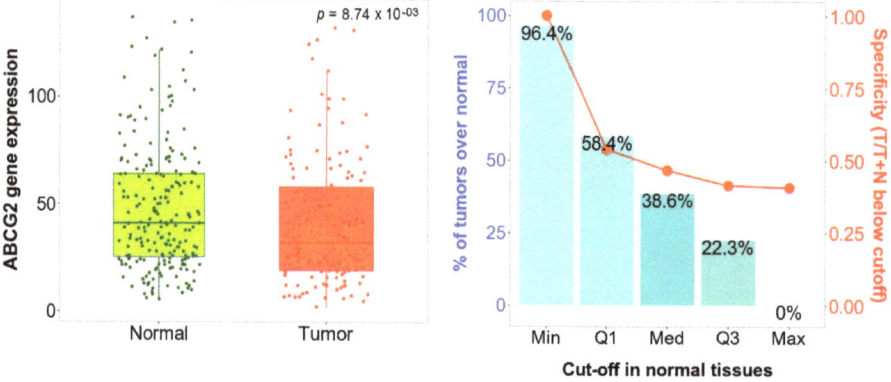

Figure 5. *ABCG2* expression level in non-paired tumour and normal tissue by TNMplot. (**A**) Gene chip data for colon cancer (**B**) RNA-Seq data for colon adenocarcinoma and rectum adenocarcinoma.

The study also evaluated the sensitivity and specificity of *ABCG2* expression as an indicator, with major cutoffs set at the base of the range of *ABCG2* expression in normal samples. The identified sensitivity and specificity are presented in the charts on the right-hand side in Figures 4 and 5. In colon cancer samples, the optimal sensitivity and specificity was found at minimum cutoff with adjacent noncancerous tissue or unpaired normal tissue used as a reference (Figures 4A and 5A). In addition, the best sensitivity (the proportions of tumour samples that show higher expression of the selected gene compared to normal samples at each of the quantile cutoff values) and specificity (calculated by dividing the number of tumour samples with the sum of tumour and normal samples below each given cutoff) were sought. Optimal sensitivity and specificity were also found for the minimum cutoff when colon and rectum adenocarcinoma tumours were analysed against unpaired healthy tissues (Figure 5B). No satisfactory cutoff point was found for the colon and rectum adenocarcinomas when adjacent non-tumour samples were considered as a reference (Figure 4B), probably because of the relatively low number of samples provided for analysis.

2.1.3. *ABCG2* Expression Is Higher in Metastatic Tissues Than in Primary Tumours of Colon Cancer

Additionally, *ABCG2* expression was compared between normal colon tissue, primary tumour and metastatic tissue (Figure 6). A significant difference in the level was found ($p = 4.42 \times 10^{-178}$). The level was substantially lower in both primary and metastatic tissue than in the normal colon ($p = 3.77 \times 10^{-176}$ and $p = 7.22 \times 10^{-14}$, respectively). However, the metastatic tissue showed higher *ABCG2* expression than the primary tumour tissue ($p = 8.37 \times 10^{-15}$).

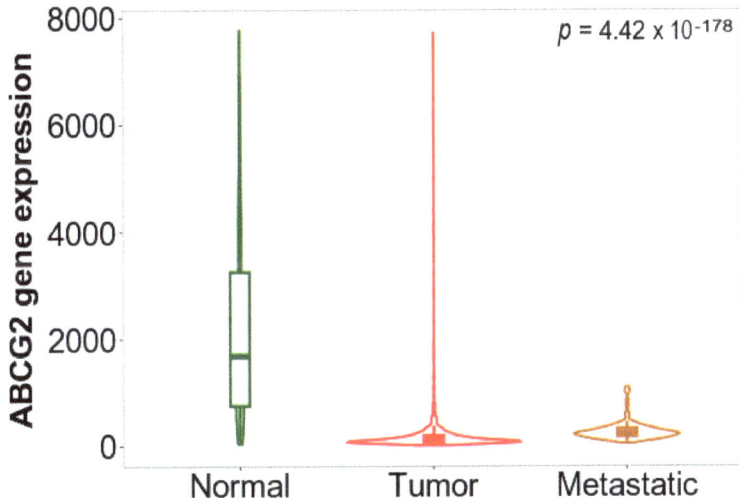

Figure 6. *ABCG2* expression level in normal, tumour and metastatic tissue by TNMplot (gene–chip data).

2.1.4. ABCG2 Protein Could Be Detected in Colon and Rectum Normal Tissue but Not in Colorectal Cancer

As the *ABCG2* mRNA expression was found to be substantially decreased in colorectal cancer, the expression and localization of ABCG2 protein in colorectal cancer and corresponding normal tissues was determined based on the immunohistochemistry staining images collected in the Human Protein Atlas (Figure 7). In both colon and rectum non-cancerous tissues, high ABCG2 protein immunostaining was revealed in the microvilli of enterocytes. In the rectum, medium-level immunostaining was detected in peripheral nerve cells and low-level staining in endothelial cells. However, no positive reaction was noted in the cancerous cells of colon or rectum adenocarcinomas.

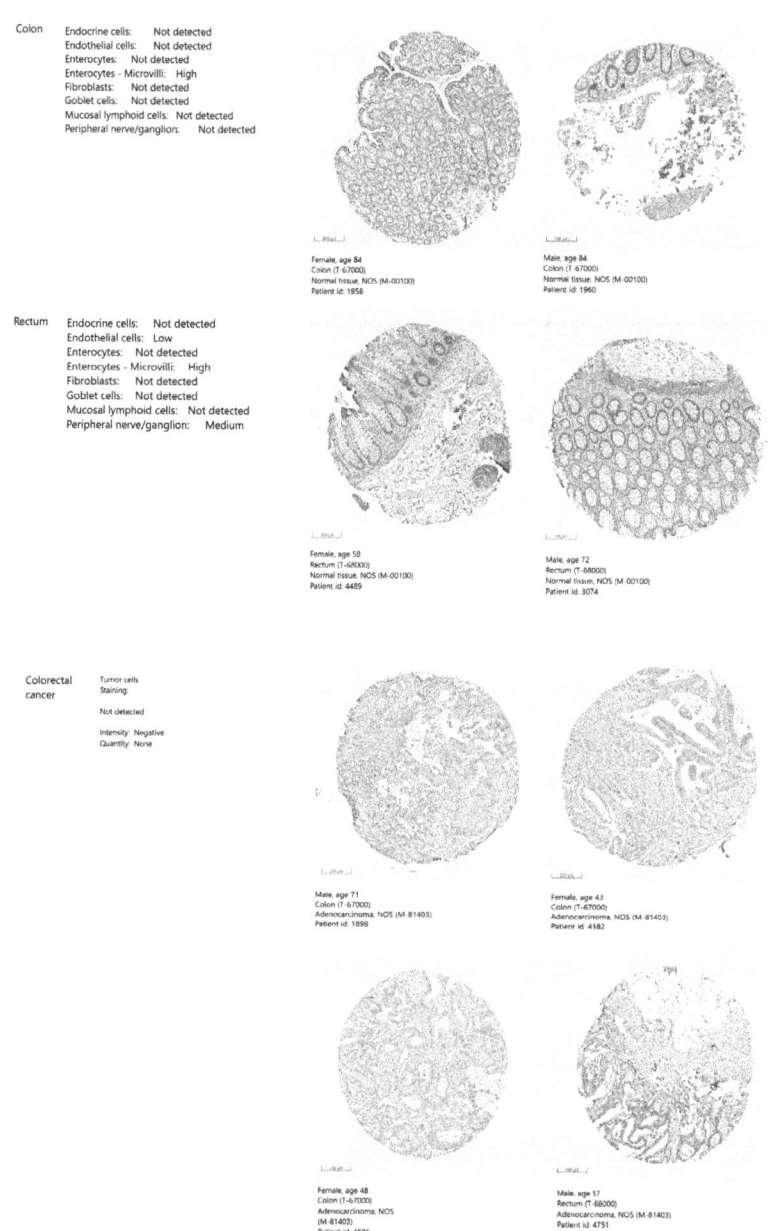

Figure 7. ABCG2 protein expression levels. The images indicate immunohistochemistry staining for normal colon and rectum tissues and colon and rectum adenocarcinomas collected with HPA. Higher antigen content (representing the level of protein expression) and distribution density is indicated by colour rendering: blue = negative; light yellow = weakly positive; brown = moderately positive; dark brown = strongly positive.

2.1.5. *ABCG2* Gene Expression Level in Colorectal Cancer Could Be Connected with Methylation Status but Not with DNA Alterations of the *ABCG2* Gene

As *ABCG2* was found to be commonly underexpressed in colorectal carcinomas, the mutational and methylation status of the gene was analysed. An Oncoprint was generated by querying 5511 patients/5285 samples from 16 studies using cBioPortal (Figure 8A). In total, *ABCG2* alterations were detected in 1.5% of colorectal cancer patients profiled for mutation, copy number changes and structural variants. With regard to histological subtypes, the highest frequencies of *ABCG2* changes were noted in mucinous adenocarcinoma of the colon and rectum (Figure 8B). Of these, the most commonly detected were mutations, with deep deletion being less common. No amplifications or structural variants were noted. Missense, truncating and splice change mutations were relatively evenly distributed along the gene (Figure 8C).

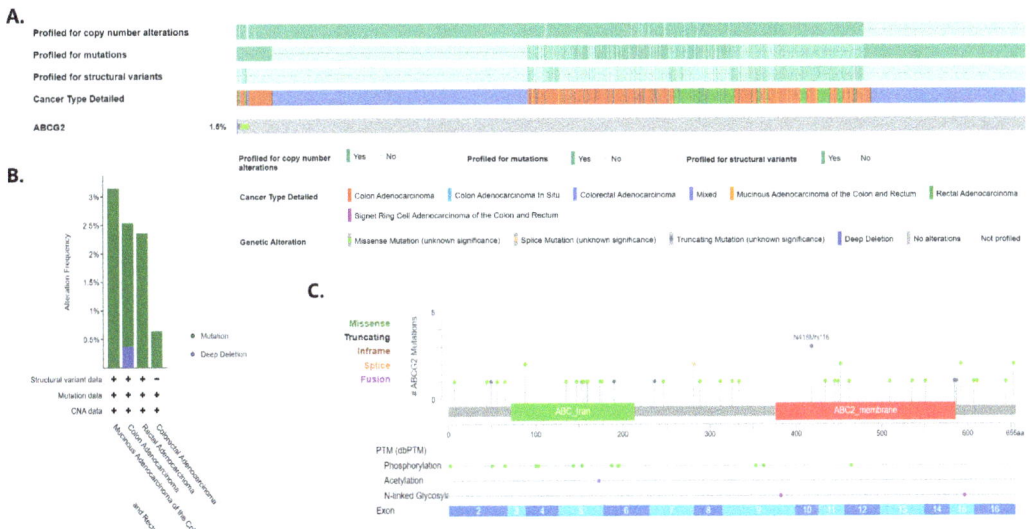

Figure 8. *ABCG2* genomic alterations in colorectal cancer according to cBioPortal. (**A**) Oncoprint of the *ABCG2* in colorectal cancer; (**B**) incidence of different alterations according to colorectal cancer types; (**C**) details of *ABCG2* mutation found in colorectal cancer.

The deep deletion mentioned above could be the possible reason for *ABCG2* underexpression. However, no increase in expression was noted when moving from loss of copy number to gain (Figure 9A): the analysis only revealed very weak and insignificant correlation coefficients (R Spearman 0.01, $p = 0.723$; R Pearson 0.07, $p = 0.829$; Figure 9B).

Changes in gene methylation occur frequently during cancerogenesis, thus influencing the expression of the genes important for transformation, the methylation level of the *ABCG2* gene was inspected in colorectal cancer. According to cBioPortal data (Figure 10A), *ABCG2* expression decreased with increased methylation. However, a statistically significant but weak Person's correlation coefficient (-0.14, $p = 0.0408$) and insignificant Spearman coefficient (-0.05, $p = 0.457$) were calculated for the association. The methylation level of the *ABCG2* was compared between colon and rectum adenocarcinoma tissue and normal samples using TCGA data provided by UALCAN (Figure 10B,C). While *ABCG2* promoter hypomethylation was noted in both adenocarcinomas and normal samples (beta values range 0.033–0.090), slightly, but significantly, lower methylation was found for both colon ($p < 0.01$) and rectum adenocarcinomas ($p = 0.0247$) in comparison to normal samples.

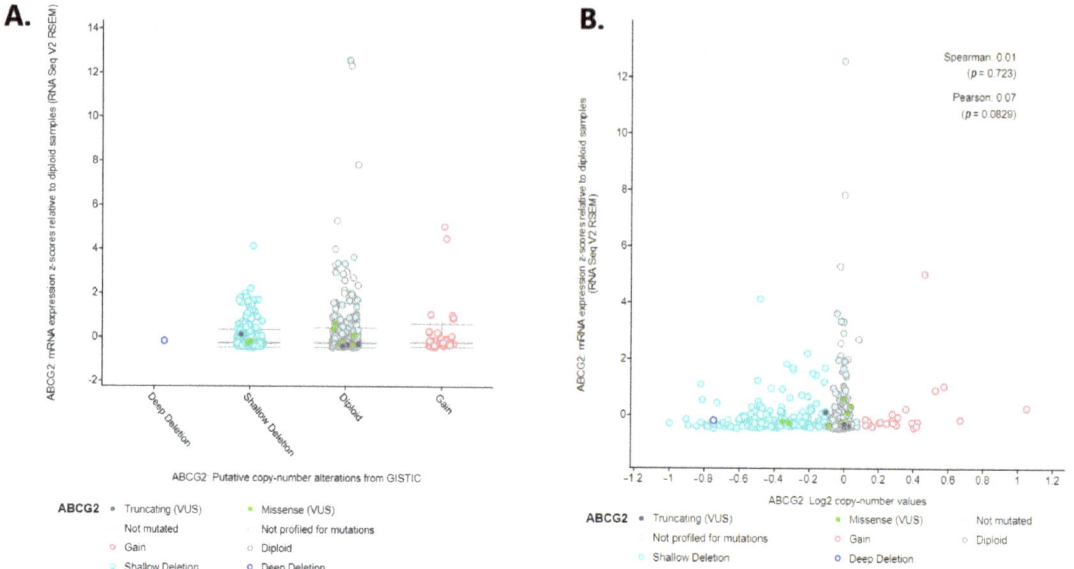

Figure 9. Association between *ABCG2* mRNA expression and (**A**) putative copy-number alteration form GISTIC; (**B**) log2 copy number value (generated by cBioPortal).

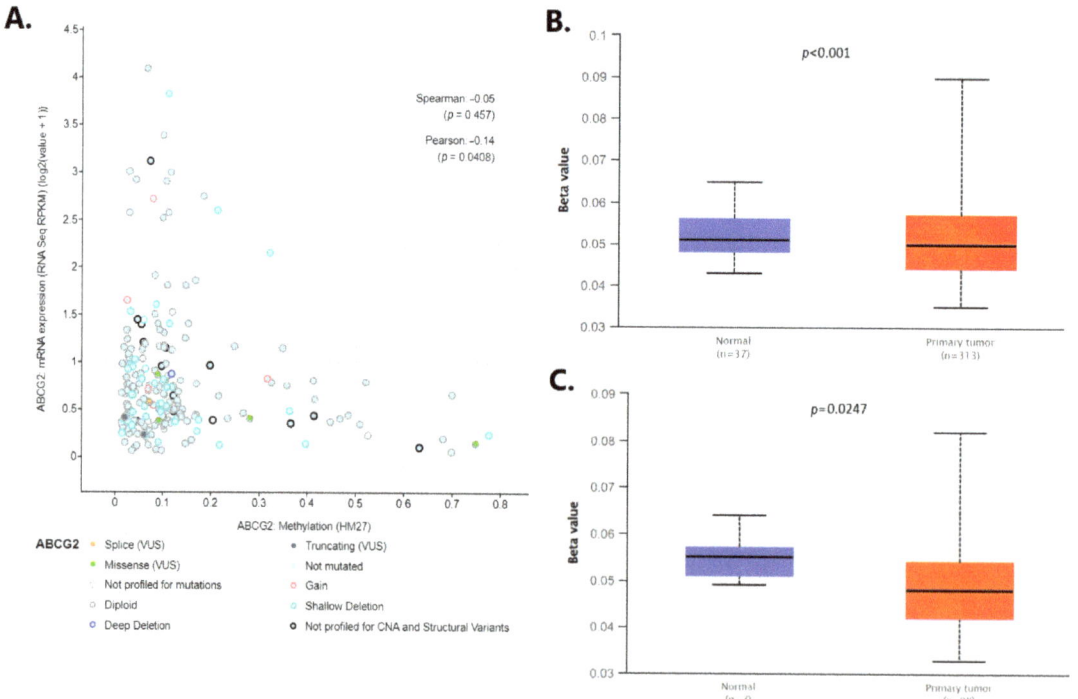

Figure 10. (**A**) Association between mRNA expression and DNA methylation profile of the *ABCG2* gene based on cBioPortal; the promoter methylation level of the *ABCG2* in (**B**) colon adenocarcinoma and (**C**) rectum adenocarcinoma in comparison to normal tissue (by UALCAN).

One of the most important factors influencing the regulation of gene expression by DNA methylation is its precise genomic location. Therefore, MEXPRESS visualization was performed of the TCGA data to determine the expression of *the studied gene* and its methylation. For the colon adenocarcinoma (Figure 11A), the level of methylation was negatively correlated with the expression for 5 of 14 probes across the *ABCG2* gene (Pearson correlation coefficients ranging from −0.132 to −0.117). For one probe (cpg location 88147879), a significant positive correlation between the methylation and expression levels was found (Pearson correlation coefficient = 0.263). Contrary to the UALCAN data shown above, no such association was found for the *ABCG2* promoter probe at location 88231061. No significant correlation between methylation and expression was detected for rectum adenocarcinoma (Figure 11B).

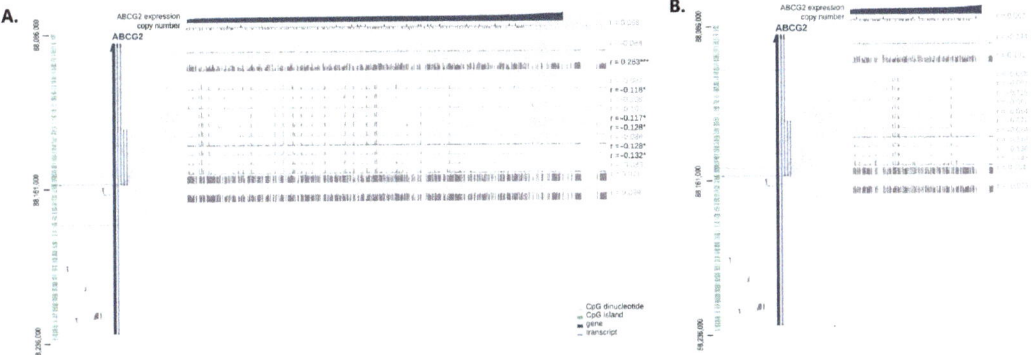

Figure 11. Association between mRNA expression and DNA methylation profile of the *ABCG2* gene by MEXPRESS in (**A**) colon adenocarcinoma (n = 557) and (**B**) rectum adenocarcinoma (n = 192). On the left side, the *ABCG2* gene together with its transcripts as well as any CpG islands and all the individual CpG dinucleotides were presented. On the right side, each row shows the DNA methylation data for a single probe with Pearson coefficients for the correlation between DNA methylation and gene expression. The promoter probe is highlighted by a black line. Significant coefficients are indicated in black, and *p*-value by using asterisks ($p \geq 0.05$, * $p < 0.05$, *** $p < 0.001$).

2.1.6. *ABCG2* Gene Expression Level in Colorectal Cancer Could Be Connected with Some Clinical Features

Various clinical factors, e.g., cancer stage, histological type of cancer or tumour localization, influence the clinical course of colorectal cancer. Therefore, the present study evaluates the clinical significance of *ABCG2* gene expression in colon and rectum adenocarcinomas. Using TCGA data and the MEXPRESS online tool, expression was compared to various clinicopathological parameters: localization of the tumour, presence of colon polyps, histological type of cancer, history of colon polyps, presence of *KRAS* mutation, loss of expression of mismatch repair proteins by IHC, microsatellite instability, new tumour event after initial treatment, non-nodal tumour deposits, pathological T, N and M, tumour stage, lymphatic, perineural and venous invasion of cancer, primary therapy outcome success, presence of residual tumour, synchronous colon cancer present, ethnicity, population type, sex and BMI. For colon adenocarcinoma (Figure 12), the only significant association was found between *ABCG2* expression level and microsatellite instability (p = 0.020). In rectum adenocarcinoma (Figure 13), *ABCG2* expression was associated with tumour localization (p = 0.014) and population type (p = 0.047).

Next, to validate and extended the analysis described above, the relationship between the *ABCG2* expression level and selected clinical features was examined with the use of the UALCAN tool (Figures 14 and 15). Although no significant correlation was found between expression and BMI, in the colon adenocarcinoma patients, those of normal weight demonstrated significantly higher expression than extremely obese patients (p = 0.0135,

Figure 14). In rectal adenocarcinoma patients of Caucasian origin, the expression level of *ABCG2* was significantly higher than in African-American patients ($p < 0.0001$, Figure 15). In both colon and rectum adenocarcinomas, expression was associated with age: the oldest colon adenocarcinoma patients (81–100 years old) showed a significantly lower level of expression than those between 21 and 40 years old ($p = 0.0328$) and between 41 and 60 years old ($p = 0.0289$). They also exhibited a slight but significantly higher expression of *ABCG2* than patients between 61 and 80 years old ($p = 0.0024$). Among rectum adenocarcinoma cases, the youngest patients (21–40 years old) had significantly lower expression levels of the *ABCG2* than patients between 61 and 80 years old ($p = 0.0496$).

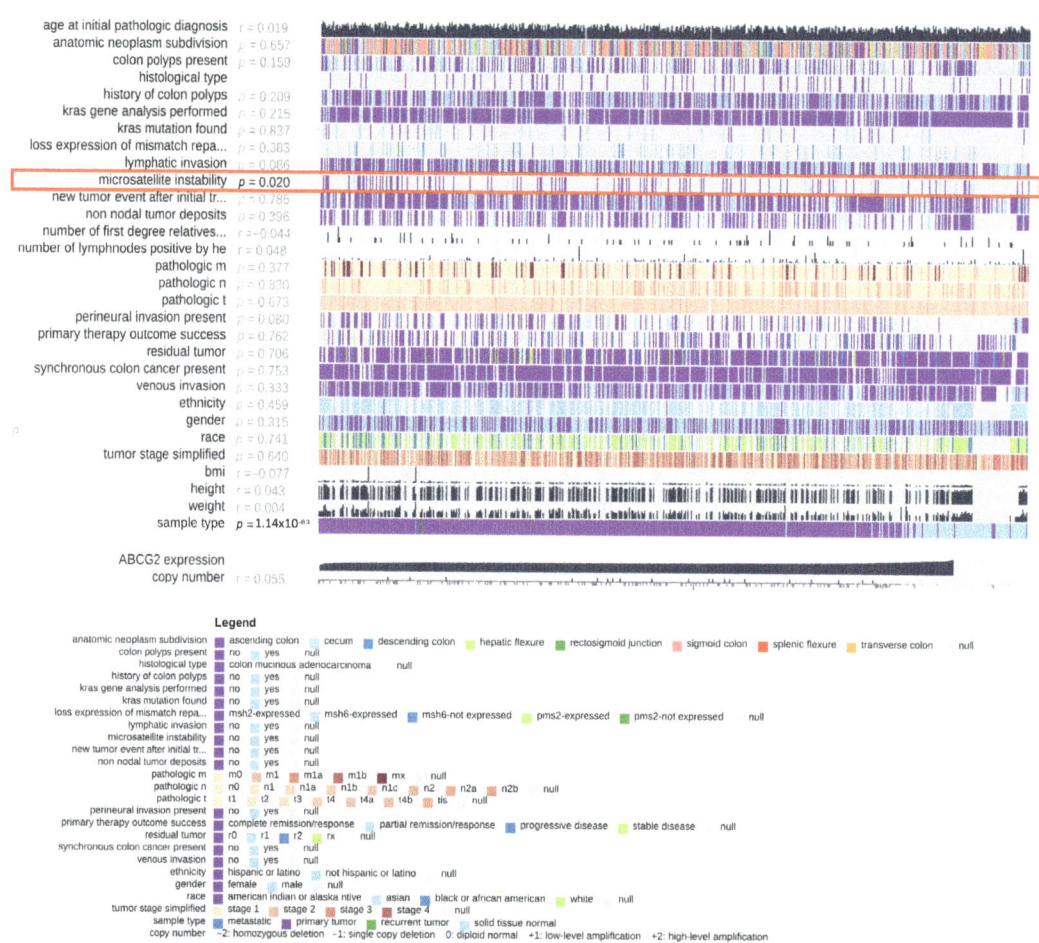

Figure 12. Association between *ABCG2* expression level and selected clinical parameters, generated by MEXPRESS for colon adenocarcinoma samples ($n = 557$). Samples are marked with vertical lines arranged in rows, which correspond to the analysed features. Samples are arranged from left to right of each row by the level of expression of the *ABCG2* gene.

2.1.7. Neither *ABCG2* Gene nor ABCG2 Protein Expression Level Is Related to a Prognosis in Colorectal Cancer

A substantial decrease in *ABCG2* mRNA and protein expression was observed in colorectal cancer, suggesting that it may play an important role in the carcinogenesis process and influence cancer progression. Therefore, GEPIA2 was used to draw Kaplan–Meier plots for the colon and rectum adenocarcinoma patients; these were divided into high-

and low-expression *ABCG2* subgroups with median expression as the threshold. Overall survival was not found to differ significantly between the mentioned subgroups for colon ($p = 0.70$) or rectum adenocarcinomas ($p = 0.99$) (Figure 16A,B). Similarly, no significant association was found between expression level and disease-free survival (COAD $p = 0.88$; READ $p = 0.38$) (Figure 16C,D).

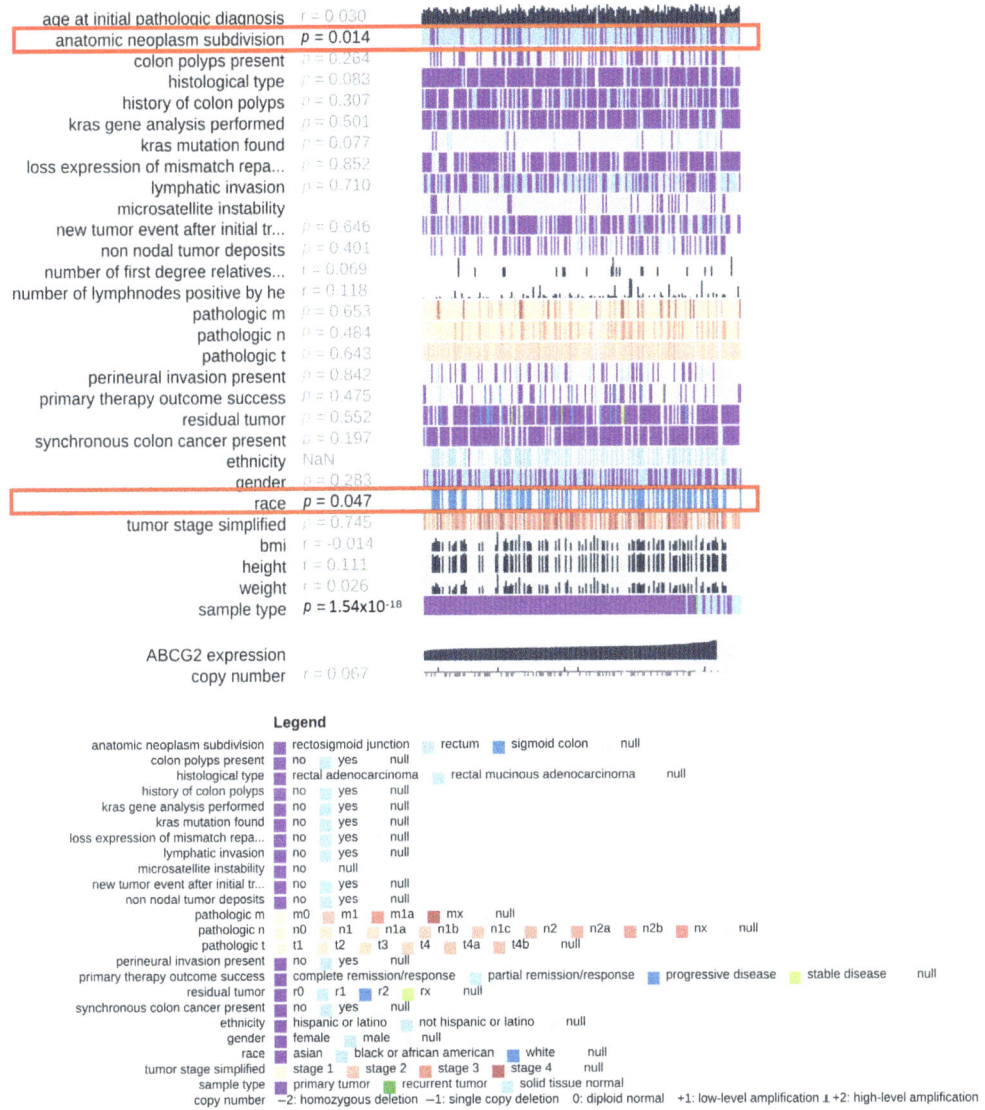

Figure 13. Connection between *ABCG2* expression level and selected clinical parameters. Generated by MEXPRESS for rectum adenocarcinoma samples ($n = 192$). Samples are marked with vertical lines arranged in rows, which correspond to the analysed features. Samples are arranged from left to right of each row by the level of expression of the *ABCG2* gene.

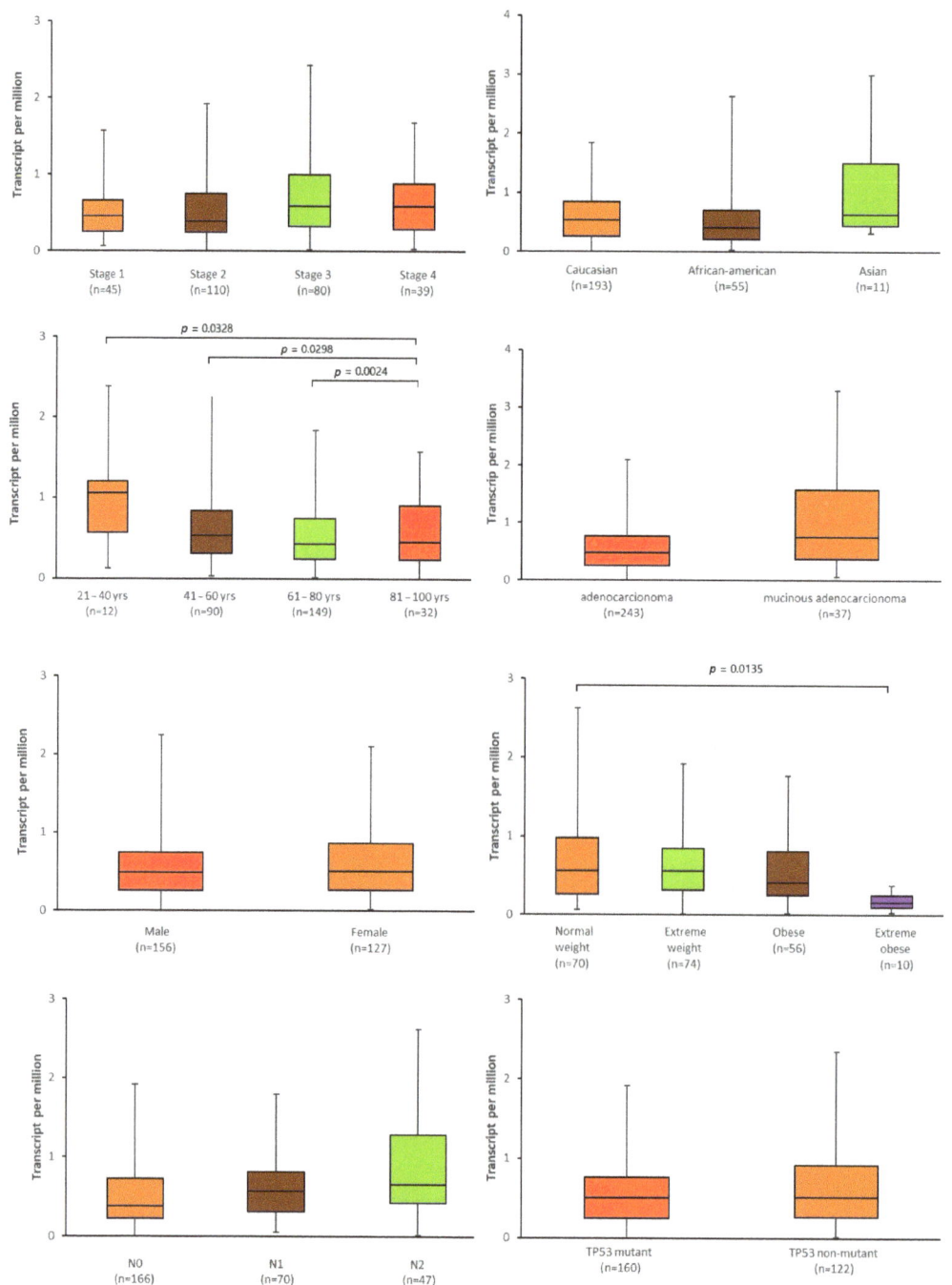

Figure 14. Association between *ABCG2* expression and selected clinical parameters: TNM stage, population affinity, sex, weight, age, cancer histological type, nodal involvement and *TP53* mutation status in colon adenocarcinoma patients and rectum carcinoma patients (UALCAN, modified).

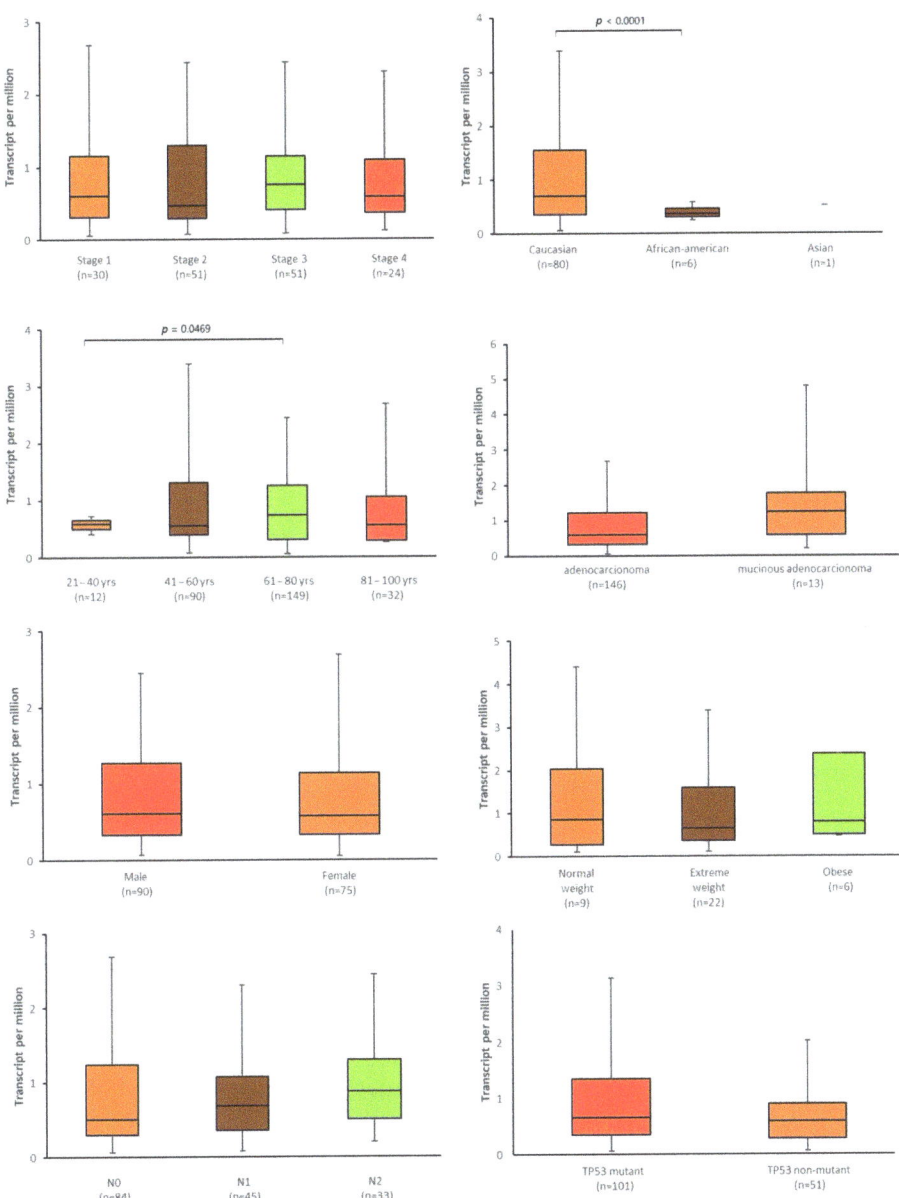

Figure 15. Association between *ABCG2* expression and selected clinical parameters: TNM stage, population affinity, sex, weight, age, cancer histological type, nodal involvement and *TP53* mutation status in rectum carcinoma patients (UALCAN, modified).

Similar results were obtained by Kaplan–Meier curve analysis of *ABCG2* gene expression in the Human Protein Atlas (Figure 17). When cancer patients were divided into two subgroups according to median *ABCG2* expression, no significant difference in overall survival probability was found between the high- and low-expression groups for colon ($p = 0.51$) or rectal adenocarcinomas ($p = 0.24$).

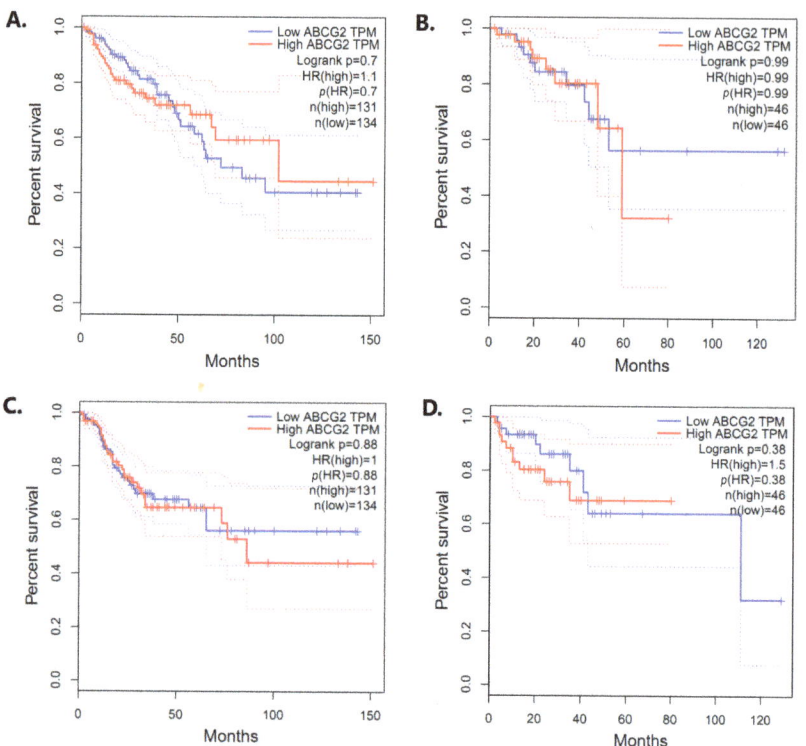

Figure 16. Kaplan–Meier survival curves according to *ABCG2* expression level by GEPIA2: overall survival of COAD (**A**) and READ (**B**) patients; disease-free survival of COAD (**C**) and READ (**D**) patients.

To validate these findings, they were compared with the survival data of colorectal cancer provided by the PrognoScan database (Table 1). Four datasets were retrieved (GSE12945, GSE17536, GSE14333, GSE17537). However, a significant association between *ABCG2* expression and overall survival was found in only one dataset (Cox *p*-value 0.0126, HR 1.45 [1.08–1.94]). In addition, a significant connection between expression and disease-specific survival was noted in only one dataset ($p = 0.0034$, HR 1.58 [1.16–2.14]).

2.1.8. ABCG2 Protein Interacts with Proteins Involved in, e.g., Leukotriene Transport, Endodermal Cell Fate Specification, and Histon Methylation and Ubiquitination

The in silico analysis was completed with the construction of an ABCG2-centered protein–protein interaction network (PPI enrichment $p < 1.0 \times 10^{-16}$) using the STRING database. Thirty-one interactors were predicted with a confidence score of at least 0.7 (Figure 18A). The top 10 functional partners of the ABCG2 protein were ATP-binding cassette protein C1 (ABCC1, score = 0.932), ATP-binding cassette protein C2 (ABCC2, score = 0.903), COMMD3-BMI1 (annotation not available, score = 0.880), polycomb complex protein BMI-1 (BMI1, score = 0.855), mitochondrial 28S ribosomal protein S7 (MRPS7, score = 0.840), solute carrier organic anion transporter family member 1B1 (SLCO1B1, score = 0.838), solute carrier organic anion transporter family member SLCO1B3-SLCO1B7 (SLCO1B3-SLCO1B7, score = 0.838), cytochrome p450 family 3 subfamily a polypeptide 4 (CYP3A4, score = 0.834), prominin-1 (PROM1, score = 0.831), and solute carrier family 2, facilitated glucose transporter member 9 (SLC2A9, score = 0.814). Within the generated PPI network, three clusters of interaction proteins were identified (Figure 18B). Functional enrichment analysis and gene ontology found the network to be mostly enriched in the following areas: leukotriene transport, xenobiotic transport across the blood–brain barrier, endodermal cell fate specification, histone h3-k4 dimethylation, urate metabolic process, sodium-independent organic anion transport, histone h3-k4 monomethylation, histone h2a-k119 monoubiquitination, bile acid and bile salt transport for biological processes; it was also significantly enriched in PRC1 complex, PcG protein complex, brush border membrane, basolateral plasma membrane and the apical plasma membrane for cellular components.

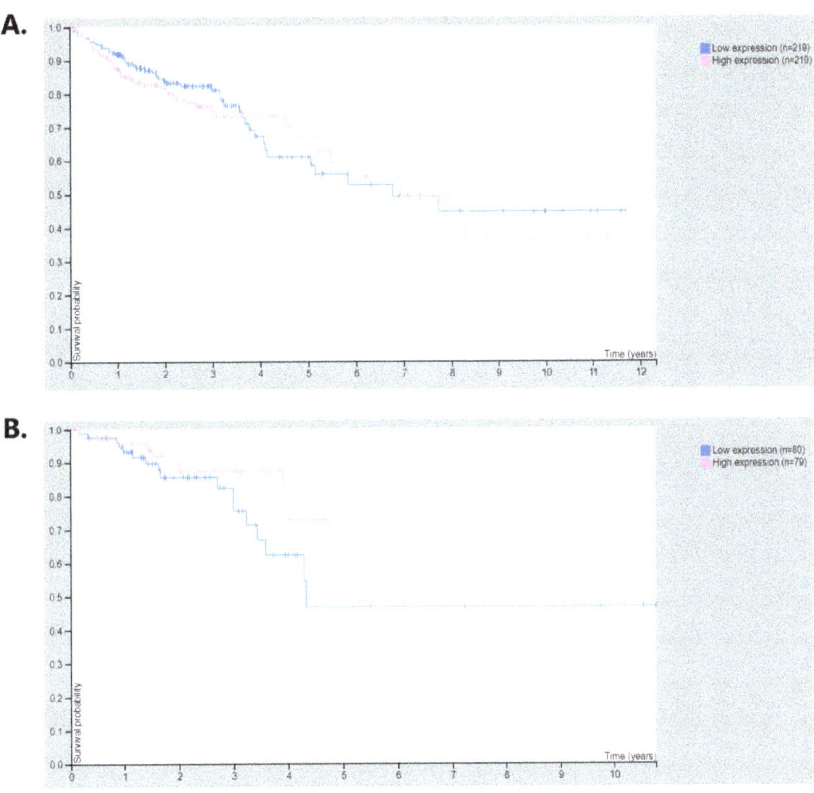

Figure 17. Kaplan–Meier survival curves according to *ABCG2* expression level (Human Protein Atlas: overall survival of COAD patients (n = 438) (**A**), READ patients (n = 159) (**B**).

2.2. ABCG2 Gene and ABCG2 Protein Expression in Colorectal Cancer Samples—Wet Validation of the In Silico Analysis Results

2.2.1. ABCG2 Protein Could Be Detected in the Cytoplasm and Membrane of Colorectal Cancer Cells

Ninety-six samples of colorectal cancer tissue were obtained during the surgical removal of the tumour from patients of the regional oncological centre. Detailed characteristics of the study group are shown in Supplementary Table S1. For immunohistochemical staining, formalin-fixed paraffin-embedded tissue blocks and the primary monoclonal anti-ABCG2 BXP-21 antibody were used. In total, 10 (10.4%) out of 96 tested samples did not express ABCG2 (0% stained cells). A total of 14 samples (14.6%) demonstrated 1–10% cell staining (trace reaction); all these were considered negative for ABCG2 expression. Samples with >10% cell staining (n = 72; 75%) were assumed positive for ABCG2 expression. A total of 33 (34.4%) samples had low ABCG2 expression (10–50% stained cells), and 39 (40.6%) samples had high expression (>50% staining). ABCG2 exhibited both cytoplasmic and membranous expression (Figure 19).

Table 1. *ABCG2* expression and survival data of colorectal cancer patients using the PrognoScan database.

Dataset	End-Point *	Probe ID	N	Cut-Point	Cox *p*-Value	HR [95% CI]
GSE12945	DFS	209735_at	51	0.75	0.3906	0.53 [0.13–2.24]
GSE12945	OS	209735_at	62	0.29	0.7889	1.07 [0.66–1.72]
GSE17536	OS	209735_at	177	0.87	0.0126	1.45 [1.08–1.94]
GSE17536	DFS	209735_at	145	0.90	0.1210	1.44 [0.91–2.28]
GSE17536	DSS	209735_at	177	0.87	0.0034	1.58 [1.16–2.14]
GSE14333	DFS	209735_at	226	0.82	0.1959	1.23 [0.90–1.69]
GSE17537	DFS	209735_at	55	0.15	0.1856	1.32 [0.87–2.00]
GSE17537	DSS	209735_at	49	0.82	0.6398	1.17 [0.61–2.21]
GSE17537	OS	209735_at	55	0.76	0.3611	1.22 [0.80–1.86]

* OS—overall survival, DSS—disease-specific survival, RFS—relapse-free survival.

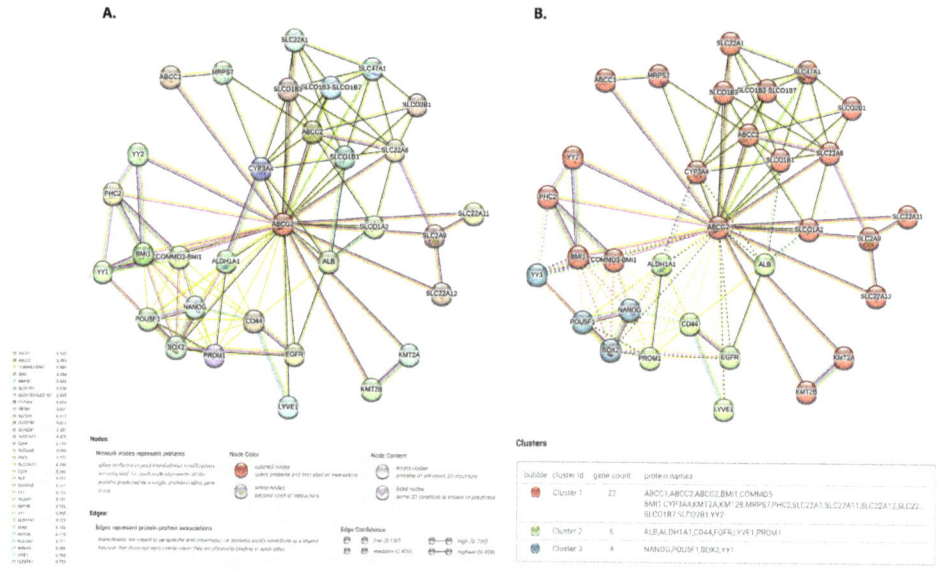

Figure 18. (**A**) The interaction network of the ABCG2 generated by STRING database, (**B**) clustered PPI network of ABCG2; edges of clusters are indicated by dotted lines.

2.2.2. *ABCG2* Gene Is Underexpressed in Nearly Two-Thirds of Colorectal Cancer Cases

In the study group, the relative *ABCG2* expression ranged from 0.01 to 731.22 (median 0.68). In 95% of cases, this level ranged from 0.02 to 50. Any outliers were excluded from further analysis (four cases). Nearly two-thirds of cases ($n = 58$, 63.7%) showed underexpression of *ABCG2* to *ACTB*. *ABCG2* expression mainly ranged from 0.51 to 1.0 (27.5%) and from 0.21 to 0.50 (18.7%).

2.2.3. No Association Was Found between *ABCG2* Gene Expression and ABCG2 Protein Levels in Colorectal Cancer Samples

The connection between *ABCG2* gene expression measured using real-time PCR and ABCG2 protein levels assessed by immunohistochemistry was analysed. First, *ABCG2* gene expression was compared in subgroups where ABCG2 protein was recorded or not in the IHC reaction, but no significant connection was found ($p = 0.381$). Second, in cases where the ABCG2 protein was detected, *ABCG2* gene expression was analysed in the high and low ABCG2 protein expression cohorts. Similar to the previous analysis, no significant association was stated ($p = 0.355$).

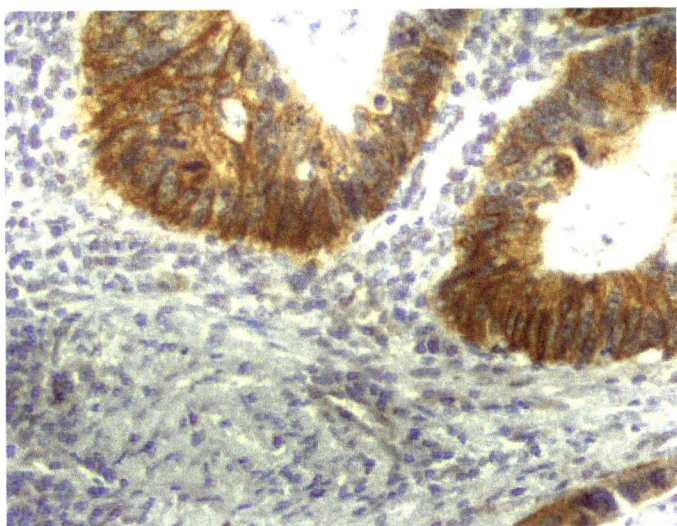

Figure 19. Positive cytoplasmatic and membranous immunohistochemical reaction with antibodies against ABCG2 in colorectal cancer tissue samples (magnification 200×).

2.2.4. Neither *ABCG2* Gene Expression Level nor ABCG2 Protein Level Is Connected with Selected Clinicopathological Factors in Colorectal Cancer Samples

Further, the association between ABCG2 protein expression and selected clinicopathological factors was investigated. Subgroups with ABCG2 protein expression were compared with those where expression was absent, and then high and low ABCG2 expression cohorts were compared (Table 2). None of the analysed clinical features was significantly correlated with either the presence of ABCG2 protein or its level, as stated in the IHC reaction.

ABCG2 gene expression level was also compared with clinicopathological features (Table 3). Similar to the protein, gene expression level was not significantly associated with any considered clinical parameters.

Table 2. The relationship between ABCG2 protein level and selected clinicopathological factors.

Feature	ABCG2 Protein Level					
	Absent	Present	p-Value	Low	High	p-Value
Age						
up to 60 y	11	34	0.906 *	16	18	0.844 *
over 60 y	13	38		17	21	
Sex						
female	13	37	0.814 *	17	20	0.984 *
male	11	35		16	19	
Tumour localization						
rectum	8	27	0.939 &	13	14	0.825 *
colon	16	44		20	24	
Histological type						
adenocarcinoma tubulare	19	64	0.389 #	31	33	0.380 #
adenocarcinoma mucinosum	5	8		2	6	
Histological grade						
G1 or G2	15	52	0.898 &	22	30	0.336 &
G3	9	20		11	19	
Depth of tumour invasion						
pT1 or pT2	5	24	0.898 &	9	15	0.316 *
pT3 or pT4	19	48		24	24	
Lymph nodes metastasis						
pN0	12	43	0.811 &	20	23	0.702 *
pN1 and pN2	12	24		10	14	

Table 2. Cont.

Feature	ABCG2 Protein Level					
	Absent	Present	p-Value	Low	High	p-Value
Distant metastases						
pM0	20	58	1.000 #	26	32	0.729 &
pM1	4	14		7	7	
Stage						
pTNM I or II	11	43	0.235 *	20	32	0.888 *
pTNM III or IV	13	29		13	16	
Lymphocyte infiltration						
absent	15	39	0.517 *	17	22	0.781 *
present	9	32		15	17	
Venous invasion						
absent	9	29	0.810 *	13	16	0.888 *
present	15	43		20	23	

* χ^2 test, # χ^2 test with Yates' correction, and & V^2 test.

Table 3. Relationship between *ABCG2* gene expression and selected clinicopathological factors.

Feature	ABCG2 Gene Expression Level			
	Min.	Median	Max.	p-Value *
Age				
up to 60 y	0.63	0.03	17.64	0.718
over 60 y	0.68	0.02	14.63	
Sex				
female	0.67	0.02	16.38	0.403
male	0.64	0.03	17.64	
Tumour localization				
rectum	0.66	0.04	14.63	0.911
colon	0.67	0.02	17.64	
Histological type				
adenocarcinoma tubulare	0.63	0.02	17.64	0.694
adenocarcinoma mucinosum	0.93	0.12	6.58	
Histological grade				
G1 or G2	0.63	0.04	16.38	0.362
G3	0.83	0.02	17.64	
Depth of tumour invasion				
pT1 or pT2	0.61	0.04	14.63	0.655
pT3 or pT4	0.67	0.02	17.64	
Lymph node metastasis				
pN0	0.65	0.03	17.64	0.773
pN1 and pN2	0.65	0.02	16.38	
Distant metastases				
pM0	0.69	0.03	17.64	0.149
pM1	0.55	0.02	8.58	
Stage				
pTNM I or II	0.67	0.03	17.64	0.799
pTNM III or IV	0.65	0.02	16.38	
Lymphocyte infiltration				
absent	0.78	0.04	16.38	0.228
present	0.58	0.02	14.60	
Venous invasion				
absent	0.67	0.03	17.64	0.798
present	0.65	0.02	11.19	

* Mann–Whitney U-test.

2.2.5. Neither *ABCG2* Gene Expression Level nor ABCG2 Protein Level Is Connected with the Overall Survival Probability of Colorectal Cancer Samples

Lastly, Kaplan–Meier curves were prepared to evaluate the influence of ABCG2 protein and gene expression on the survival time of colorectal cancer patients (Figure 20). No significant difference in the survival probability was found between groups with ABCG2 protein present and absent in tumour tissue ($p = 0.236$; Figure 20A). Among the patients with protein expression, overall survival was better in those with high ABCG2 expression, but not significantly ($p = 0.077$; Figure 20B). Similarly, favourable survival was associated with higher levels of *ABCG2* gene expression (above median expression level in the whole group), but, again, the relationship was not statistically significant ($p = 0.080$; Figure 20C).

Significantly better overall survival was connected with a lower depth of tumour invasion ($p = 0.041$), an absence of nodal and distant metastases ($p = 0.001$ and $p < 0.000$, respectively) and the presence of lymphocyte infiltration ($p = 0.036$). The number of deaths and log-rank p-values for all analysed parameters are summarized in Table 4.

Table 4. Overall survival concerning clinicopathological features, ABCG2 protein level and *ABCG2* gene expression.

Feature	Overall Survival	
	Number of Deaths (%)	p-Value *
Age		
up to 60 y	22 (48.9)	0.288
over 60 y	30 (60.0)	
Sex		
female	27 (54.0)	0.763
male	25 (55.6)	
Tumour localization		
rectum	24 (68.6)	0.141
colon	28 (47.5)	
Histological type		
adenocarcinoma tubulare	45 (54.9)	0.915
adenocarcinoma mucinosum	7 (53.9)	
Histological grade		
G1 or G2	33 (50.0)	0.112
G3	19 (65.5)	
Depth of tumour invasion		
pT1 or pT2	12 (41.4)	0.041
pT3 or pT4	40 (61.6)	
Lymph node metastasis		
pN0	23 (41.8)	0.001
pN1 and pN2	25 (71.4)	
Distant metastases		
pM0	34 (44.2)	<0.001
pM1	18 (100.0)	
Stage		
pTNM I or II	22 (40.7)	<0.001
pTNM III or IV	30 (73.2)	
Lymphocyte infiltration		
absent	34 (63.0)	0.036
present	17 (42.5)	
Venous invasion		
absent	17 (44.7)	0.070
present	35 (61.4)	
ABCG2 protein expression		
absent	10 (43.5)	0.236
present	42 (58.3)	
low	24 (72.7)	0.077
high	18 (46.2)	
ABCG2 expression level		
low	36 (63.2)	0.080
high	14 (42.4)	

* Log-rank test.

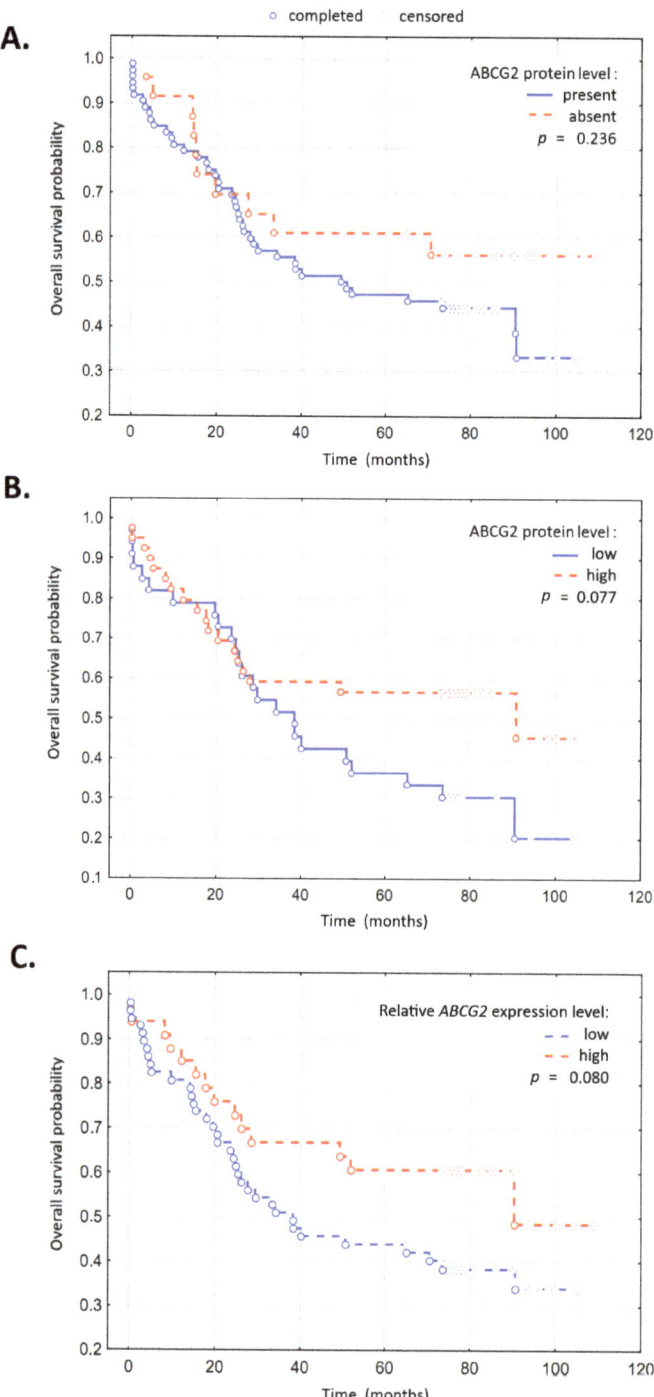

Figure 20. Kaplan–Meier curves for overall survival among colorectal cancer patients with regard to (**A**) the presence of the ABCG2 protein, (**B**) the level of ABCG2 protein and (**C**) *ABCG2* gene expression in tumour tissue samples (*p*-values calculated by log-rank test).

3. Discussion

ABCG2 was first described by Doyle et al. [47] in MCF7/AdVp3000 human breast cancer cells. Because it caused high adriamycin resistance, it was originally named breast cancer resistance protein (BCRP). Since then, the role of *ABCG2* mRNA and protein overexpression in multidrug resistance has been well established in various cancer cell types. This overexpression may serve as a defence against toxic substances such as antitumour drugs.

The present study assessed the *ABCG2* gene expression in a series of diverse malignancies using publicly available big data. Most of the analysed cancer types showed a downregulation of *ABCG2* gene expression. Indeed, decreased gene expression was noted in cancers of distinct tissue origins such as colorectal, bladder, breast, endometrial and lung cancers compared to neighbouring noncancerous tissue. Significantly lower *ABCG2* mRNA level was reported in cancer of 12 organs by Gupta et al. [26]. However, some exceptions were also noted in our analysis; for example, elevated expression was noted in renal clear cell carcinoma. Hence, it appears that *ABCG2* expression level could depend on the cancer type and specificity of tissue origin, and its changes can reflect its role in the carcinogenesis process.

Andersen et al. [48] assessed the role of ABCG2 in the normal–adenoma–carcinoma sequence and found *ABCG2* expression level to be altered in mild/moderate dysplasia, suggesting that this protein is involved in the early steps of carcinogenesis. *ABCG2* mRNA levels were significantly lower in adenomas and carcinomas compared to unaffected tissue from the same individuals and to tissue from healthy; however, the adjacent normal tissue of cancer patients demonstrated higher *ABCG2* expression than the tissue from healthy individuals. The authors suggested that dysfunctions in transport across the epithelial barrier during the transition from mild to moderate dysplasia could enhance the accumulation of carcinogens, thus promoting carcinogenesis in the colon and rectum. Similar results were published by Havlata et al. [49] regarding the primary tumour of colorectal mucosa and paired distant unaffected mucosa. Our present findings strongly support this hypothesis. Our TNMplot analysis revealed that *ABCG2* is underexpressed in both colon and rectum cancer compared to adjacent noncancerous tissue and unpaired noncancerous tissue from healthy individuals. Sensitivity and specificity analysis found that *ABCG2* expression could be a good discriminator between cancerous and adjacent noncancerous tissues in both colon and rectum adenocarcinomas, and it may hence be potentially useful as a colorectal cancer biomarker.

The decrease in *ABGC2* expression level observed in primary colorectal tumours raises the question of whether *ABCG2* is also underexpressed in metastatic tissue. Liu HG et al. [46] reported higher-intensity immunohistochemical ABCG2 protein staining in colorectal cancer cases with positive lymph nodes compared to those with negative nodes. Additionally, ABCG2-positive cells were positioned mainly in the front of carcinomatous tissue or between the carcinomatous and non-carcinomatous margin tissue, which supports the hypothesis that ABCG2 plays an essential role in cancer progression. In our analysis, *ACBG2* expression was significantly higher in colon metastatic tumours than in tumours from the primary location. In contrast, however, Candeil et al. [50] reported that *ABCG2* was highly expressed in the normal colon, and that this expression was dramatically lower in tumoral cells, i.e., colon tumour cells, as well as in untreated hepatic metastases. However, unlike our present findings, they did not detect any significant difference in *ABCG2* expression between cancerous tissue from primary and metastatic locations collected from the same 42 patients, although our present analysis was performed on a much greater number of samples, which were not paired. It could be speculated that while the observed global increase in *ABCG2* expression in metastatic tissue can result from cancer progression, it may also be influenced by the type of therapy. Candeil et al. [50] reported higher *ABCG2* expression in hepatic metastases after irinotecan-based chemotherapy than in irinotecan-naïve metastases.

The frequent deregulation of *ABCG2* expression in various cancers prompted our search for the molecular mechanisms underlying the decrease in *ABCG2* expression in colorectal cancer, namely the sequence changes and methylation of the *ABCG2* gene. In the present study, the data provided by the cBioPortal indicated that *ABCG2* sequence changes are rare events in colorectal cancer. In 5285 analysed colorectal cancer samples, the combined frequency of structural variants, copy number alterations and point mutations was only 1.5%, with the relatively highest frequency in mucinous adenocarcinoma of the colon (about 3%). It is reasonable to assume that the gene expression level should reflect its copy number; however, no increase in *ABCG2* expression level was observed between lower and higher *ABCG2* copy numbers. The low occurrence of the *ACBG2* sequence and copy number changes in colorectal cancer indicates that they are unlikely to be responsible for *ABCG2* underexpression, that another molecular mechanism is responsible for regulating the transcription of this gene in colorectal cancer.

In renal carcinoma cell lines, *ABCG2* gene inactivation was found to be connected with the formation of a repressor complex in the CpG island, which was dependent on DNA methylation [51]. In addition, in multiple myeloma cell lines and ex vivo plasma cells, Turner et al. [52] found the expression of *ABCG2* to be regulated, at least partially, by the methylation of its promoter. Furthermore, differences in the methylation of the promoter upstream region, promoter region and first exon region of the *ABCG2* gene were found between healthy men in China using stool samples [53]. Our present findings indicate significantly lower promoter methylation levels in both colon and rectum adenocarcinomas in comparison to noncancerous tissues; however, only a weak negative correlation was found between *ABCG2* expression and methylation level. Although no significant correlation was observed for the promoter region probe location in either colon or rectum adenocarcinomas, *ABCG2* expression was found to be related to methylation level in other locations in colon adenocarcinoma samples: a negative correlation was noted in five positions and a positive correlation in one. Surprisingly, no such relationship was stated for rectal adenocarcinoma. Hence, it appears that in the *ABCG2* gene, some sites other than the promoter can influence its expression, and that this phenomenon can be restricted to certain localizations of the colorectal tumour.

Studies have indicated that lowered mRNA transcription of *ABCG2* resulted in lowered ABCG2 protein levels. Gupta et al. [26] reported decreased expression of both the ABCG2 mRNA and protein in the luminal surface of colorectal cancer, as well as its liver metastasis, compared to the colorectal epithelium and hepatic tissue in the same patient. Additionally, both *ABCG2* gene expression and ABCG2 protein level were downregulated in colon adenoma with low-grade intraepithelial neoplasia in humans and mice compared to adjacent healthy tissue [9]. Our screening of ABCG2 protein expression in human colon and rectum adenocarcinoma samples deposited in the Human Protein Atlas revealed an absence of ABCG2-specific immunohistochemical staining in the cancerous tissue. However, Maliepaard et al. [54] reported the presence of the protein in healthy colon and rectum enterocytes on the apical membrane of the colon, rectum, jejunum and duodenum. In contrast, higher expression of ABCG2 protein has been reported in colorectal cancer tissue than in non-carcinomatous margin tissues [46]. In addition, elevated expression was noted in about half of the metastatic colorectal tumours studied by Lin P-Ch et al. [55]; however, this group comprised cases ranging from zero to strong expression, with half demonstrating expression in 25–75% of cells. ABCG2 expression was weaker in the normal mucosa than in cancer tissue.

Both the intensity of ABCG2 expression and the proportion of cells expressing it were significantly connected with response to FOLOX [55]. ABCG2 protein expression was observed in 87.1% of cases of CRC tissue from III stage CC [56]. Wang et al. [30] reported ABCG2 protein expression in 96.7% of a large group of colorectal cases, where positivity was considered as more than 10% of tumour cells with an intensity score of at least 1 (weak staining). Assuming 10% positive staining as a minimal cutoff for positivity in our wet analysis, our present findings confirm ABCG2 protein expression in three-quarters of colorectal cancer patients. The discrepancy between the mentioned results may be due to differences in methodology and tissue material.

Our data also indicate both membranous but also cytoplasmatic staining of the cancer cells, which corroborates some previous findings. Gupta et al. [26] reported that ABCG2 was localized at the brush border membrane of normal epithelial cells, and cancer cells showed markedly diminished expression. However, Wang et al. [30] detected the protein in the cytoplasm of over 80% of studied colorectal cancer tissue samples, and in the cell membrane of about two-thirds of cases, where the normal mucosa exhibited strong staining of the apical membrane. Kang et al. [57] reported both cytoplasmatic and membranous ABCG2 expression in over 60% of studied colorectal cancer samples. Both localizations were also detected by Hu J et al. [24] in right-sided colorectal cancer tissues. Palshof et al. [58] reported recently that in addition to the cytoplasm, ABCG2 expression was also present in both the apical/luminal and basolateral membranes of the colorectal cancer cells. It could be speculated that subcellular localization of the ABCG2 can be associated with specific function or loss of function of the transporter during colorectal carcinogenesis. The PI3K/Akt signalling pathway was also found to regulate the translocation of ABCG2 to the plasma membrane and side population phenotype in a mouse model [59]. Altered ABCG2 expression and function could result from EGFR-mediated activation of MAPK cascade [60].

The clinical significance of the *ABCG2* gene and ABCG2 protein expression remains unclear. Some negative findings were published. No association has been found between ABCG2 expression and clinicopathological parameters [56], or between the expression of ABCG2 protein (basolateral, apical or cytoplasmatic) and age, sex, WHO performance status, location of the primary tumour, number of metastatic sites or liver or lung metastases in colorectal cancer [58]. Gupta et al. [26] indicated no significant correlation between *ABCG2* mRNA level and age, sex, population type, grade, stage or localization, and Halavata et al. [49] reported no connection between *ABCG2* expression with the grade, primary localization, T, N, M, age at diagnosis or sex. No difference in *ABCG2* gene expression was found between mucinous and nonmucinous colorectal cancer [44].

In contrast, some significant associations have been reported. In one study, neither cytoplasmatic nor membranous expression of ABCG2 protein was found to be connected with age, sex, tumour site or TNM stage [57]; however, higher expression in both localizations was linked with more pathologically differentiated lesions. No connection was noted between ABCG2 protein positivity and age, sex, tumour size or tumour shape, but higher TNM stage, poor differentiation and positive lymphovascular invasion were found to be associated with greater ABCG2 expression [24]. Additionally, the ABCG2 protein was detected more frequently in cases without perineural invasion [57].

Considering these conflicting reports, the present study analysed the relationships between various clinicopathological factors and *ABCG2* expression using publicly available TCGA datasets. From the large number of factors analysed, only a few were found to be connected with *ABCG2* expression, and different associations were observed for distinct anatomic cancer locations. *ABCG2* expression was significantly associated with microsatellite instability and patient weight in colon carcinoma, and with anatomical organ subdivision, patient age and population type in rectum adenocarcinoma. Unfortunately, our validation analysis in colorectal cancer patient cohort did not identify any significant association between *ABCG2* expression, at the mRNA or protein level, and clinicopathological parameters.

As our present findings, and some previous studies, found ABCG2 gene and/or protein expression to be associated with colorectal cancer clinical parameters, the present study also attempted to translate these associations into patient survival. The existing literature was again divided. High ABCG2 protein expression was associated with poor prognosis [30,45,46]. Hu, J. et al. [24] showed that ABCG2 positive staining of right-sided colorectal cancer was associated with a decreased 5-year survival rate, whereas the opposite was reported by Gupta et al. [26]. Moreover, Palshof et al. [58] reported no association of ABCG2 protein with RFS or OS. Silvestris et al. [61] did not find any connection between ABCG2 expression and patient survival in metastatic colorectal cancer patients.

In our in silico analysis, no significant connection was found between *ABCG2* expression and disease-free or overall survival in either colon or rectum adenocarcinoma patients. Moreover, overall survival did not correlate with ABCG2 protein or *ABCG2* gene expression in our colorectal cancer cohort. Some reports have indicated that cell localization of ABCG2 could determine its influence on survival. Kang et al. [57] found high expression of membranous ABCG2 to be associated with better overall and disease-specific survival; however, no such association was detected for cytoplasmatic ABCG2. After stratification of patients according to TNM stage, only stages II and III demonstrated an association with OS and DFS, and high membranous expression was an independent prognostic factor of OS and DFS. This may be due to the transportation activity of the epithelium and the protective function of membranous ABCG2, which could influence survival time.

Kim et al. [62] reported that ABCG2 protein expression was associated with favourable disease-free survival but not overall survival. However, it was not an independent indicator of OS and DFS. In line with these findings, Han et al. [56] noted that ABCG2 protein positivity was connected with prolonged overall and disease-free survival of CIII stage patients treated postoperatively with FOLFOX-4 chemotherapy. Positivity for ABCG2 was an independent prognostic positive indicator of OS, and ABCG2 negativity was connected with an almost three-times-higher risk of death. In contrast, Wang et al. [30] showed that strong membranous expression of ABCG2 correlated with the lymph node and distant metastasis and Dukes stage, while the cytoplasmic expression was connected with tumour stage only. However, strong membranous expression was linked with shortened survival, but cytoplasmatic expression was not. This contradicts the suggestion that ABCG2 protects cancer cells from harmful substances and prolongs the life of cancer cells; however, this could be connected with some other properties of ABCG2. Giampieri et al. [45] correlated a panel of stemness markers with clinical outcome in resected stage II and III colon cancer patients; *ABCG2* was found to be among those genes with a higher "weight" in determining different prognoses: patients with higher expression of ABCG2 have a worse prognosis (time to relapse).

In the absence of a clear connection with clinical parameters and prognosis, significant alterations in *ABCG2* gene and protein expression in colorectal cancer may suggest that ABCG2 has a complex role in tumorigenesis that is not directly or solely related to its transport function. It is possible that this may be a result of its interaction with other cellular components. Therefore, in the last part of the in silico analysis, a functional protein–protein interaction network was built to identify the molecular partners of ABCG2 that could mediate or enhance the carcinogenic function of the transporter. STRING analysis revealed that ABCG2 collaborates with proteins grouped into three main clusters. The largest cluster comprised various SLC and ABC transporters, which are critical for the absorption, distribution, metabolism and elimination of different drugs and endo-/exogenous toxins. Some of these proteins are involved in the regulation of the physiological molecular signalling network between the intestines, liver and kidneys (ABCC2, SLC22A1, SLC22A8, SLCO1B1) [63]. In addition, the same elements of the ABCG2 network are considered together as important predictive factors during assessing the effectiveness of single drugs (e.g., irinotecan, 5-fluorouracil) or full therapeutic regimens (e.g., FOLFIRI, FOLFOX) [64].

The second network cluster contains e.a. molecules important for cell interaction and signalling. CD44 is a major cell surface receptor for hyaluronic acid (HA), and its expression enhances CSC aggregation. Additionally, the level of phosphorylated transmembrane tyrosine kinases (e.g., ERBB2) and its interactions with other signalling factors in colon cancer cell lines may depend on endogenous HA and CD44 interaction [65]. In other types of cancer, HA-CD44 binding also plays a role in triggering signals from later receptors in the tyrosine kinase family (such as EGFR), leading to PI3K/Akt or MAPK pathway activation [66]. Monoclonal antibodies against EGFR are commonly used in the treatment of metastatic colorectal cancer, and some of these agents synergistically inhibit both EGFR phosphorylation and ABCG2 drug efflux activity [67–69]. EGFR was also found to exert a post-transcriptional effect on ABCG2 expression via the PI3K/AKT and RAS/RAF/MEK/ERK signalling pathways [63–65]. Bleau et al. [70] reported that PTEN/PI3K/Akt signalling regulates ABCG2 activity in mouse and human gliomas. Mutual regulation has also been confirmed in other studies, indicating that increased expression of both *ABCG2* and *EGFR* (metastatic marker) is positively correlated with resistance to anoikis [71] and metastatic potential [72] in the colorectal cancer cell population.

The third cluster of the built PPI network is well represented by *transcriptional factors* e.g., such as SOX2, NANOG and POU5F1/OCT4, which are *considered cancer stem cell (CSC) markers*. Some phenotypic markers (e.g., CD44 or *BMI-1*) and other stemness-related factors (e.g., ALDH1) [73] can also be found in the other clusters of the network. CSCs often demonstrate resistance against chemotherapeutics due to high expression of ABC transporter genes. Similarly, cancer stem-like side population cells, which may be identified or mediated, among others, by ABCG2 transporter activity, show an increased tendency to proliferation, colony formation, invasiveness and multipotent differentiation; in addition, they may be more tumorigenic and resistant to chemotherapeutic drugs. The side population of colon cancer cell line SW480 exhibits high *ABCG2* mRNA and transporter expression, accompanied by high *CD44* mRNA and protein levels, regarded as a key marker of solid tumour CSCs [74]. Another important marker of colorectal CSCs is BMI-1. Both the CD44v6 isoform and BMI-1 alone identify CSCs [75].

Another group of CSC markers comprises pluripotency transcription factors. Spheroid culture from the HT-29 cell line, a more realistic colorectal cancer in vitro model, shows significantly higher expression of *ABCG2*, *NANOG*, *SOX2* and *POU5F1* compared to 2D cell culture conditions [76]. It has been found that the E1A isoform of the *ABCG2* transcript, whose expression in human embryonic stem cell lines correlates with the level of *POU5F1* and *NANOG*, may be responsible for the increased level of total *ABCG2* mRNA in CSCs [77]. Moreover, in mouse embryonic stem cell lines, transfection-mediated inhibition of *ABCG2* downregulates the expression of Nanog, possibly leading to a subsequent reduction in its downstream target POU5F1/Oct-4. This phenomenon may be mediated by changes in the nuclear level of TP53; it could also contribute to cell arrest in the G1 phase of the cell cycle, and thus the removal of such cells from the self-renewal pool [78]. The activity of ALDH1, a member of the second network cluster, is another characteristic feature of both normal and cancer stem cells [79]. As previously mentioned, CSCs are not only small, pluripotent cells that can enter a reversible cell cycle arrest, but they are also the most drug-resistant subpopulation of tumour cells. They are certainly promoted by the mutual co-expression of *ABCG2*, *ALDH1A1* and *CYP3A4* (a member of the first network cluster) observed, e.g., in CSCs of the COLO 205 line [80]. Increased ALDH1A1, a key ALDH isozyme in stem cells, decreases the reactive oxygen species (ROS) level, prevents apoptosis, provides radioresistant properties and has a protective function against cytotoxic drugs [81]. Taken together, the string network brings new information on potentially important partners of ABCG2, which may explain its role in carcinogenesis. However, because the network of interactions is created mainly based on the co-expression of particular genes, further multifaceted research is required to understand the nature of the mechanism of the association between network members.

4. Materials and Methods
4.1. In Silico Analysis
4.1.1. ABCG2 Gene Expression and ABCG2 Protein Level Analysis
Oncomine

ABCG2 mRNA expression level was analysed in a variety of human cancers using the Oncomine database [82] (https://www.oncomine.org, accessed on 1 January 2022). The following threshold settings were used: gene ranking of the top 10%, change ≥ 2, p-value $\leq 1 \times 10^{-4}$. All statistical methods and statistical values were obtained directly from the mentioned database.

TIMER2.0

The differential expression of the *ABCG2* gene in TCGA tumours was compared between tumour and adjacent normal tissues using the Gene_DE module of the Tumor Immune Estimation Resource 2.0 [83] (http://timer.cistrome.org, accessed on 1 January 2022). The distributions of gene expression levels are displayed using box plots. The statistical significance (*p*-value) was computed by the Wilcoxon test.

TMNplot

The TMNplot web tool [84] (https://tnmplot.com, accessed on 1 January 2022) was used (1) to display pan-cancer changes in *ABCG2* expression based on RNA-seq data from TCGA, genotype-tissue expression (GTEX), therapeutically applicable research to generate effective treatment (TARGET) (significant differences are given in red and marked with an asterisk), (2) to compare *ABCG2* expression level in colorectal cancer and non-tumour colon and rectum tissues based on RNA-seq and DNA chip data, and (3) to compare the *ABCG2* expression in normal colon tissue, tumours and metastatic tissue of colon cancer based on DNA chip data. The normal and tumour samples were compared by the Mann–Whitney U-test, and matched tissues with adjacent samples were compared using the Wilcoxon test. Normal–tumorous–metastatic tissue comparison was done using the Kruskal–Wallis test and Dunn's test.

Human Protein Atlas

Example images of immunohistochemistry staining of normal colon and rectum tissues, as well as the colon and rectum adenocarcinomas, were obtained from the Human Protein Atlas [85] (https://www.proteinatlas.org/, accessed on 29 March 2023). The methods of obtaining and analysing the available data are described in detail on the HPA websites: https://www.proteinatlas.org/humanproteome/tissue/method (accessed on 22 May 2023); https://www.proteinatlas.org/humanproteome/pathology/method#the_pathology_section___methods_summary (accessed on 22 May 2023).

4.1.2. Analysis of DNA Alteration and Methylation of the *ABCG2* Gene

cBioPortal

The genomic characteristics of *ABCG2* in colorectal cancers were analysed using the cBioPortal for Cancer Genomics [86] (v3.7.28; http://www.cbioportal.org, accessed on 4 February 2023). The query comprised 5511 patients/5285 samples from 16 studies. The incidence of different alterations of the studied gene was assessed in colorectal cancer cases and, specifically, in colorectal cancer histological types. Additionally, the association between *ABCG2* mRNA expression level and copy number alteration and between the mRNA level of the gene and methylation beta-value (HM27) was analysed. Spearman's and Pearson's correlation coefficients were calculated.

UALCAN

The association between *ABCG2* expression and *ABCG2* promoter methylation in the colon and rectum adenocarcinomas was determined using Ualcan TCGA data available on the UALCAN portal [87] (http://ualcan.path.uab.edu/index.html, accessed on 1 January 2022). The results were presented in box-whisker plots with the minimum, q1, median, q3 and maximum values. The presented beta-value is the ratio of the methylated probe intensity and the overall intensity (sum of methylated and unmethylated probe intensities). The significance of the difference was estimated by Student's *t*-test considering unequal variance.

MEXPRESS

The relationship between TCGA expression and DNA methylation data for the *ABCG2* gene was determined using the MEXPRESS visualization tool (https://www.mexpress.be/, accessed on 22 May 2023) [88]. Pearson correlation coefficients and Benjamini-Hochberg-adjusted *p*-values were calculated for the comparison between the methylation level for each specific probe and the *ABCG2* expression level.

4.1.3. Analysis of Connection of *ABCG2* and Clinicopathological Features

MEXPRESS

The connection between TCGA expression and clinical data for the *ABCG2* gene was determined with the MEXPRESS visualization tool (https://www.mexpress.be/, accessed on 22 May 2023) [88]. Pairs of continuous variables were compared using Pearson's correlation coefficient, while continuous and categorical variables were compared using a *t*-test or ANOVA. Benjamini-Hochberg-adjusted *p*-values are provided.

UALCAN

The association between *ABCG2* expression and selected clinical features in colon adenocarcinoma and rectal adenocarcinoma was validated using TCGA data available on the UALCAN portal [87] (http://ualcan.path.uab.edu/index.html, accessed on 29 March 2023). The results were presented in box-whisker plots with the minimum, q1, median, q3 and maximum values. The significance of the difference was estimated by Student's *t*-test considering unequal variance.

4.1.4. Prognosis and Survival Analysis

GEPIA2

The GEPIA2 [89] (http://gepia2.cancer-pku.cn/#survival, accessed on 29 March 2023) was applied to evaluate the prognostic value of *ABCG2* expression for overall survival and disease-free survival in colon and rectal adenocarcinomas. Kaplan–Meier plots were drawn using "ABCG2" as an input query, and patients were split by median; the hazard ratio was calculated based on the Cox PH model.

Human Protein Atlas

The prognostic value of ABCG2 protein expression regarding overall survival in colon adenocarcinoma and rectal adenocarcinoma was evaluated using data from the Human Protein Atlas [85] (https://www.proteinatlas.org/, accessed on 29 March 2023). Patients were split by median *ABCG2* expression, i.e., the median FPKM value calculated from the gene expression (FPKM) data from all patients in the dataset. Log-rank *p*-values for Kaplan–Meier plots were provided.

PrognoScan

The association between *ABCG2* expression level and overall or relapse-free survival in colon and rectal adenocarcinomas was determined using PrognoScan [90] (http://dna00.bio.kyutech.ac.jp/PrognoScan/index.html, accessed on 1 January 2022). Cox *p*-values and hazard ratios with a 95% confidence interval were calculated according to *ABCG2* mRNA level (high vs. low).

4.1.5. Protein–Protein Interaction Analysis

STRING

A protein–protein interaction (PPI) network querying the protein "ABCG2" and organism "Homo sapiens" was created using the STRING database [91] (https://string-db.org/, accessed on 1 January 2023). The main parameters were set as follows: the minimum required interaction score was 0.7 and no more than 50 interactors to show. K-means clustering of the generated PPI network was performed with a pre-set of three clusters.

4.2. ABCG2 Gene Expression and ABCG2 Protein Analysis in Colorectal Cancer Samples

4.2.1. Patients and Tissue Samples

A total of 96 patients of the Oncological Center of Łódź, Poland, with colorectal carcinomas were enrolled in the study. Cancer tissue samples were obtained from the patients during the surgical removal of the tumour. Detailed characteristics of the study group are shown in Supplementary Table S1.

Tumour tissues intended for molecular analysis were frozen immediately after collection in liquid nitrogen and stored at −80 °C until analysis. In addition, tissues for immunohistochemical analysis were fixed in 10% PBS-buffered formalin and embedded in paraffin blocks. Histological diagnosis and clinical staging were performed for each patient. All experiments were carried out with the local ethical committee approval (RNN/83/20/KE) and the patient's informed consent.

4.2.2. ABCG2 Protein Level Analysis by Immunohistochemistry

Briefly, 4 μm sections of formalin-fixed, paraffin-embedded tissue were placed on SuperFrost Plus slides (Menzel-Glaser, Braunschweig, Germany). These were deparaffinized in xylenes and rehydrated through graded alcohol. Then, the sections were microwaved in 0.01 M sodium citrate buffer, pH 6.0, twice for 10 min at 360 W for epitope retrieval. The slides were then washed with TRIS buffered saline, pH 7.4, and incubated for 1 h at room temperature with the primary monoclonal antibody anti-ABCG2 (clone BXP-21, 1:25 dilution, Chemicon International, Temecula, CA, USA) and processed with EnVision+ (DAKO, Glostrup, Denmark) system. Sections were counterstained with haematoxylin, dehydrated with ethanol and cleared in xylene. Negative controls were obtained by omitting the application of the monoclonal antibody. Expression was assessed by counting the positive cell reactions. Depending on the number of cells, the cases were divided into four classes: 0% of cells stained—no expression, 1–10% of cells stained—trace expression, 11–50% of cells stained—low expression, 51–100% of cells stained—high expression; the cases with more than 10% of cells with a positive reaction were considered positive (adopted after [92]).

4.2.3. RNA Isolation and cDNA Synthesis

Total RNA was isolated from frozen tissue sections (50–100 mg) with TRI Reagent (Sigma-Aldrich, St. Louis, MO, USA) according to the manufacturer's instructions. The obtained RNA was stored at −80 °C until further analysis. Reverse transcription was performed according to the Enhanced Avian protocol HS RT-PCR Kit, Two-Step Reaction (Sigma-Aldrich, USA) using 400 ng of total RNA. The obtained cDNA was stored at −20 °C until further analyses.

4.2.4. Real-Time PCR Reaction

The reaction mixture consisted of 12.5 μL of the mixture SYBR®Green JumpStart™ Taq ReadyMix™ (Sigma-Aldrich, USA), 0.5 μL of each primer (final concentration: 0.2 μM), 9 μL of sterile, nuclease-free water and 2.5 μL of previously prepared cDNA. Together, negative control samples were also reacted with the test samples, which contained all components of the reaction mixture as the test samples except cDNA. They were replaced with 2.5 μL of sterile, nuclease-free water. All reactions were made in triplicate. After each reaction, the melting curve of the obtained products was determined. The reaction was carried out in a MiniOpticon™ System thermocycler (Bio-Rad Laboratories, Hercules, CA, USA). The primer sequences and reaction conditions are as follows: *ABCG2* Forward 5′CCT TAG TTA TGT TAT CTT TGT G3′; *ABCG2* Reverse 5′GTG GGG CGC CCC AGG CAC CA3′; *ACTB* Forward 5′GTG GGG CGC CCC AGG CAC CA3′, *ACTB* Reverse 5′CTC CTT AAT GTC ACG CAC GAT TTC3′; 35 cycles: 94 °C-15 s; 59 °C-45 s; 72 °C-45 s. The relative expression of the *ABCG2* gene was determined according to Pfaffl [93].

4.2.5. Statistical Analysis

Statistical analysis was performed using Dell Statistica version 13, Dell Inc. (2016). To investigate the relationship between qualitative or quantitative characteristics in nominal scales, the χ^2 test, χ^2 test with Yates' correction, and V^2 tests were used. The normality of the distribution of the continuous variables was determined using the Shapiro–Wilk W test. The nonparametric Mann–Whitney U-test was used to determine the significance of differences in continuous variables between the two groups. Overall survival analysis (time between surgery and death) was performed using Kaplan–Meier curves. Observed differences in survival probabilities were tested by the test log rank (univariate analysis). In all analyses, statistical significance was assumed for $p < 0.05$.

5. Conclusions

The findings from the in silico analysis and wet experiments indicate that *ABCG2* gene expression is commonly deregulated in cancerogenesis, and a decrease in the expression of the gene is a general feature of colorectal cancer cells. This downregulation is not driven by *ABCG2* gene sequence or copy number changes, but it can be connected with the methylation level of some sites in the gene. The role of ABCG2 in colorectal cancerogenesis could be linked with the transport function of the protein, but it could also indicate its participation some signalling pathways or protein interactors, which may determine the role of ABCG2 in cancer cell self-renewal and behaviour. As these ABCG2 partners could also influence the clinical significance of ABCG2, simple analyses of *ABCG2* or ABCG2 expression alone cannot yield clear conclusions. These interactions require further in-depth research to reveal the significance of *ABCG2* and its protein expression in colorectal cancer.

Supplementary Materials: The supporting information can be downloaded at: https://www.mdpi.com/article/10.3390/ijms241310539/s1.

Author Contributions: Conceptualization, A.S.-K. and E.B.; investigation, A.S.-K., D.Z., L.S., R.K.; writing—original draft preparation, A.S.-K. and A.J.; writing—review and editing, A.S.-K., A.J. and E.B.; supervision, A.S.-K. All authors have read and agreed to the published version of the manuscript.

Funding: This research was funded by the Medical University of Lodz, grant number 503/3-015-02/503-31-001.

Institutional Review Board Statement: Not applicable.

Informed Consent Statement: Informed consent was obtained from all subjects involved in the study.

Data Availability Statement: Links to publicly archived datasets analysed: https://www.oncomine.org (accessed on 1 January 2022), http://timer.cistrome.org (accessed on 1 January 2022), https://tnmplot.com (accessed on 1 January 2022), http://ualcan.path.uab.edu/index.html (accessed on 29 March 2023), http://dna00.bio.kyutech.ac.jp/PrognoScan/index.html (accessed on 1 January 2022), http://www.cbioportal.org (accessed on 4 February 2023), https://string-db.org/ (accessed on 1 January 2023), http://gepia2.cancer-pku.cn/ (accessed on 29 March 2023), https://www.proteinatlas.org/ (accessed on 29 March 2023), https://www.mexpress.be/ (accessed on 22 May 2023).

Acknowledgments: The authors would like to thank Mariusz Panczyk, Medical University of Warsaw, for his help in creating Figure 1.

Conflicts of Interest: The authors declare no conflict of interest.

References

1. The Global Cancer Observatory; International Agency for Research on Cancer; World Health Organization. Colorectal Cancer-Fact Sheet. 2020. Available online: https://gco.iarc.fr/today/data/factsheets/cancers/10_8_9-Colorectum-fact-sheet.pdf (accessed on 1 May 2023).
2. The Global Cancer Observatory; International Agency for Research on Cancer; World Health Organization. Cancer Tomorrow. 2020. Available online: https://gco.iarc.fr/tomorrow/en (accessed on 1 May 2023).
3. Gottesman, M.M.; Fojo, T.; Bates, S.E. Multidrug resistance in cancer: Role of ATP-dependent transporters. *Nat. Rev. Cancer* **2002**, *2*, 48–58. [PubMed]
4. Nielsen, D.L.; Palshof, J.A.; Brünner, N.; Stenvang, J.; Viuff, B.M. Implications of ABCG2 Expression on Irinotecan Treatment of Colorectal Cancer Patients: A Review. *Int. J. Mol. Sci.* **2017**, *18*, 1926. [CrossRef] [PubMed]
5. Dawson, R.J.; Hollenstein, K.; Locher, K.P. Uptake or extrusion: Crystal structures of full ABC transporters suggest a common mechanism. *Mol. Microbiol.* **2007**, *65*, 250–257. [CrossRef] [PubMed]
6. Higgins, C.F.; Linton, K.J. The ATP switch model for ABC transporters. *Nat. Struct. Mol. Biol.* **2004**, *11*, 918–926.
7. Linton, K.J. Structure and function of ABC transporters. *Physiology* **2007**, *22*, 122–130.

8. Hollenstein, K.; Dawson, R.J.; Locher, K.P. Structure and mechanism of ABC transporter proteins. *Curr. Opin. Struct. Biol.* **2007**, *17*, 412–418. [CrossRef]
9. Dietrich, C.G.; Vehr, A.K.; Martin, I.V.; Gassler, N.; Rath, T.; Roeb, E.; Schmitt, J.; Trautwein, C.; Geier, A. Downregulation of breast cancer resistance protein in colon adenomas reduces cellular xenobiotic resistance and leads to accumulation of a food-derived carcinogen. *Int. J. Cancer* **2011**, *129*, 546–552.
10. Alvarez, A.I.; Real, R.; Pérez, M.; Mendoza, G.; Prieto, J.G.; Merino, G. Modulation of the activity of ABC transporters (P-glycoprotein, MRP2, BCRP) by flavonoids and drug response. *J. Pharm. Sci.* **2010**, *99*, 598–617.
11. Uno, S.; Uraki, M.; Ito, A.; Shinozaki, Y.; Yamada, J.; Kawase, A.; Iwaki, M. Changes in mRNA expression of ABC and SLC transporters in liver and intestines of the adjuvant-induced arthritis rat. *Biopharm. Drug Dispos.* **2009**, *30*, 49–54.
12. Englund, G.; Jacobson, A.; Rorsman, F.; Artursson, P.; Kindmark, A.; Rönnblom, A. Efflux transporters in ulcerative colitis: Decreased expression of BCRP (ABCG2) and Pgp (ABCB1). *Inflamm. Bowel Dis.* **2007**, *13*, 291–297.
13. Mosaffa, F.; Kalalinia, F.; Lage, H.; Afshari, J.T.; Behravan, J. Pro-inflammatory cytokines interleukin-1 beta, interleukin 6, and tumor necrosis factor-alpha alter the expression and function of ABCG2 in cervix and gastric cancer cells. *Mol. Cell. Biochem.* **2012**, *363*, 385–393. [CrossRef]
14. Deuring, J.J.; de Haar, C.; Koelewijn, C.L.; Kuipers, E.J.; Peppelenbosch, M.P.; van der Woude, C.J. Absence of ABCG2-mediated mucosal detoxification in patients with active inflammatory bowel disease is due to impeded protein folding. *Biochem. J.* **2012**, *441*, 87–93.
15. Albermann, N.; Schmitz-Winnenthal, F.H.; Z'graggen, K.; Volk, C.; Hoffmann, M.M.; Haefeli, W.E.; Weiss, J. Expression of the drug transporters MDR1/ABCB1, MRP1/ABCC1, MRP2/ABCC2, BCRP/ABCG2, and PXR in peripheral blood mononuclear cells and their relationship with the expression in intestine and liver. *Biochem. Pharmacol.* **2005**, *70*, 949–958.
16. Sarkadi, B.; Homolya, L.; Hegedűs, T. The ABCG2/BCRP transporter and its variants-from structure to pathology. *FEBS Lett.* **2020**, *594*, 4012–4034.
17. To, K.K.; Zhan, Z.; Litman, T.; Bates, S.E. Regulation of ABCG2 expression at the 3' untranslated region of its mRNA through modulation of transcript stability and protein translation by a putative microRNA in the S1 colon cancer cell line. *Mol. Cell. Biol.* **2008**, *28*, 5147–5161. [CrossRef]
18. Campa, D.; Pardini, B.; Naccarati, A.; Vodickova, L.; Novotny, J.; Försti, A.; Hemminki, K.; Barale, R.; Vodicka, P.; Canzian, F. A gene-wide investigation on polymorphisms in the ABCG2/BRCP transporter and susceptibility to colorectal cancer. *Mutat. Res.* **2008**, *645*, 56–60.
19. Kopp, T.I.; Andersen, V.; Tjonneland, A.; Vogel, U. Polymorphisms in ATP-binding cassette transporter genes and interaction with diet and life style factors in relation to colorectal cancer in a Danish prospective case-cohort study. *Scand. J. Gastroenterol.* **2015**, *50*, 1469–1481. [CrossRef]
20. Andersen, V.; Ostergaard, M.; Christensen, J.; Overvad, K.; Tjonneland, A. Polymorphisms in the xenobiotic transporter Multidrug Resistance 1 (MDR1) gene and interaction with meat intake in relation to risk of colorectal cancer in a Danish prospective case-cohort study. *BMC Cancer* **2009**, *9*, 407.
21. Haraguchi, N.; Utsunomiya, T.; Inoue, H.; Tanaka, F.; Mimori, K.; Barnard, G.F.; Mori, M. Characterization of a side population of cancer cells from human gastrointestinal system. *Stem Cells* **2006**, *24*, 506–513.
22. Xie, Z.Y.; Lv, K.; Xiong, Y.; Guo, W.H. ABCG2-meditated multidrug resistance and tumor-initiating capacity of side population cells from colon cancer. *Oncol. Res. Treat.* **2014**, *37*, 666–668, 670–672.
23. Ma, L.; Li, T.; Jin, Y.; Wei, J.; Yang, Y.; Zhang, H. ABCG2 is required for self-renewal and chemoresistance of CD133-positive human colorectal cancer cells. *Tumour. Biol.* **2016**, *37*, 12889–12896. [PubMed]
24. Hu, J.; Li, J.; Yue, X.; Wang, J.; Liu, J.; Sun, L.; Kong, D. Expression of the cancer stem cell markers ABCG2 and OCT-4 in right-sided colon cancer predicts recurrence and poor outcomes. *Oncotarget* **2017**, *8*, 28463–28470. [PubMed]
25. Krishnamurthy, P.; Ross, D.D.; Nakanishi, T.; Bailey-Dell, K.; Zhou, S.; Mercer, K.E.; Sarkadi, B.; Sorrentino, B.P.; Schuetz, J.D. The stem cell marker Bcrp/ABCG2 enhances hypoxic cell survival through interactions with heme. *J. Biol. Chem.* **2004**, *279*, 24218–24225. [PubMed]
26. Gupta, N.; Martin, P.M.; Miyauchi, S.; Ananth, S.; Herdman, A.V.; Martindale, R.G.; Podolsky, R.; Ganapathy, V. Down-regulation of BCRP/ABCG2 in colorectal and cervical cancer. *Biochem. Biophys. Res. Commun.* **2006**, *343*, 571–577.
27. Chen, J.S.; Pardo, F.S.; Wang-Rodriguez, J.; Chu, T.S.; Lopez, J.P.; Aguilera, J.; Altuna, X.; Weisman, R.A.; Ongkeko, W.M. EGFR regulates the side population in head and neck squamous cell carcinoma. *Laryngoscope* **2006**, *116*, 401–406.
28. Bhatia, P.; Bernier, M.; Sanghvi, M.; Moaddel, R.; Schwarting, R.; Ramamoorthy, A.; Wainer, I.W. Breast cancer resistance protein (BCRP/ABCG2) localises to the nucleus in glioblastoma multiforme cells. *Xenobiotica* **2012**, *42*, 748–755. [CrossRef]
29. Liang, S.C.; Yang, C.Y.; Tseng, J.Y.; Wang, H.L.; Tung, C.Y.; Liu, H.W.; Chen, C.Y.; Yeh, Y.C.; Chou, T.Y.; Yang, M.H.; et al. ABCG2 localizes to the nucleus and modulates CDH1 expression in lung cancer cells. *Neoplasia* **2015**, *17*, 265–278.
30. Wang, X.; Xia, B.; Liang, Y.; Peng, L.; Wang, Z.; Zhuo, J.; Wang, W.; Jiang, B. Membranous ABCG2 expression in colorectal cancer independently correlates with shortened patient survival. *Cancer Biomark.* **2013**, *13*, 81–88. [CrossRef]
31. Benderra, Z.; Faussat, A.M.; Sayada, L.; Perrot, J.Y.; Chaoui, D.; Marie, J.P.; Legrand, O. Breast cancer resistance protein and P-glycoprotein in 149 adult acute myeloid leukemias. *Clin. Cancer Res.* **2004**, *10*, 7896–7902.
32. Uggla, B.; Ståhl, E.; Wågsäter, D.; Paul, C.; Karlsson, M.G.; Sirsjö, A.; Tidefel, U. BCRP mRNA expression v. clinical outcome in 40 adult AML patients. *Leuk. Res.* **2005**, *29*, 141–146. [CrossRef]

3. Yoh, K.; Ishii, G.; Yokose, T.; Minegishi, Y.; Tsuta, K.; Goto, K.; Nishiwaki, Y.; Kodama, T.; Suga, M.; Ochiai, A. Breast cancer resistance protein impacts clinical outcome in platinum-based chemotherapy for advanced non-small cell lung cancer. *Clin. Cancer Res.* **2004**, *10*, 1691–1697.
4. Kim, Y.H.; Ishii, G.; Goto, K.; Ota, S.; Kubota, K.; Murata, Y.; Mishima, M.; Saijo, N.; Nishiwaki, Y.; Ochiai, A. Expression of breast cancer resistance protein is associated with a poor clinical outcome in patients with small-cell lung cancer. *Lung Cancer* **2009**, *65*, 105–111. [CrossRef]
5. Hang, D.; Dong, H.C.; Ning, T.; Dong, B.; Hou, D.L.; Xu, W.G. Prognostic value of the stem cell markers CD133 and ABCG2 expression in esophageal squamous cell carcinoma. *Dis. Esophagus* **2012**, *25*, 638–644.
6. Huang, L.; Lu, Q.; Han, Y.; Li, Z.; Zhang, Z.; Li, X. ABCG2/V-ATPase was associated with the drug resistance and tumor metastasis of esophageal squamous cancer cells. *Diagn. Pathol.* **2012**, *7*, 180.
7. Tsunoda, S.; Okumura, T.; Ito, T.; Kondo, K.; Ortiz, C.; Tanaka, E.; Watanabe, G.; Itami, A.; Sakai, Y.; Shimada, Y. ABCG2 expression is an independent unfavorable prognostic factor in esophageal squamous cell carcinoma. *Oncology* **2006**, *71*, 251–258.
8. Lee, S.H.; Kim, H.; Hwang, J.H.; Lee, H.S.; Cho, J.Y.; Yoon, Y.S.; Han, H.S. Breast cancer resistance protein expression is associated with early recurrence and decreased survival in resectable pancreatic cancer patients. *Pathol. Int.* **2012**, *62*, 167–175.
9. Yuan, Y.; Yang, Z.; Miao, X.; Li, D.; Liu, Z.; Zou, Q. The clinical significance of FRAT1 and ABCG2 expression in pancreatic ductal adenocarcinoma. *Tumour. Biol.* **2015**, *36*, 9961–9968.
10. Shen, B.; Dong, P.; Li, D.; Gao, S. Expression and function of ABCG2 in head and neck squamous cell carcinoma and cell lines. *Exp. Ther. Med.* **2011**, *2*, 1151–1157.
11. Yamada, A.; Ishikawa, T.; Ota, I.; Kimura, M.; Shimizu, D.; Tanabe, M.; Chishima, T.; Sasaki, T.; Ichikawa, Y.; Morita, S.; et al. High expression of ATP-binding cassette transporter ABCC11 in breast tumors is associated with aggressive subtypes and low disease-free survival. *Breast Cancer Res. Treat.* **2013**, *137*, 773–782.
12. Xiang, L.; Su, P.; Xia, S.; Liu, Z.; Wang, Y.; Gao, P.; Zhou, G. ABCG2 is associated with HER-2 expression, lymph node metastasis and clinical stage in breast invasive ductal carcinoma. *Diagn. Pathol.* **2011**, *6*, 90.
13. Larbcharoensub, N.; Sornmayura, P.; Sirachainan, E.; Wilasrusmee, C.; Wanmoung, H.; Janvilisri, T. Prognostic value of ABCG2 in moderately and poorly differentiated intrahepatic cholangiocarcinoma. *Histopathology* **2011**, *59*, 235–246. [PubMed]
14. Glasgow, S.C.; Yu, J.; Carvalho, L.P.; Shannon, W.D.; Fleshman, J.W.; McLeod, H.L. Unfavourable expression of pharmacologic markers in mucinous colorectal cancer. *Br. J. Cancer* **2005**, *92*, 259–264. [PubMed]
15. Giampieri, R.; Scartozzi, M.; Loretelli, C.; Piva, F.; Mandolesi, A.; Lezoche, G.; Del Prete, M.; Bittoni, A.; Faloppi, L.; Bianconi, M.; et al. Cancer stem cell gene profile as predictor of relapse in high risk stage II and stage III, radically resected colon cancer patients. *PLoS ONE* **2013**, *8*, e72843.
16. Liu, H.G.; Pan, Y.F.; You, J.; Wang, O.C.; Huang, K.T.; Zhang, X.H. Expression of ABCG2 and its significance in colorectal cancer. *Asian Pac. J. Cancer Prev.* **2010**, *11*, 845–848. [PubMed]
17. Doyle, L.A.; Yang, W.; Abruzzo, L.V.; Krogmann, T.; Gao, Y.; Rishi, A.K.; Ross, D.D. A multidrug resistance transporter from human MCF-7 breast cancer cells. *Proc. Natl. Acad. Sci. USA* **1998**, *95*, 15665–15670. [CrossRef]
18. Andersen, V.; Vogel, L.K.; Kopp, T.I.; Sæbø, M.; Nonboe, A.W.; Hamfjord, J.; Kure, E.H.; Vogel, U. High ABCC2 and low ABCG2 gene expression are early events in the colorectal adenoma-carcinoma sequence. *PLoS ONE* **2015**, *10*, e0119255.
19. Hlavata, I.; Mohelnikova-Duchonova, B.; Vaclavikova, R.; Liska, V.; Pitule, P.; Novak, P.; Bruha, J.; Vycital, O.; Holubec, L.; Treska, V.; et al. The role of ABC transporters in progression and clinical outcome of colorectal cancer. *Mutagenesis* **2012**, *27*, 187–196.
20. Candeil, L.; Gourdier, I.; Peyron, D.; Vezzio, N.; Copois, V.; Bibeau, F.; Orsetti, B.; Scheffer, G.L.; Ychou, M.; Khan, Q.A.; et al. ABCG2 overexpression in colon cancer cells resistant to SN38 and in irinotecan-treated metastases. *Int. J. Cancer* **2004**, *109*, 848–854.
21. To, K.K.; Zhan, Z.; Bates, S.E. Aberrant promoter methylation of the ABCG2 gene in renal carcinoma. *Mol. Cell. Bio.* **2006**, *26*, 8572–8585. [CrossRef]
22. Turner, J.G.; Gump, J.L.; Zhang, C.; Cook, J.M.; Marchion, D.; Hazlehurst, L.; Munster, P.; Schell, M.J.; Dalton, W.S.; Sullivan, D.M. ABCG2 expression, function, and promoter methylation in human multiple myeloma. *Blood* **2006**, *108*, 3881–3889.
23. Peng, Y.; Xu, B.; Tang, J.; Wan, Z.; Sun, H.; Wang, G.; Zhu, Y.S. Analysis of ABCG2 methylation in stool samples of Chinese healthy males by pyrosequencing. *Pharmazie* **2016**, *71*, 447–454.
24. Maliepaard, M.; Scheffer, G.L.; Faneyte, I.F.; van Gastelen, M.A.; Pijnenborg, A.C.; Schinkel, A.H.; van De Vijver, M.J.; Scheper, R.J.; Schellens, J.H. Subcellular localization and distribution of the breast cancer resistance protein transporter in normal human tissues. *Cancer Res.* **2001**, *61*, 3458–3464.
25. Lin, P.C.; Lin, H.H.; Lin, J.K.; Lin, C.C.; Yang, S.H.; Li, A.F.; Chen, W.S.; Chang, S.C. Expression of ABCG2 associated with tumor response in metastatic colorectal cancer patients receiving first-line FOLFOX therapy—Preliminary evidence. *Int. J. Biol. Markers* **2013**, *28*, 182–186.
26. Han, S.H.; Kim, J.W.; Kim, M.; Kim, J.H.; Lee, K.W.; Kim, B.H.; Oh, H.K.; Kim, D.W.; Kang, S.B.; Kim, H.; et al. Prognostic implication of ABC transporters and cancer stem cell markers in patients with stage III colon cancer receiving adjuvant FOLFOX-4 chemotherapy. *Oncol. Lett.* **2019**, *17*, 5572–5580.
27. Kang, D.; Park, J.M.; Jung, C.K.; Lee, B.I.; Oh, S.T.; Choi, M.G. Prognostic impact of membranous ATP-binding cassette Sub-family G member 2 expression in patients with colorectal carcinoma after surgical resection. *Cancer Biol. Ther.* **2015**, *16*, 1438–1444.

58. Palshof, J.A.; Cederbye, C.N.; Høgdall, E.V.S.; Poulsen, T.S.; Linnemann, D.; Nygaard, S.B.; Stenvang, J.; Christensen, I.J.; Jensen, B.V.; Pfeiffer, P.; et al. ABCG2 Protein Levels and Association to Response to First-Line Irinotecan-Based Therapy for Patients with Metastatic Colorectal Cancer. *Int. J. Mol. Sci.* **2020**, *21*, 5027.
59. Mogi, M.; Yang, J.; Lambert, J.F.; Colvin, G.A.; Shiojima, I.; Skurk, C.; Summer, R.; Fine, A.; Quesenberry, P.J.; Walsh, K. Akt signaling regulates side population cell phenotype via Bcrp1 translocation. *J. Biol. Chem.* **2003**, *278*, 39068–39075.
60. Meyer zu Schwabedissen, H.E.; Grube, M.; Dreisbach, A.; Jedlitschky, G.; Meissner, K.; Linnemann, K.; Fusch, C.; Ritter, C.A.; Völker, U.; Kroemer, H.K. Epidermal growth factor-mediated activation of the map kinase cascade results in altered expression and function of ABCG2 (BCRP). *Drug Metab. Dispos.* **2006**, *34*, 524–533.
61. Silvestris, N.; Simone, G.; Partipilo, G.; Scarpi, E.; Lorusso, V.; Brunetti, A.E.; Maiello, E.; Paradiso, A.; Mangia, A. CES2, ABCG2, TS and Topo-I primary and synchronous metastasis expression and clinical outcome in metastatic colorectal cancer patients treated with first-line FOLFIRI regimen. *Int. J. Mol. Sci.* **2014**, *15*, 15767–15777. [CrossRef]
62. Kim, B.H.; Oh, H.K.; Kim, D.W.; Kang, S.B.; Choi, Y.; Shin, E. Clinical Implications of Cancer Stem Cell Markers and ABC Transporters as a Predictor of Prognosis in Colorectal Cancer Patients. *Anticancer. Res.* **2020**, *40*, 4481–4489. [CrossRef]
63. Rosenthal, S.B.; Bush, K.T.; Nigam, S.K. A Network of SLC and ABC Transporter and DME Genes Involved in Remote Sensing and Signaling in the Gut-Liver-Kidney Axis. *Sci. Rep.* **2019**, *9*, 11879. [PubMed]
64. De Mattia, E.; Toffoli, G.; Polesel, J.; D'Andrea, M.; Corona, G.; Zagonel, V.; Buonadonna, A.; Dreussi, E.; Cecchin, E. Pharmacogenetics of ABC and SLC transporters in metastatic colorectal cancer patients receiving first-line FOLFIRI treatment. *Pharm. Genom.* **2013**, *23*, 549–557.
65. Ghatak, S.; Misra, S.; Toole, B.P. Hyaluronan constitutively regulates ErbB2 phosphorylation and signaling complex formation in carcinoma cells. *J. Biol. Chem.* **2005**, *280*, 8875–8883. [PubMed]
66. Misra, S.; Toole, B.P.; Ghatak, S. Hyaluronan constitutively regulates activation of multiple receptor tyrosine kinases in epithelial and carcinoma cells. *J. Biol. Chem.* **2006**, *281*, 34936–34941. [CrossRef] [PubMed]
67. Ge, X.J.; Jiang, J.Y.; Wang, M.; Li, M.Y.; Zheng, L.M.; Feng, Z.X.; Liu, L. Cetuximab enhances the efficiency of irinotecan through simultaneously inhibiting the MAPK signaling and ABCG2 in colorectal cancer cells. *Pathol. Res. Pract.* **2020**, *216*, 152798.
68. Pick, A.; Wiese, M. Tyrosine kinase inhibitors influence ABCG2 expression in EGFR-positive MDCK BCRP cells via the PI3K/Akt signaling pathway. *ChemMedChem* **2012**, *7*, 650–662.
69. Ma, H.; Yao, Q.; Zhang, A.M.; Lin, S.; Wang, X.X.; Wu, L.; Sun, J.G.; Chen, Z.T. The effects of artesunate on the expression of EGFR and ABCG2 in A549 human lung cancer cells and a xenograft model. *Molecules* **2011**, *16*, 10556–10569.
70. Bleau, A.M.; Hambardzumyan, D.; Ozawa, T.; Fomchenko, E.I.; Huse, J.T.; Brennan, C.W.; Holland, E.C. PTEN/PI3K/Akt pathway regulates the side population phenotype and ABCG2 activity in glioma tumor stem-like cells. *Cell Stem Cell* **2009**, *4*, 226–235.
71. Guha, D.; Saha, T.; Bose, S.; Chakraborty, S.; Dhar, S.; Khan, P.; Adhikary, A.; Das, T.; Sa, G. Integrin-EGFR interaction regulates anoikis resistance in colon cancer cells. *Apoptosis* **2019**, *24*, 958–971.
72. Sogawa, C.; Eguchi, T.; Namba, Y.; Okusha, Y.; Aoyama, E.; Ohyama, K.; Okamoto, K. Gel-Free 3D Tumoroids with Stem Cell Properties Modeling Drug Resistance to Cisplatin and Imatinib in Metastatic Colorectal Cancer. *Cells* **2021**, *10*, 344.
73. Zhao, W.; Li, Y.; Zhang, X. Stemness-Related Markers in Cancer. *Cancer Transl. Med.* **2017**, *3*, 87–95.
74. Xiong, B.; Ma, L.; Hu, X.; Zhang, C.; Cheng, Y. Characterization of side population cells isolated from the colon cancer cell line SW480. *Int. J. Oncol.* **2014**, *45*, 1175–1183.
75. Hervieu, C.; Christou, N.; Battu, S.; Mathonnet, M. The Role of Cancer Stem Cells in Colorectal Cancer: From the Basics to Novel Clinical Trials. *Cancers* **2021**, *13*, 1092.
76. Gheytanchi, E.; Naseri, M.; Karimi-Busheri, F.; Atyabi, F.; Mirsharif, E.S.; Bozorgmehr, M.; Ghods, R.; Madjd, Z. Morphological and molecular characteristics of spheroid formation in HT-29 and Caco-2 colorectal cancer cell lines. *Cancer Cell Int.* **2021**, *21*, 204.
77. Sándor, S.; Jordanidisz, T.; Schamberger, A.; Várady, G.; Erdei, Z.; Apáti, Á.; Sarkadi, B.; Orbán, T.I. Functional characterization of the ABCG2 5′ non-coding exon variants: Stem cell specificity, translation efficiency and the influence of drug selection. *Biochim. Biophys. Acta* **2016**, *1859*, 943–951.
78. Susanto, J.; Lin, Y.H.; Chen, Y.N.; Shen, C.R.; Yan, Y.T.; Tsai, S.T.; Chen, C.H.; Shen, C.N. Porphyrin homeostasis maintained by ABCG2 regulates self-renewal of embryonic stem cells. *PLoS ONE* **2008**, *3*, e4023.
79. Alowaidi, F.; Hashimi, S.M.; Alqurashi, N.; Alhulais, R.; Ivanovski, S.; Bellette, B.; Meedenyia, A.; Lam, A.; Wood, S. Assessing stemness and proliferation properties of the newly established colon cancer 'stem' cell line, CSC480 and novel approaches to identify dormant cancer cells. *Oncol. Rep.* **2018**, *39*, 2881–2891. [CrossRef]
80. Olszewski, U.; Liedauer, R.; Ausch, C.; Thalhammer, T.; Hamilton, G. Overexpression of CYP3A4 in a COLO 205 Colon Cancer Stem Cell Model in vitro. *Cancers* **2011**, *3*, 1467–1479.
81. Tomita, H.; Tanaka, K.; Tanaka, T.; Hara, A. Aldehyde dehydrogenase 1A1 in stem cells and cancer. *Oncotarget* **2016**, *7*, 11018–11032.
82. Rhodes, D.R.; Yu, J.; Shanker, K.; Deshpande, N.; Varambally, R.; Ghosh, D.; Barrette, T.; Pandeyb, A.; Chinnaiyan, A.M. ONCOMINE: A cancer microarray database and integrated data-mining platform. *Neoplasia* **2004**, *6*, 1–6.
83. Li, T.; Fu, J.; Zeng, Z.; Cohen, D.; Li, J.; Chen, Q.; Li, B.; Liu, X.S. TIMER2.0 for analysis of tumor-infiltrating immune cells. *Nucleic Acids Res.* **2020**, *48*, W509–W514. [PubMed]

84. Bartha, Á.; Győrffy, B. TNMplot.com: A web tool for the comparison of gene expression in normal, tumor and metastatic tissues. *Int. J. Mol. Sci.* **2021**, *22*, 2622. [CrossRef] [PubMed]
85. Uhlén, M.; Fagerberg, L.; Hallström, B.M.; Lindskog, C.; Oksvold, P.; Mardinoglu, A.; Sivertsson, Å.; Kampf, C.; Sjöstedt, E.; Asplund, A.; et al. Proteomics. Tissue-based map of the human proteome. *Science* **2015**, *347*, 1260419. [PubMed]
86. Cerami, E.; Gao, J.; Dogrusoz, U.; Gross, B.E.; Sumer, S.O.; Aksoy, B.A.; Jacobsen, A.; Byrne, C.J.; Heuer, M.L.; Larsson, E.; et al. The cBio cancer genomics portal: An open platform for exploring multidimensional cancer genomics data. *Cancer Discov.* **2012**, *2*, 401–404. [PubMed]
87. Chandrashekar, D.S.; Bashel, B.; Balasubramanya, S.A.H.; Creighton, C.J.; Ponce-Rodriguez, I.; Chakravarthi, B.V.S.K.; Varambally, S. UALCAN: A portal for facilitating tumor subgroup gene expression and survival analyses. *Neoplasia* **2017**, *19*, 649–658.
88. Koch, A.; De Meyer, T.; Jeschke, J.; Van Criekinge, W. MEXPRESS: Visualizing expression, DNA methylation and clinical TCGA data. *BMC Genom.* **2015**, *16*, 636.
89. Tang, Z.; Kang, B.; Li, C.; Chen, T.; Zhang, Z. GEPIA2: An enhanced web server for large-scale expression profiling and interactive analysis. *Nucleic Acids Res.* **2019**, *47*, W556–W560.
90. Mizuno, H.; Kitada, K.; Nakai, K.; Sarai, A. PrognoScan: A new database for meta-analysis of the prognostic value of genes. *BMC Med. Genom.* **2009**, *2*, 18.
91. Szklarczyk, D.; Gable, A.L.; Nastou, K.C.; Lyon, D.; Kirsch, R.; Pyysalo, S.; Doncheva, N.T.; Legeay, M.; Fang, T.; Bork, P.; et al. The STRING database in 2021: Customizable protein-protein networks, and functional character-ization of user-uploaded gene/measurement sets. *Nucleic Acids Res.* **2021**, *49*, D605–D612.
92. Diestra, J.E.; Scheffer, G.L.; Català, I.; Maliepaard, M.; Schellens, J.H.; Scheper, R.J.; Germà-Lluch, J.R.; Izquierdo, M.A. Frequent expression of the multi-drug resistance-associated protein BCRP/MXR/ABCP/ABCG2 in human tumours detected by the BXP-21 monoclonal antibody in paraffinembedded material. *J. Pathol.* **2002**, *198*, 213–219. [CrossRef]
93. Pfaffl, M.W. A new mathematical model for relative quantification in real-time RT-PCR. *Nucleic Acids Res.* **2001**, *29*, e45.

Disclaimer/Publisher's Note: The statements, opinions and data contained in all publications are solely those of the individual author(s) and contributor(s) and not of MDPI and/or the editor(s). MDPI and/or the editor(s) disclaim responsibility for any injury to people or property resulting from any ideas, methods, instructions or products referred to in the content.

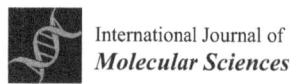

Communication

Analysis of Circulating Tumor DNA in Synchronous Metastatic Colorectal Cancer at Diagnosis Predicts Overall Patient Survival

José María Sayagués [1,2,*,†], Juan Carlos Montero [1,2,†], Andrea Jiménez-Pérez [1,2], Sofía del Carmen [3], Marta Rodríguez [1,2], Rosario Vidal Tocino [4], Enrique Montero [5], Julia Sanz [6] and Mar Abad [1,2,*]

1. Department of Pathology and IBSAL, University Hospital of Salamanca, University of Salamanca, 37007 Salamanca, Spain; jcmon@usal.es (J.C.M.); abjimenez@saludcastillayleon.es (A.J.-P.); martarodriguez@saludcastillayleon.es (M.R.)
2. Biomedical Research Networking Centers-Oncology (CIBERONC), 28029 Madrid, Spain
3. Department of Pathology, University Hospital of Marqués de Valdecilla, 39008 Santander, Spain; sofia.delcarmen@scsalud.es
4. Department of Oncology and IBSAL, University Hospital of Salamanca, 37007 Salamanca, Spain; mrvidal@saludcastillayleon.es
5. Department of Pathology, University Hospital of Zamora, 49071 Zamora, Spain; emonteroma@saludcastillayleon.es
6. Department of Pathology, Puerto Real University Hospital, 11510 Cadiz, Spain; jsrepetto@saludcastillayleon.es
* Correspondence: ppmari@usal.es (J.M.S.); marabad@usal.es (M.A.)
† These authors contributed equally to this work.

Abstract: Sporadic colorectal cancer (sCRC) initially presents as metastatic tumors in 25–30% of patients. The 5-year overall survival (OS) in patients with metastatic sCRC is 50%, falling to 10% in patients presenting with synchronous metastatic disease (stage IV). In this study, we systematically analyzed the mutations of *RAS*, *PIK3CA* and *BRAF* genes in circulating tumor DNA (ctDNA) and tumoral tissue DNA (ttDNA) from 51 synchronous metastatic colorectal carcinoma (SMCC) patients by real-time PCR, and their relationship with the clinical, biological and histological features of disease at diagnosis. The highest frequency of mutations detected was in the *KRAS* gene, in tumor biopsies and plasma samples, followed by mutations of the *PIK3CA*, *NRAS* and *BRAF* genes. Overall, plasma systematically contained those genetic abnormalities observed in the tumor biopsy sample from the same subject, the largest discrepancies detected between the tumor biopsy and plasma from the same patient being for mutations in the *KRAS* and *PIK3CA* genes, with concordances of genotyping results between ttDNA and ctDNA at diagnosis of 75% and 84%, respectively. Of the 51 SMCC patients in the study, 25 (49%) showed mutations in at least 1 of the 4 genes analyzed in patient plasma. From the prognostic point of view, the presence and number of the most common mutations in the *RAS*, *PIK3CA* and *BRAF* genes in plasma from SMCC patients are independent prognostic factors for OS. Determination of the mutational status of ctDNA in SMCC could be a key tool for the clinical management of patients.

Keywords: synchronous metastatic colorectal cancer; liquid biopsy; *KRAS*; *NRAS*; *PIK3CA*; *BRAF*; anti-EGFR; anti-VEGF

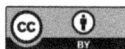

1. Introduction

Approximately 25–30% of patients with sporadic colorectal cancer (sCRC) initially present as metastatic tumors (stage IV). Of the other patients, who are mainly diagnosed in stages II or III, 40% will progress to more advanced stages and metastatic processes, the liver being the most common site for metastatic spread of the primary tumor [1]. Overall, the 5-year overall survival (OS) in patients with metastatic CRC is 50%, falling to 10% in stage IV patients (synchronous metastatic disease) [1].

It is well known that the pathogenesis of sCRC is due to the sequential appearance of abnormalities at the genetic level that, from a preneoplastic stage, lead to a generalized alteration of the genome by the clonal expansion of cells carrying mutations that frequently affect *APC*, *RAS*, *TP53* and/or *DCC* genes [2]. However, genetic alterations participating in the metastatic process, through which tumor cells of the primary tumor can colonize other tissues, remain to be identified. Recent genetic studies of metastatic tumors carried out by our research group suggest that the metastatic potential resides in the primary tumor itself [3]. Thus, we and other researchers have recently shown specific genomic alterations that are already present in the primary tumor of metastatic sCRC patients (e.g., del(17p) and del(22q)), as well as the differential expression of 28 genes (e.g., dysregulated transcripts of *ADH1B*, *BST2* and *FER1L4* genes) between metastatic and non-metastatic sCRC tumors [4].

Various therapeutic protocols based on general chemotherapeutic agents have been applied for the treatment of metastatic sCRC, and, more recently, new protocols have been implemented that consist of the combined use of chemotherapy with monoclonal antibodies against specific oncogenic targets. Although at the beginning of the 1980s the median survival of patients with disseminated disease was 6 months, this was extended to 1 year with the appearance of regimens based on 5-fluorouracil. Subsequently, this was extended to as much as 20 months by the addition of irinotecan and oxaliplatin. More recently, and as a result of oncology entering the molecular era, the following monoclonal antibodies have been included in clinical practice: bevacizumab, anti-vascular endothelial growth factor (VEGF), and cetuximab and panitumumab, two anti-epithelial growth factor receptors (EGFRs) that, combined with cytostatic and surgical treatment, extend patient survival to approximately 24 months. However, these two anti-EGFRs are only active when the tumor cells of the patient do not present mutations at the level of the *RAS*, *PIK3CA* and *BRAF* genes. Therefore, triple-negative patients (*KRAS*, *BRAF* and *PI3KCA*; "wild type") are those who would benefit the most from these therapies [5].

Currently, mutations of these genes are evaluated in DNA from formalin-fixed, paraffin-embedded tumor tissue (tumor resection or biopsies). However, it is not always possible to extract sufficient DNA of adequate quality for mutational studies [6]. DNA fragmentation is very frequent in paraffin samples, which can affect the integrity of the molecule. In recent years, the analysis of circulating tumor DNA (ctDNA) has opened up a new avenue for the study and monitoring of patient tumor burden. ctDNA can be isolated from plasma or serum and has the potential to be a viable starting material for identifying genetic markers for disease diagnosis and recurrence. In addition, ctDNA analysis provides a real-time assessment of the mutational status (presence of pathogenic mutations) of genes involved in disease pathogenesis. On the other hand, ctDNA mutational analysis may also provide a better representation of the tumor because it has the potential to generate information about all subclones of a tumor, which may contain DNA fragments from the primary tumor and the distant metastatic tumors [7].

In the present study, we investigated the prognostic value of the mutational status of the *KRAS*, *NRAS*, *PIK3CA* and *BRAF* genes detected in tumor biopsies and plasma samples from 51 synchronous metastatic colorectal cancer (SMCC) patients. Overall, our results show that *KRAS* mutations, determined both in tumor tissue and in patient plasma, showed a significant adverse influence on OS in univariate analysis. However, in the multivariate analysis, only the mutations identified in the plasma of the SMCC patients maintained statistical significance, behaving as an independent prognostic factor for OS.

2. Results

2.1. Frequency, Type and Concordance of KRAS, NRAS, PIK3CA and BRAF Mutations Detected in Tumor Tissue and Plasma of 51 Patients with Synchronous Metastatic Colorectal Cancer (SMCC)

The highest frequency of mutations occurred in the *KRAS* gene, in the tumor biopsy (45% of cases) and plasma (43% of patients), the G12V and G13D mutations being the most frequently detected (Figure 1), followed by mutations of the *PIK3CA* (24% in tumor biopsy and 16% in plasma), *NRAS* (2% and 6%) and *BRAF* genes (2% and 4%), and the ES45X, Q61R/K and V600E mutations (Figure 1).

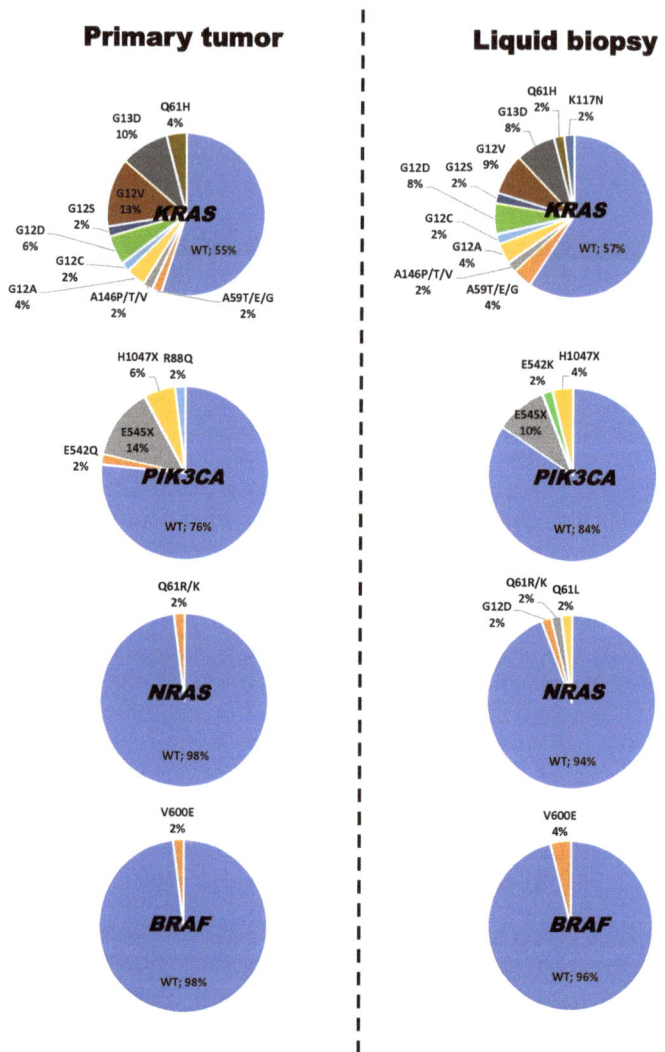

Figure 1. Frequency and type of mutations detected in the *KRAS*, *NRAS*, *PIK3CA* and *BRAF* genes in paired primary tumor and plasma (liquid biopsy) samples from 51 patients with synchronous metastatic colorectal cancer (SMCC) at diagnosis.

We also observed a statistically significant correlation among the mutational status of the *KRAS*, *NRAS*, *PIK3CA* and *BRAF* genes detected in plasma and tumoral tissue at diagnosis of the disease (Table 1). Overall, plasma systematically contained those genetic abnormalities observed in the tumor biopsy sample from the same subject. However, tumor biopsies from many cases (up to 5 out of 51) showed *KRAS* mutations that were not found in their corresponding plasma, while the plasma from 4 cases displayed *KRAS* mutations that were not detected in their corresponding tumoral biopsy sample (Figure 1 and Supplementary Table S1). Two patients showed *NRAS* mutations in the plasma, but not in their tumor biopsy sample, while only one patient showed such a discrepancy for

BRAF gene mutations (Table 1). The concordances of genotyping results between tDNA and ctDNA at diagnosis were 75%, 96%, 98% and 84% for the KRAS, NRAS, BRAF and PIK3CA genes, respectively.

Table 1. Clinical, biological and genetic characteristics of synchronous metastatic colorectal cancer (SMCC) patients with positive (n = 26) and negative (n = 25) liquid biopsy at diagnosis. Patients with a positive liquid biopsy were considered when at least one mutation in the KRAS, NRAS, PIK3CA and/or BRAF genes was detected in the patient's plasma.

Variable	Negative Liquid Biopsy Patients (n = 25)	Positive Liquid Biopsy Patients (n = 26)	p	Total (n = 51)
Age (years) *	65 (43–83)	67 (50–81)	0.89	66 (43–83)
Gender				
Female	5 (20%)	9 (35%)	0.51	14 (27%)
Male	20 (80%)	17 (55%)		37 (63%)
Site of PT				
Right colon	7 (28%)	11 (42%)		18 (35%)
Left colon	1 (4%)	3 (12%)	0.11	4 (8%)
Rectum	17 (68%)	12 (46%)		29 (57%)
Treatment type				
Chemotherapy + anti-EGFR	19 (76%)	5 (19%)		24 (47%)
Chemotherapy + anti-VEGF	2 (8%)	16 (62%)	<0.001	18 (35%)
Chemotherapy	4 (16%)	5 (19%)		9 (18%)
CEA serum levels *				
≤7.5 ng/mL	10 (40%)	1 (4%)	0.002	11 (22%)
>7.5 ng/mL	15 (60%)	25 (96%)		40 (78%)
Mutational status of PT				
Mutated	16 (64%)	3 (12%)	<0.001	19 (27%)
Wild type	9 (36%)	23 (89%)		32 (63%)
Number of deaths	15 (60%)	21 (81%)	0.009	36 (71%)
Overall survival (months)	52 (38–67)	24 (16–31)	<0.001	40 (30–51)

Results are expressed as the number of cases (percentage) or * as the median (range). PT: primary tumor; CEA: carcinoembryogenic antigen. A primary tumor was considered to be mutated when at least one mutation in the KRAS, NRAS, PIK3CA and/or BRAF genes was detected in the patient's primary tumor.

2.2. Association between Mutational Status Detected in Patient Plasma and Other Features of the Disease

Of the 51 SMCC patients included in the present study, 26 (51%) displayed mutations for at least 1 of the 4 genes analyzed in the plasma (positive biopsy). Overall, most patients with a positive biopsy had a tumor in the right colon or rectum with abnormally high CEA serum levels (>7.5 ng/mL; p = 0.002), and they showed a higher frequency of deaths (p = 0.009) in association with significantly shortened patient overall survival (OS) (median of 24 months; $p \leq 0.001$). As expected, a significant correlation was detected between the mutations detected in plasma and those identified in the primary tumor. In contrast, no significant differences were found between positive and negative biopsy SMCC patients, having taken gender and patient age into account (Table 1).

2.3. Impact of Liquid Biopsy on Patient OS

From the prognostic point of view, the clinical, biological and pathological characteristics of the disease that displayed a significant adverse influence on OS in the univariate analysis included increased (>7.5 ng/mL) CEA serum levels (p = 0.073), KRAS mutations determined in both primary tumor and plasma (p = 0.05 and p = 0.004, respectively), positive liquid biopsy at diagnosis (p = 0.05) and, interestingly, the number of mutations detected in plasma at diagnosis ($p \leq 0.001$) (Table 2), the determination of the KRAS mutation in plasma being a good prognostic factor in the univariate analysis. However, multivariate analysis of the prognostic factors for OS showed that the presence and number of mutations detected in the plasma at diagnosis were the only independent variables that predicted an adverse outcome (Table 1 and Figure 2).

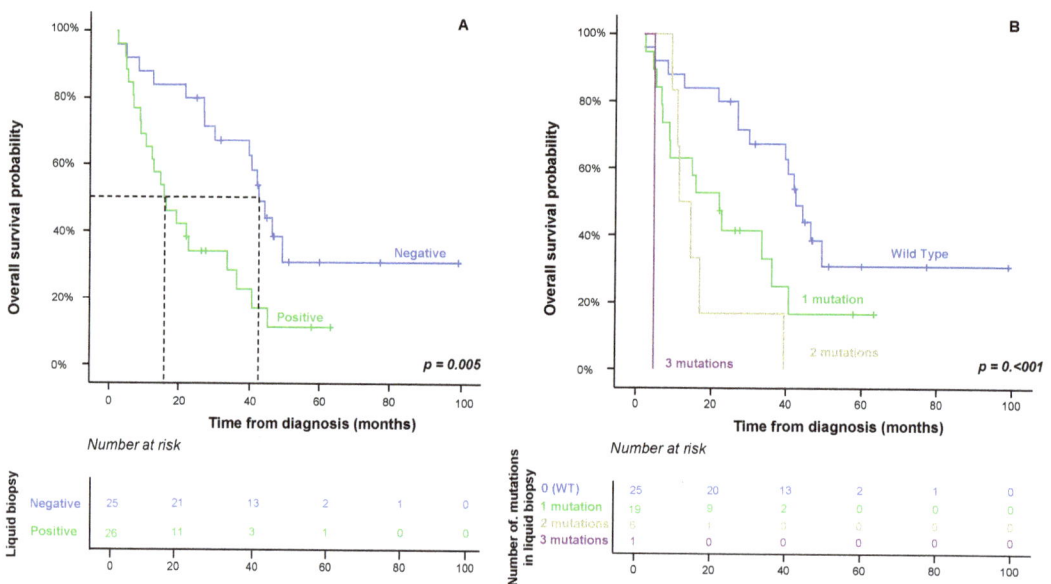

Figure 2. Identification of at least one mutation in the *KRAS*, *NRAS*, *PIK3CA* and/or *BRAF* genes in the plasma of synchronous metastatic colorectal cancer patients (positive liquid biopsy) at diagnosis (Panel **A**), and the increase in the number of mutations detected (Panel **B**), show a significant impact on overall survival in the univariate ($p \leq 0.005$) and multivariate ($p \leq 0.007$) analyses.

Table 2. Clinical, biological and genetic characteristics of synchronous metastatic colorectal cancer (SMCC) patients ($n = 51$) and their association with overall survival (OS).

Variable	N *	Univariate Analysis	Multivariate Analysis	HR (95% CI)
Age				
<66 years	26 (51%)	0.889		
≥66 years	25 (49%)			
Gender				
Male	37 (76%)	0.879		
Female	14 (24%)			
Site of PT				
Right colon	18 (35%)			
Left colon	4 (8%)	0.114		
Rectum	29 (57%)			
CEA serum levels				
<7.5 ng	11 (22%)	0.073	NS	
≥7.5 ng	40 (78%)			
Treatment type				
Chemotherapy + anti-EGFR	24 (47%)			
Chemotherapy + anti-VEGF	18 (35%)	0.053	NS	
Chemotherapy	9 (18%)			
Microsatellite instability				
No	50 (98%)	0.879		
Yes	1 (2%)			
KRAS mutation in PT				
Yes	23 (45%)	0.050	NS	
No	28 (55%)			
NRAS mutation in PT				
Yes	1 (2%)	0.487		
No	50 (98%)			
BRAF mutation in PT				
Yes	1 (2%)	0.937		
No	50 (98%)			
PIK3CA mutation in PT				
Yes	12 (24%)	0.728		
No	39 (76%)			

Table 2. Cont.

Variable	N *	Univariate Analysis	Multivariate Analysis	HR (95% CI)
KRAS mutation in plasma				
Yes	23 (45%)	0.004	NS	
No	28 (55%)			
NRAS mutation in plasma				
Yes	3 (6%)	0.420		
No	48 (94%)			
PIK3CA mutation in plasma				
Yes	8 (16%)	0.185		
No	43 (84%)			
BRAF mutation in plasma				
Yes	2 (4%)	0.472		
No	49 (96%)			
Liquid biopsy at diagnosis				
Positive	26 (53%)	0.005	0.007	0.388 (0.196–0.768)
Negative	25 (47%)			
Mutations in liquid biopsy				
Wild type	25 (49%)			
1 mutation	19 (37%)		0.001	2.018 (0.316–3.095)
2 mutations	6 (12%)			
3 mutations	1 (2%)			

* Results are expressed as the number of cases (percentage). PT: primary tumor. A liquid biopsy was considered to be positive when at least one mutation in the KRAS, NRAS, PIK3CA and/or BRAF genes was detected in the patient's plasma. NS: not statistically significant ($p > 0.05$).

3. Discussion

The chances of a cure for patients with sporadic colorectal cancer (sCRC) who develop distant metastases to the liver and other organs at the time of diagnosis are dramatically low. Even though we now have a much better understanding of the genetic mechanisms that control the early stages of disease, the factors involved in metastatic processes remain poorly understood. In this context, it is of utmost importance to develop methods capable of identifying patients at high risk for an adverse outcome or of predicting the onset of metastasis, the main cause of death of sCRC patients. In recent years, various studies have demonstrated the prognostic value of cfDNA in sCRC, raising the possibility that their analysis might identify patients with localized tumors who are at risk of recurrence [8]. Other studies have shown that molecular analysis of the tumor through liquid biopsies provides information about the changes in the RAS mutational status due to tumoral heterogeneity and selective pressure by targeted therapies throughout the course of the disease [9,10]. However, the significance of liquid biopsy in the clinical management of patients with synchronous metastases remains to be elucidated.

In this study, we describe the frequency and type of mutations found in biopsies of tumor tissue and in peripheral blood at the time of diagnosis of the disease to determine the most appropriate therapy for each synchronous metastatic colorectal cancer (SMCC) patient: chemotherapy alone or combined with monoclonal antibodies, anti-epidermal growth factor receptor (EGFR) or anti-vascular endothelial growth factor receptor (VEGFR). In turn, we show how the presence of mutations and their accumulation influence the overall survival (OS) of the patient, regardless of the medical treatment received. To the best of our knowledge, this is the first report demonstrating that the co-occurrence of mutations in genes involved in the EGFR signaling pathway in peripheral blood from SMCC patients is associated with a significantly short OS. Consistent with our observations, Kawazoe et al. [11], in a retrospective observational study, described the mutational status of KRAS, NRAS, BRAF or PIK3CA in tissue biopsies from 264 patients with mCRC, demonstrating that patients with any mutation in these genes had a shorter survival outcome after receiving treatments with monoclonal antibodies. However, the series of patients studied was not homogeneous since it included patients with synchronous and metachronous metastases. In addition, they did not determine the mutational status of the genes using liquid biopsy techniques, which could resolve the possible genetic heterogeneity present in this type of tumor and find other genetic lesions present in the metastatic samples [12]. In this regard, several studies that have explored ctDNA levels in mCRC have indicated that elevated ctDNA levels are correlated with poorer survival. Thus, Yang et al. [7] analyzed ctDNA levels in 47 CRC patients in early or late cancer stages and found that stage IV patients had significantly higher ctDNA concentrations than stage I patients. Similarly, Güttlein's work [13] also supports the utility of *KRAS*, *NRAS* and *BRAF* analysis in liquid biopsy from CRC patients with synchronous and metachronous metastases, finding an association between *RAS/BRAF*-mutated patients and a shorter OS. These studies support the implication that ctDNA characteristics could help in the clinical management of metastatic patients.

In the present study, all patients in our cohort had both tissue and plasma available at diagnosis. The concordance between tissue and plasma was approximately 75% when the *KRAS* gene was analyzed, as previously observed. In an earlier study, Rodon et al. [12] found a 76.5% concordance of genotyping results using NGS in 18 tissue and blood samples of patients with locally advanced CRC or mCRC. Similarly, Erve et al. [14] observed a 93% concordance between tumoral tissue DNA (ttDNA) and liquid biopsy *RAS/BRAF* ctDNA in their analysis of 100 sCRC patients with liver metastases. Kagawa et al. [15] investigated the concordance of the RAS status between Digital PCR (OncoBEAM™) and tissue biopsies in 221 mCRC patients, and found concordance ratios between 64% and 91%, depending on whether the metastatic site was the liver, peritoneum or lung. Discrepant results could be explained by the acquisition of the mutation during the disease's progression to the liver. However, *KRAS* mutation occurs in early stages of carcinogenesis [16], although it is not uncommon for the *KRAS* mutation to be acquired after metastasis. In our series, 4 (8%) patients had a *KRAS* mutation that was detected in liquid biopsy, but not in the tumoral biopsy. Taniguchi et al. [17] demonstrated that metastatic lesions harbored diverse acquired mutations of *KRAS* in primary tumors.

The results of our study show that the best method for predicting the disease prognosis is the mutational characterization of the EGFR signaling pathway genes in the patient's plasma (vs. tumor tissue). Testing ctDNA in peripheral blood (liquid biopsy) has emerged as a new and useful tool in the diagnosis and follow-up of sCRC patients. Detection of the mutational status of genes involved in the EGFR signaling pathway genes in ctDNA from blood samples seems to be a simple and non-invasive alternative to testing primary tumors. In addition, it is an easy and inexpensive technique to perform in clinical laboratories, and it can be carried out easily at different times during the course of the disease, providing information about dynamic changes in the genotype of mCRC cells [18], successfully resolving the possible spatial and temporal heterogeneity present in this type of tumor [19]. The absolute amount of ctDNA depends on the stage [20] and location [17] of the tumor. Surgery and medical treatment both modify ctDNA levels, which act as a surrogate biomarker of the response to anti-EGFR treatments and progression-free survival (PFS) in sCRC patients with localized disease. However, the clinical significance and impact of anti-angiogenics (anti-VEGFR agents) [21] in synchronous metastatic disease remain to be elucidated. Most studies have focused on the progression of the primary tumor after its surgical resection. In the metastatic process of sCRC, tumor hypoxia produces overexpression of the hypoxia-inducible factor-1 (HIF-1) and release of the VEGF, which stimulates neoangiogenesis to ensure the survival of the tumor cells [22]. In addition, VEGF expression under hypoxic conditions can also be stimulated by the EGFR signaling pathway, which, in turn, is frequently activated by the appearance of mutations in the *KRAS*, *NRAS*, *BRAF* or *PIK3CA* genes [23]. Currently, the decision to administer a treatment is based solely on the molecular information obtained from the initial tumor biopsy. However, published results show that metastatic disease can undergo mutational variations that can condition the choice of treatment by the selection of resistant clones after administering systemic therapy [19,24,25]. In fact, the study carried out by Erik et al. suggests that analysis of plasma-derived ctDNA in patients with mCRC may identify additional RAS mutations that would improve patient selection for anti-EGFR therapies [25]. Klein et al. [9] demonstrated that although systemic therapies kill many tumor cells, resistant tumor cell clones are selected, avoiding the cytotoxic action of the administered therapy. It has been hypothesized that the tumor hypoxia produced in the metastatic process could also contribute to this selection of clones capable of surviving in conditions of low oxygen supply. Half of the patients analyzed by Gazzaniga et al. [26] changed their mutational status to become RAS wild-type after receiving antiangiogenic therapy. Garcia et al. [27] detected a RAS mutational change in 74% of patients after a median of 3 months of bevacizumab treatment. Even traditional chemotherapy has been linked to the modification of the RAS mutational status. Therefore, the study of molecular profiling using liquid biopsy could be a key tool for predicting OS in patients with SMCC treated with anti-EGFR and anti-VEGFR drugs. It should be noted that several studies of genome sequencing have observed that one in five healthy individuals may carry disease-related genetic mutations [16,28]. However, none of the mutations detected in these studies were present in the genes studied here.

Limited information is available on the feasibility and clinical potential of ctDNA analysis in non-metastatic CRC cancer and/or in early stage of the disease. The results of these studies are difficult to interpret and compare, especially due to significant heterogeneity regarding the patient's series analyzed. While Tie et al. [29] reported that ctDNA significantly outperforms standard clinicopathologic characteristics as a prognostic marker in stage II patients, Sclafani et al. [30] failed to predict the prognosis with the detection of *KRAS* mutation in ctDNA of locally advanced rectal cancer patients. Larger series are needed to better address the role of ctDNA as a prognostic or predictive tool in this regard.

In summary, our results show that the presence of mutations in the *RAS*, *PIK3CA* and/or *BRAF* genes in the plasma of patients with SMCC is an independent prognostic factor for OS. The data also provide evidence that the number of mutations is negatively correlated with the OS of patients, regardless of the treatment they receive. Molecular information obtained by ctDNA analysis could be useful in our daily clinical practice to improve prognostic assessments and to guide clinical decision making in SMCC patients. Additional prospective studies are required in larger series to confirm the utility of the proposed predictive model.

4. Materials and Methods

4.1. Patients and Samples

Peripheral blood and endoscopically acquired tumor tissue biopsies from the primary tumor were obtained from 51 consecutive patients with synchronous metastatic colorectal cancer (SMCC) between June 2014 and September 2017 in the Department of Surgery of the University Hospital of Salamanca (Salamanca, Spain), before administering any cytotoxic therapy and after each subject had given their informed consent, in accordance with the Declaration of Helsinki. In total, 37 were men and 14 women, with a median age 66 years (range 43–83 years). Diagnosis and classification of the tumor were made according to the AJCC criteria [31]. All cases were adenocarcinomas. Median follow-up at the close of the study was 40 months (range 30–50 months). Patient clinical, laboratory and follow-up data are summarized in Table 3.

Table 3. Correlation between the mutational status of the *KRAS*, *NRAS*, *PIK3CA* and *BRAF* genes detected in the plasma and primary tumor of patients ($n = 51$) with synchronous metastatic colorectal cancer (SMCC).

Primary Tumor	Plasma											
	KRAS			NRAS			BRAF			PIK3CA		
	WT ($n = 29$)	Mutated ($n = 22$)	R/p	WT ($n = 48$)	Mutated ($n = 3$)	R/p	WT ($n = 49$)	Mutated ($n = 2$)	R/p	WT ($n = 43$)	Mutated ($n = 8$)	R/p
KRAS												
WT ($n = 28$)	24 (86)	4 (14)	0.65/<0.001									
Mutated ($n = 23$)	5 (22)	18 (78)										
NRAS												
WT ($n = 50$)				48 (96)	2 (4)	0.57/0.05						
Mutated ($n = 1$)				0 (0)	1 (100)							
BRAF												
WT ($n = 50$)							49 (98)	1 (2)	0.77/<0.001			
Mutated ($n = 1$)							0 (0)	1 (100)				
PIK3CA												
WT ($n = 39$)										37 (95)	2 (5)	0.53/0.001
Mutated ($n = 12$)										6 (50)	6 (50)	

Results expressed as number of cases (percentage); WT: wild type; R, correlation coefficient; *p*, probability.

The study was approved by the local ethics committee of the University Hospital of Salamanca (Salamanca, Spain).

4.2. Tissue-Based RAS, BRAF and PIK3CA Mutation Analysis

Tumor tissue biopsies were collected and mutations were sought at diagnosis. Hematoxylin-eosin (HE)-stained slides were reviewed. The DNA was isolated from a paraffin block containing at least 70% of tumor cells. One or two 10 μm-thick formalin-fixed paraffin-embedded (FFPE) tumor tissue sections were deparaffinized with xylene for 5 min at room temperature (RT), dehydrated in absolute alcohol for 5 min at RT and allowed to air-dry completely for 10 min. Later, DNA was isolated using the Cobas DNA Sample Preparation Kit (Roche, Branchburg, NJ, USA) following the manufacturer's instructions.

4.3. Blood-Based RAS, BRAF and PIK3CA Mutation Analysis

In parallel, cfDNA was isolated from 2 mL of plasma obtained from each patient ($n = 51$) at diagnosis, using a Cobas® cfDNA Sample Preparation Kit (Roche, Branchburg, NJ, USA) and following the manufacturer's instructions.

A Nanodrop UV spectrophotometer (Thermo Fisher Scientific, Wilmington, DE, USA) was used to verify the quality and quantity of the extracted DNA from both tumor tissue and patient plasma. Amplification and detection were performed with an Automated Cobas z480 analyzer instrument (Roche Molecular System Inc., Pleasanton, CA, USA). The real-time PCR tests examined the most common mutations in codons 12, 13, 59, 61, 117 and 146 in the *KRAS* and *NRAS* genes; the V600E *BRAF* mutation; and in exons 2, 5, 8, 10 and 21 of *PIK3CA* mutations. The tests to detect these mutations both in tumor tissue and in the patient's peripheral blood were purchased from Roche (Branchburg, NJ, USA): the KRAS v2 mutation test (LSR), BRAF/NRAS mutation test (LSR) and the Cobas mutation test PIK3CA. Data were analyzed according to the manufacturer's instructions by uploading the .ixo files to the online LSR Data Analysis tool: https://lifescience.roche.com/en_nl/brands/oncology-research-kits.html (accession on 18 January 2023).

4.4. Statistical Analyses

The mean, standard deviation (SD) and range of all continuous variables were calculated, and dichotomous variables were reported as frequencies and percentages. To evaluate the statistical significance of group differences, Student's *t*-test and the Mann–Whitney U test were used for normally and non-normally distributed continuous variables, respectively. For dichotomous variables, the X^2 test was used. Overall survival (OS) curves were plotted according to the Kaplan–Meier method, and the log-rank test (one-sided) was used to determine the statistical significance of the differences between survival curves. Multivariate analysis of prognostic factors for OS were identified by multivariate stepwise Cox regression, using forward selection and considering only those variables that showed a significant association with OS in the univariate analysis. All analyses were carried out using IBM SPSS Statistics v.22 (IBM Corp., Armonk, NY, USA). Statistical significance was concluded for values of p (Pearson-corrected where appropriate) of <0.05.

Supplementary Materials: The following supporting information can be downloaded at: https://www.mdpi.com/article/10.3390/ijms24098438/s1.

Author Contributions: Conceptualization, J.M.S. and M.A.; methodology, A.J.-P., J.C.M. and S.d.C.; formal analysis, J.M.S.; investigation, R.V.T., J.C.M. and M.R.; writing—original draft preparation, J.M.S., J.C.M., J.S. and E.M.; writing—review and editing, J.C.M. and M.A.; funding acquisition, M.A. All authors have read and agreed to the published version of the manuscript.

Funding: This work was partially supported by a grant from the Gerencia Regional de Salud de Castilla y León, Valladolid, Spain (GRS 2626/A/22). We also want to thank the laboratory technicians, Ruth Gervas, Belen Rivas, Saray Muñoz and Raquel Díaz for their support with the technical processes carried out in the present study.

Institutional Review Board Statement: The study was conducted in accordance with the Declaration of Helsinki and approved by the Local Ethics Committee of the University Hospital of Salamanca (PI 2022 07 1092; Salamanca, Spain), approved on 8 July 2022.

Informed Consent Statement: Informed consent was obtained from all subjects involved in the study.

Data Availability Statement: All study data can be viewed in the manuscript.

Conflicts of Interest: The authors declare no potential conflict of interest with respect to the research, authorship or publication of this article.

References

1. Van Cutsem, E.; Cervantes, A.; Adam, R.; Sobrero, A.; van Krieken, J.H.; Aderka, D.; Aguilar, E.A.; Bardelli, A.; Benson, A.; Bodoky, G.; et al. ESMO consensus guidelines for the management of patients with metastatic colorectal cancer. *Ann. Oncol.* **2016**, *27*, 1386–1422. [CrossRef] [PubMed]
2. Del Carmen, S.; Sayagués, J.M.; Bengoechea, O.; Anduaga, M.F.; Alcazar, J.A.; Gervas, R.; García, J.; Orfao, A.; Bellvis, L.M.; Sarasquete, M.E.; et al. Spatio-temporal tumor heterogeneity in metastatic CRC tumors: A mutational-based approach. *Oncotarget* **2018**, *9*, 34279–34288. [CrossRef] [PubMed]
3. Muñoz-Bellvis, L.; Fontanillo, C.; González-González, M.; Garcia, E.; Iglesias, M.; Esteban, C.; Gutierrez, M.L.; Abad, M.M.; Bengoechea, O.; Rivas, J.D.L.; et al. Unique genetic profile of sporadic colorectal cancer liver metastasis versus primary tumors as defined by high-density single-nucleotide polymorphism arrays. *Mod. Pathol.* **2012**, *25*, 590–601. [CrossRef] [PubMed]
4. González-González, M.; Muñoz-Bellvís, L.; Mackintosh, C.; Fontanillo, C.; Gutiérrez, M.L.; Abad, M.M.; Bengoechea, O.; Teodosio, C.; Fonseca, E.; Fuentes, M.; et al. Prognostic Impact of del(17p) and del(22q) as Assessed by Interphase FISH in Sporadic Colorectal Carcinomas. *PLoS ONE* **2012**, *7*, e42683. [CrossRef]
5. Martini, G.; Ciardiello, D.; Napolitano, S.; Martinelli, E.; Troiani, T.; Latiano, T.P.; Avallone, A.; Normanno, N.; Di Maio, M.; Maiello, E.; et al. Efficacy and safety of a biomarker-driven cetuximab-based treatment regimen over 3 treatment lines in mCRC patients with RAS/BRAF wild type tumors at start of first line: The CAPRI 2 GOIM trial. *Front. Oncol.* **2023**, *13*, 1069370. [CrossRef]
6. Witt, J.; Haupt, S.; Ahadova, A.; Bohaumilitzky, L.; Fuchs, V.; Ballhausen, A.; Przybilla, M.J.; Jendrusch, M.; Seppälä, T.T.; Fürst, D.; et al. A simple approach for detecting *HLA-A* *02 alleles in archival formalin-fixed paraffin-embedded tissue samples and an application example for studying cancer immunoediting. *Hla* **2023**, *101*, 24–33. [CrossRef]
7. Yang, Y.C.; Wang, D.; Jin, L.; Yao, H.W.; Zhang, J.H.; Wang, J.; Zhao, X.M.; Shen, C.Y.; Chen, W.; Wang, X.L.; et al. Circulating tumor DNA detectable in early- and late-stage colorectal cancer patients. *Biosci. Rep.* **2018**, *38*, BSR20180322. [CrossRef]
8. Allegretti, M.; Cottone, G.; Carboni, F.; Cotroneo, E.; Casini, B.; Giordani, E.; Amoreo, C.A.; Buglioni, S.; Diodoro, M.; Pescarmona, E.; et al. Cross-sectional analysis of circulating tumor DNA in primary colorectal cancer at surgery and during post-surgery follow-up by liquid biopsy. *J. Exp. Clin. Cancer Res.* **2020**, *39*, 69. [CrossRef]
9. Klein, C.A. Selection and adaptation during metastatic cancer progression. *Nature* **2013**, *501*, 365–372. [CrossRef]
10. Bádon, E.S.; Mokánszki, A.; Mónus, A.; András, C.; Méhes, G. Clonal diversity in KRAS mutant colorectal adenocarcinoma under treatment: Monitoring of cfDNA using reverse hybridization and DNA sequencing platforms. *Mol. Cell. Probes* **2023**, *67*, 101891. [CrossRef]
11. Kawazoe, A.; Shitara, K.; Fukuoka, S.; Kuboki, Y.; Bando, H.; Okamoto, W.; Kojima, T.; Fuse, N.; Yamanaka, T.; Doi, T.; et al. A retrospective observational study of clinicopathological features of KRAS, NRAS, BRAF and PIK3CA mutations in Japanese patients with metastatic colorectal cancer. *BMC Cancer* **2015**, *15*, 258. [CrossRef]
12. Font, N.R.; Garbarino, Y.N.; Castello, O.D.; Amoros, J.M.; Sánchez, P.B.; Lletget, D.C.; Cabello, M.A.L.; Marcet, J.B.; Meca, S.M.; Escape, I.; et al. Concordance analysis between liquid biopsy (ctDNA) and tumor DNA molecular profiles from panel-based next-generation sequencing. *Rev. Española De Patol.* **2022**, *55*, 156–162. [CrossRef]
13. Güttlein, L.; Luca, M.R.; Esteso, F.; Fresno, C.; Mariani, J.; Otero Pizarro, M.; Brest, E.; Starapoli, S.; Kreimberg, K.; Teves, P.; et al. Liquid biopsy for *KRAS*, *NRAS* and *BRAF* mutation testing in advanced colorectal cancer patients: The Argentinean experience. *Future Oncol. Lond. Engl.* **2022**, *18*, 3277–3287. [CrossRef]
14. Van't Erve, I.; Greuter, M.J.; Bolhuis, K.; Vessies, D.C.; Leal, A.; Vink, G.R.; van den Broek, D.; Velculescu, V.E.; Punt, C.J.A.; Meijer, G.A.; et al. Diagnostic Strategies toward Clinical Implementation of Liquid Biopsy RAS/BRAF Circulating Tumor DNA Analyses in Patients with Metastatic Colorectal Cancer. *J. Mol. Diagn.* **2020**, *22*, 1430–1437. [CrossRef]
15. Kagawa, Y.; Elez, E.; García-Foncillas, J.; Bando, H.; Taniguchi, H.; Vivancos, A.; Akagi, K.; García, A.; Denda, T.; Ros, J.; et al. Combined Analysis of Concordance between Liquid and Tumor Tissue Biopsies for *RAS* Mutations in Colorectal Cancer with a Single Metastasis Site: The METABEAM Study. *Clin. Cancer Res.* **2021**, *27*, 2515–2522. [CrossRef]
16. Watson, R.; Liu, T.-C.; Ruzinova, M.B. High frequency of KRAS mutation in early onset colorectal adenocarcinoma: Implications for pathogenesis. *Hum. Pathol.* **2016**, *56*, 163–170. [CrossRef]

17. Taniguchi, F.; Nyuya, A.; Toshima, T.; Yasui, K.; Mori, Y.; Okawaki, M.; Kishimoto, H.; Umeda, Y.; Fujiwara, T.; Tanioka, H.; et al. Concordance of acquired mutations between metastatic lesions and liquid biopsy in metastatic colorectal cancer. *Futur. Sci. OA* **2021**, *7*, FSO757. [CrossRef]
18. Yamada, T.; Matsuda, A.; Koizumi, M.; Shinji, S.; Takahashi, G.; Iwai, T.; Takeda, K.; Ueda, K.; Yokoyama, Y.; Hara, K.; et al. Liquid Biopsy for the Management of Patients with Colorectal Cancer. *Digestion* **2018**, *99*, 39–45. [CrossRef]
19. McGranahan, N.; Swanton, C. Clonal Heterogeneity and Tumor Evolution: Past, Present, and the Future. *Cell* **2017**, *168*, 613–628. [CrossRef] [PubMed]
20. Liebs, S.; Keilholz, U.; Kehler, I.; Schweiger, C.; Haybäck, J.; Nonnenmacher, A. Detection of mutations in circulating cell-free DNA in relation to disease stage in colorectal cancer. *Cancer Med.* **2019**, *8*, 3761–3769. [CrossRef]
21. Hrebien, S.; Citi, V.; Garcia-Murillas, I.; Cutts, R.; Fenwick, K.; Kozarewa, I.; McEwen, R.; Ratnayake, J.; Maudsley, R.; Carr, T.; et al. Early ctDNA dynamics as a surrogate for progression-free survival in advanced breast cancer in the BEECH trial. *Ann. Oncol.* **2019**, *30*, 945–952. [CrossRef] [PubMed]
22. Zheng, J.; Sun, X.; Wang, W.; Lu, S. Hypoxia-inducible factor-1alpha modulates the down-regulation of the homeodomain protein CDX2 in colorectal cancer. *Oncol. Rep.* **2010**, *24*, 97–104. [PubMed]
23. Singh, D.; Attri, B.K.; Gill, R.K.; Bariwal, J. Review on EGFR Inhibitors: Critical Updates. *Mini. Rev. Med. Chem.* **2016**, *16*, 1134–1166. [CrossRef] [PubMed]
24. Klein-Scory, S.; Wahner, I.; Maslova, M.; Al-Sewaidi, Y.; Pohl, M.; Mika, T.; Ladigan, S.; Schroers, R.; Baraniskin, A. Evolution of RAS Mutational Status in Liquid Biopsies During First-Line Chemotherapy for Metastatic Colorectal Cancer. *Front. Oncol.* **2020**, *10*, 1115. [CrossRef] [PubMed]
25. Van Helden, E.J.; Angus, L.; Menke-van der Houven van Oordt, C.W.; Heideman, D.A.M.; Boon, E.; van Es, S.C.; Radema, S.A.; van Herpen, C.M.L.; de Jan, J.A.D.; de Vries, E.G.E.; et al. RAS and BRAF mutations in cell-free DNA are predictive for outcome of cetuximab monotherapy in patients with tissue-tested RAS wild-type advanced colorectal cancer. *Mol. Oncol.* **2019**, *13*, 2361–2374. [CrossRef] [PubMed]
26. Gazzaniga, P.; Raimondi, C.; Urbano, F.; Cortesi, E. EGFR Inhibitor as Second-Line Therapy in a Patient with Mutant RAS Metastatic Colorectal Cancer: Circulating Tumor DNA to Personalize Treatment. *JCO Precis. Oncol.* **2018**, *2*, 1–6. [CrossRef]
27. De Santiago, B.G.; López-Gómez, M.; Delgado-López, P.D.; Gordo, A.J.; Neria, F.; Thuissard-Vasallo, I.J.; Gómez-Raposo, C.; Tevar, F.Z.; Moreno-Rubio, J.; Hernández, A.M. RAS Mutational Status in Advanced Colorectal Adenocarcinoma Treated with Anti-angiogenics: Preliminary Experience with Liquid Biopsy. *In Vivo* **2021**, *35*, 2841–2844. [CrossRef]
28. Vassy, J.L.; Christensen, K.D.; Schonman, E.F.; Blout, C.L.; Robinson, J.O.; Krier, J.B.; Diamond, P.M.; Lebo, M.; Machini, K.; Azzariti, D.R.; et al. The Impact of Whole-Genome Sequencing on the Primary Care and Outcomes of Healthy Adult Patients: A Pilot Randomized Trial. *Ann. Intern. Med.* **2017**, *167*, 159–169. [CrossRef]
29. Tie, J.; Wang, Y.; Tomasetti, C.; Li, L.; Springer, S.; Kinde, I.; Silliman, N.; Tacey, M.; Wong, H.-L.; Christie, M.; et al. Circulating tumor DNA analysis detects minimal residual disease and predicts recurrence in patients with stage II colon cancer. *Sci. Transl. Med.* **2016**, *8*, 346ra92. [CrossRef]
30. Sclafani, F.; Chau, I.; Cunningham, D.; Hahne, J.C.; Vlachogiannis, G.; Eltahir, Z.; Lampis, A.; Braconi, C.; Kalaitzaki, E.; De Castro, D.G.; et al. KRAS and BRAF mutations in circulating tumour DNA from locally advanced rectal cancer. *Sci. Rep.* **2018**, *8*, 1445. [CrossRef]
31. Weiser, M.R. AJCC 8th Edition: Colorectal Cancer. *Ann. Surg. Oncol.* **2018**, *25*, 1454–1455. [CrossRef]

Disclaimer/Publisher's Note: The statements, opinions and data contained in all publications are solely those of the individual author(s) and contributor(s) and not of MDPI and/or the editor(s). MDPI and/or the editor(s) disclaim responsibility for any injury to people or property resulting from any ideas, methods, instructions or products referred to in the content.

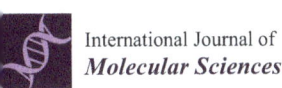

Article

Muscarinic Acetylcholine Receptor M3 Expression and Survival in Human Colorectal Carcinoma—An Unexpected Correlation to Guide Future Treatment?

Leonard A. Lobbes [1,*,†], Marcel A. Schütze [1,†], Raoul Droeser [2], Marco Arndt [1], Ioannis Pozios [1], Johannes C. Lauscher [1], Nina A. Hering [1] and Benjamin Weixler [1]

[1] Department of General and Visceral Surgery, Charité—Universitätsmedizin Berlin, Corporate Member of Freie Universität Berlin and Humboldt-Universität zu Berlin, Hindenburgdamm 30, 12203 Berlin, Germany
[2] Clarunis, Department of Visceral Surgery, University Centre for Gastrointestinal and Liver Diseases, St. Clara Hospital and University Hospital Basel, CH-4058 Basel, Switzerland
* Correspondence: leonard.lobbes@charite.de
† These authors contributed equally to this work.

Abstract: Muscarinic acetylcholine receptor M3 (M3R) has repeatedly been shown to be prominently expressed in human colorectal cancer (CRC), playing roles in proliferation and cell invasion. Its therapeutic targetability has been suggested in vitro and in animal models. We aimed to investigate the clinical role of MR3 expression in CRC for human survival. Surgical tissue samples from 754 CRC patients were analyzed for high or low immunohistochemical M3R expression on a clinically annotated tissue microarray (TMA). Immunohistochemical analysis was performed for established immune cell markers (CD8, TIA-1, FOXP3, IL 17, CD16 and OX 40). We used Kaplan–Meier curves to evaluate patients' survival and multivariate Cox regression analysis to evaluate prognostic significance. High M3R expression was associated with increased survival in multivariate (hazard ratio (HR) = 0.52; 95% CI = 0.35–0.78; $p = 0.001$) analysis, as was TIA-1 expression (HR = 0.99; 95% CI = 0.94–0.99; $p = 0.014$). Tumors with high M3R expression were significantly more likely to be grade 2 compared to tumors with low M3R expression (85.7% vs. 67.1%, $p = 0.002$). The 5-year survival analysis showed a trend of a higher survival rate in patients with high M3R expression (46%) than patients with low M3R expression CRC (42%) ($p = 0.073$). In contrast to previous in vitro and animal model findings, this study demonstrates an increased survival for CRC patients with high M3R expression. This evidence is highly relevant for translation of basic research findings into clinically efficient treatments.

Keywords: colorectal cancer (CRC); muscarinic acetylcholine receptor M3 (M3R) expression; human colorectal cancer survival; tissue microarray; immune cell markers; TIA-1; therapeutic target

1. Introduction

Colorectal cancer (CRC) is one of the most prevalent cancer types, causing approximately 1.15 million new cases and 577,000 deaths globally in 2020 [1]. Its incidence in patients aged 20–50 is observably increasing, particularly in the left-sided colon and rectum [2,3]. Concurrently, a rise in high-risk and metastasized (Union for International Cancer Control (UICC) stages II, III and IV) early-onset CRC cases can be observed [4], which require especially precise and efficient adjuvant therapies [5]. However, the selection of adjuvant therapy regimens is currently mainly based on criteria such as tumor extent, tumor grade, lymph-node status, and lymphatic and venous invasion [6], which are not sufficient to describe tumor aggressiveness, prognosis and targetability [6,7]. Hence, further characterization is needed to increase prognostic predictability and to provide new targets for improved therapies [8,9]. While the number of potential prognostic markers is growing, their clinical role often remains unclear [10–14]. Recently, through advanced techniques such as gene and proteome analysis, many new biomarkers of CRC have been suggested in vitro, for example, immune checkpoint molecules such as OX40, receptors such as CXCR4 and CX3CR1 and kinases such as FJX1 (four-jointed box kinase 1), as well as micro-RNAs [10,13,15–19]. Data on the respective clinical expression and efficacy of these biomarkers is lacking. Muscarinic receptor subtype M3 (M3R) has been described as a promotor of cell proliferation in CRC and may serve as a new prognostic and predictive marker [20]. Muscarinic acetylcholine receptors are G-protein-coupled receptors comprising five subtypes (M1-M5), which correspond to the genes CHRM1-5 [20]. Of the known muscarinic receptor subtypes, M3 has been shown to be expressed exclusively in the HT29 colon cancer cell line, which suggests its potential benefit for prognosis and therapy for human CRC [21]. Furthermore, muscarinic receptor antagonists were reported to inhibit unstimulated H508 colon cancer cells by approximately 40%, while acetylcholinesterase inhibitors increased proliferation by 2 to 2.5-fold [22]. The effects of M3R activation in CRC tissue are seemingly not limited to proliferation but may also play an important role in cell invasion. Acetylcholine increased the expression of matrix metalloproteinase 1 (MMP-1) and stimulated the invasion of HT29 and H508 colon cancer cells into human umbilical vein endothelial cell monolayers [23]. All these findings suggest that the overexpression of M3R may lead to an increase in proliferation and invasiveness in CRC. We recently demonstrated the efficacy of MR3 inhibition by darifenacin in vitro and in vivo via a CRC xenograft mouse model [24].

However, data about the prognostic significance of M3R expression in CRC are scarce. In particular, its role in human CRC remains unclear. The goal of this study was to assess the prognostic significance of M3R expression in human CRC and its correlation with established prognostic immune cell markers on the basis of the findings of our previous publication [24].

2. Results

Results are presented following the reporting recommendations for tumor marker prognostic studies (REMARK) [25].

2.1. Clinicopathological Patient Characteristics

Tissue samples of 754 patients with CRC were analyzed. The median age was 70 years (range: 30–96) (Table 1). A total of 407 patients were female, and 347 were male. The mean tumor size was 50.8 mm, with a range of 5–170 mm. Tumor location was the left hemicolon in 520 cases and the right hemicolon in 232 cases. Of all cases, 288 were rectal cancer. A total of 97 cases were UICC stage I, 288 cases were UICC stage II and 342 cases were UICC stage III. The tumor border configuration was infiltrative in 516 specimens and pushing in 221. Vascular invasion was present in 207 specimens and not present in 532. The TMA contained 658 mismatch repair (MMR)-proficient specimens and 96 MMR-deficient specimens.

Table 1. Clinicopathological characteristics of the CRC patient cohort [1,2].

Patient Characteristic		N or Mean	Percentage or Range
Age, years (median, mean)		70, 68.8	30–96
Tumor size in mm (median, mean)		50, 50.8	5–170
Sex	Female	407	50%
	Male	347	43%
Anatomic site of the tumor	Left-sided	520	64%
	Right-sided	232	29%

Table 1. *Cont.*

Patient Characteristic		N or Mean	Percentage or Range
UICC stage	Stage IB, T2N0	71	9%
	Stage IIA, T3N0	254	31%
	Stage IIB-C, T4N0	34	4%
	Stage III, >N0	342	42%
Tumor border configuration	Infiltrative	516	63%
	Pushing	221	27%
Vascular invasion	No	532	65%
	Yes	207	25%
Microsatellite stability	Proficient	658	81%
	Deficient	96	96%
Rectal cancers		288	35%
Rectosigmoid cancers		50	6%
Overall survival time (months)		58.9	1–152
5-year survival % (95% CI)		0.45	0.42–0.49

[1] Percentages may not add up to 100% due to missing values for some variables. [2] Abbreviations: N = total number of observations; UICC = Union for International Cancer Control; T = size or extension of primary tumor; N = degree of spread to regional lymph nodes; M = presence of distant metastasis.

2.2. Association of M3 Low and High Expression with Clinicopathological Features in CRC

Clinicopathological features in CRC under examination in this study and their relation to the two subgroups of low and high M3R expression samples are shown in Table 2. After immunohistochemical processing, a total of 635 punches remained for the evaluation of M3R expression (Figure 1). Of these, 568 showed a high expression of M3R, and 67 showed a low expression of M3R (Figure 2).

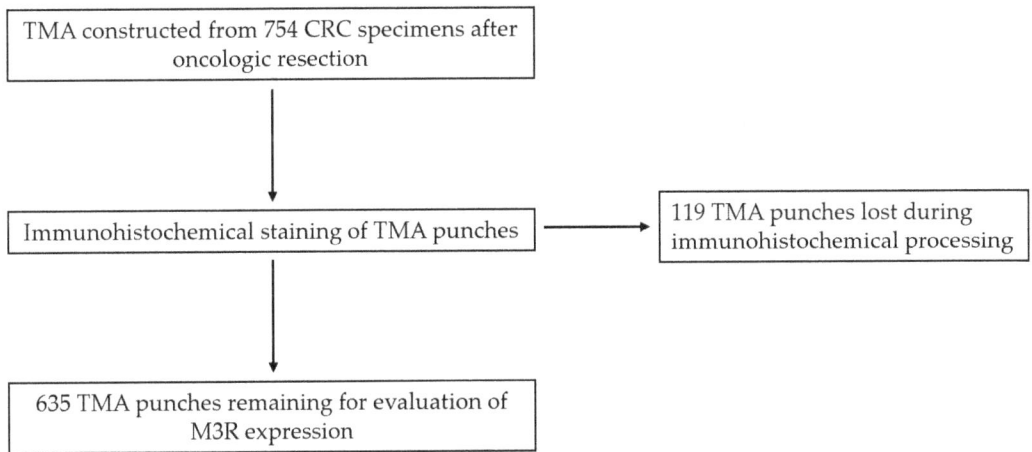

Figure 1. Transition from total number of tissue samples to remaining number of tissue microarrays (TMAs) after immunohistochemical processing. Abbreviations: TMA = tissue microarray; CRC = colorectal cancer.

Table 2. [1,2]: Association of M3 low and high expression with clinicopathological features in CRC.

Parameter		M3R-Low	M3R-High	p-Value
		N = 67 (10.6%)	N = 568 (89.5%)	
Age	Years, mean ± SD	67.3 ± 11.9	68.8 ± 11.4	0.418
Tumor diameter	mm, mean ± SD	50.5 ± 22.1	50.9 ± 20.1	0.760
Gender	Female Male	33 (49.3%) 31 (46.3%)	294 (51.7%) 244 (42.9%)	0.640
Tumor location	Left-sided Right-sided	42 (62.7%) 22 (32.8%)	379 (66.7%) 157 (27.6%)	0.401
Histologic subtype	Mucinous Non-mucinous	6 (9.0%) 61 (91.0%)	22 (3.9%) 546 (96.1%)	<0.001
pT stage	pT1–2 pT3–4	14 (20.9%) 44 (65.7%)	105 (18.5%) 425 (74.8%)	0.436
pN stage	pN0 pN1–2	32 (47.8%) 31 (46.3%)	279 (49.1%) 243 (42.8%)	0.690
Tumor grade	G1 G2 G3	3 (4.5%) 45 (67.1%) 10 (14.9%)	14 (2.5%) 487 (85.7%) 29 (5.1%)	0.002
Vascular invasion	Absent Present	39 (58.2%) 19 (28.4%)	387 (68.1%) 143 (25.2%)	0.350
Tumor border	Pushing Infiltrating	12 (17.9%) 46 (68.7%)	171 (30.1%) 357 (62.9%)	0.068
PTL inflammation	Absent Present	47 (70.2%) 11 (16.4%)	406 (71.5%) 124 (21.8%)	0.446
Microsatellite stability	Deficient Proficient	8 (11.9%) 56 (83.6%)	60 (10.6%) 478 (84.2%)	0.747
5-year survival rate	(95% CI)	42% (0.30–0.54)	46% (0.41–0.50)	0.073

[1] Percentages may not add up to 100% due to missing values of some variables; age and tumor size were evaluated using the Kruskal–Wallis test. Gender, anatomical site, T stage, N stage, grade, vascular invasion and tumor border configuration were analyzed using the χ^2 test. Survival analysis was performed using the Kaplan–Meier method. [2] Abbreviations: M3R-low = CRC specimens with low M3R (muscarinic acetylcholine receptor M3) expression; M3R-high = CRC specimens with high M3R (muscarinic acetylcholine receptor M3) expression; N = total number of observations; SD = standard deviation; mm = millimeters; pT = histopathological size or extension of primary tumor; pN = histopathological degree of spread to regional lymph nodes; G = tumor grade; PTL inflammation = peritumoral lymphocytic inflammation.

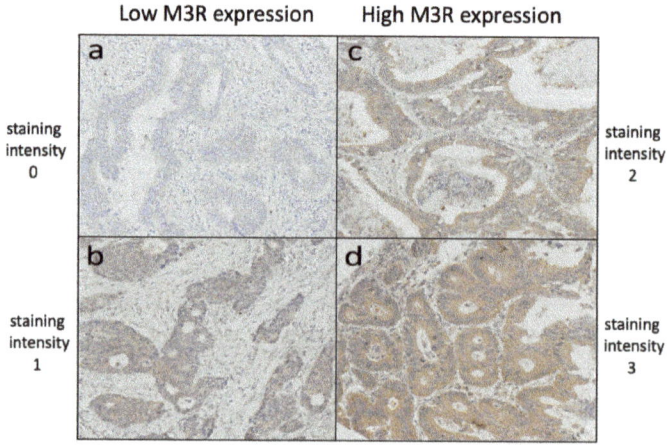

Figure 2. Staining intensities of CRC TMAs after immunohistochemical staining using an anti-M3R primary antibody, revealing low M3R expression (**a**,**b**) and high M3R expression (**c**,**d**). Abbreviations: TMA = tissue microarray; CRC = colorectal cancer; M3R = muscarinic acetylcholine receptor M3.

CRC tissues with a high M3R expression were significantly more likely to be of the non-mucinous histologic subtype as compared to the mucinous subtype than specimens with a low M3R expression (Table 2). CRC specimens with high M3R expression were also more likely to be tumor grade G2 (85.7% of specimens with high M3R expression) compared to CRC with low M3R expression (67.1% of specimens with low M3R expression). Specimens with low M3R expression had a higher proportion of tumor grade G3 (14.9%) compared to specimens with a high M3R expression (5.1%) (Table 2).

2.3. Immune Cell Density According to M3 Low and High Expression

We further tested for immune cell infiltration with different well-established immune cell markers in CRC and their relation to the two subgroups of low and high M3R expression (Table 3). In patients with a low expression of M3R, a significantly higher density of CD8 and TIA-1-positive immune cells was observed (Table 3). No correlation was found for FOXP3, IL 17, CD16 and OX 40.

Table 3. [1] Immune cell density according to M3 low and high expression.

	M3-Low	M3-High	p-Value
	Mean ± SD	Mean ± SD	
CD8	18.9 ± 32.6	8.67 ± 16.8	0.018
FOXP3	30.3 ± 34.9	34.0 ± 39.4	0.638
IL17	10.3 ± 15.6	15.8 ± 29.1	0.141
TIA-1	4.5 ± 8.0	2.7 ± 6.9	0.047
CD16	30.0 ± 32.1	32.9 ± 32.1	0.292
OX40	37.3 ± 49.0	45.5 ± 60.5	0.380

[1] Abbreviations: CD8 = cluster of differentiation 8; FOXP3 = forkhead box P3; IL17 = interleukin 17 family; TIA-1 = TIA1 cytotoxic granule-associated RNA-binding protein; CD16 = cluster of differentiation 16; OX40 = tumor necrosis factor receptor superfamily, member 4.

2.4. Survival Analysis

The mean overall survival time was 58.9 months (range 1–152 months). The five-year survival rate was 45% (95% CI = 49.8–57.4). The 5-year survival rate for patients with high M3R expression (46%) showed a trend of higher survival than patients with low-M3R-expression CRC (42%) (p = 0.073) (Figure 3).

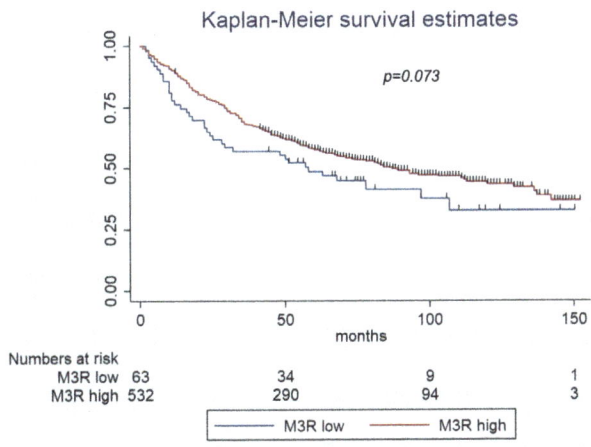

Figure 3. Kaplan–Meier survival estimates for low MR3 expression and high MR3 expression. The 5-year survival rate showed a trend of higher survival for patients with high-M3R CRC (46%) than patients with low-M3R CRC (42%) (p = 0.073). Abbreviations: M3R-low = CRC specimens with low M3R (muscarinic acetylcholine receptor M3) expression; M3R-high = CRC specimens with high M3R (muscarinic acetylcholine receptor M3) expression.

2.5. Uni- and Multivariate Cox Regression Survival Analysis of Low and High Expression of M3R

In univariate Cox regression survival analysis, high expression of M3R (hazard ratio (HR), 0.73; 95% CI, 0.52–1.03; p = 0.075) and CD8 (HR per immune cell, 0.99; 95% CI, 0.98–1.0; p = 0.014) were associated with increased survival, whereas male gender (HR, 1.28; 95% CI, 1.05–1.56; p = 0.015), age > 60 (HR, 1.03; 95% CI, 1.02–1.04; p < 0.001), vascular invasion (HR, 2.57; 95%, CI 2.09–3.16; p < 0.001), invasive margin configuration (HR, 2.02; 95% CI, 1.58–2.59; p < 0.001), MMR proficiency (HR, 1.61; 95% CI, 1.15–2.56; p = 0.005), higher T stage (HR, 3.02; 95% CI, 19–4.35, p < 0.001) and lymph-node positivity (HR, 2.82; 95% CI, 2.28–3.47; p < 0.001) were associated with worse survival (Table 4).

Table 4. [1] Uni- and multivariate Cox regression analysis.

Variable	Univariate Regression		Multivariate Regression	
	OR (95% CI)	p-Value	OR (95% CI)	p-Value
Sex				
Female	Reference		Reference	
Male	1.28 (1.05–1.56)	0.015	1.35 (1.05–1.74)	0.017
Age				
<60	Reference		Reference	
>60	1.03 (1.02–1.04)	<0.001	1.04 (1.03–1.05)	<0.001
Vascular invasion				
Absent	Reference		Reference	
Present	2.57; 2.09–3.16;	<0.001	2.03 (1.55–2.66)	<0.001
Invasive tumor margin configuration				
Pushing	Reference		Reference	
Infiltrative	2.02 (1.58–2.59)	<0.001	1.34 (0.96–1.84)	0.07
Microsatellite stability				
Deficient	Reference		Reference	
Proficient	1.61 (1.15–2.56)	0.005	1.59 (1.01–2.49)	0.043
pT Stage				
pT 1–2	Reference		Reference	
pT 3–4	3.09 (2.19–4.35)	<0.001	2.30 (1.47–3.60)	<0.001
pN Stage				
pN 0	Reference		Reference	
pN > 0	2.82 (2.28–3.47)	<0.001	2.26 (1.72–2.96)	<0.001
Grade				
G0-G1	Reference		Reference	
G2-G3	6.06. (1.94–18.87)	0.002	2.58 (0.62–10.80)	0.193
M3R expression				
low	Reference		Reference	
high	0.73 (0.52–1.03)	0.075	0.52 (0.35–0.78)	0.001
CD8 expression				
low	Reference		Reference	
high	0.99 (0.98–1.0) [2]	0.014	1.00 (0.99–1.01) [2]	0.609
TIA-1 expression				
Low	Reference		Reference	
High	0.99 (0.98–1.0) [2]	0.24	0.97 (0.94–0.99) [2]	0.014

[1] Abbreviations: OR = odds ratio; CI = confidence interval; pT = histopathological size or extension of primary tumor; pN = histopathological degree of spread to regional lymph nodes; G = tumor grade; M3R = M3R (muscarinic acetylcholine receptor M3) expression of CRC specimens, CD8 = cluster of differentiation 8; TIA-1 = TIA1 cytotoxic granule-associated RNA-binding protein. [2] Odds ratio calculated per immune cell, subsequently indicating that, e.g., 10 additional immune cells in a sample would generate an HR of 0.991010 = 0.9 or, in the case of 20 more cells, 0.992020 = 0.82.

In multivariate Cox regression survival analysis, high M3R expression was significantly associated with a risk for increased survival (HR, 0.52; 95% CI, 0.35–0-78; $p = 0.001$), as was TIA-1 expression (HR per immune cell = 0.97; 95% CI = 0.94–0.99; $p = 0.014$). In contrast, male sex (HR, 1.35; 95% CI, 1.05–1.74; $p = 0.017$), age > 60 (HR, 1.04; 95% CI, 1.03–1.05; $p < 0.001$), vascular invasion (HR, 2.03; 95% CI, 1.55–2.66; $p < 0.001$), MMR proficiency (HR, 1.59; 95% CI, 1.01–2.49; $p = 0.043$), higher T stage (HR, 2.30; 95% CI, 1.47–3.60; $p < 0.001$) and higher N stage (HR, 2.26; 95% CI, 1.72–2.96; $p < 0.001$) were associated with a risk for poorer survival (Table 4).

Neither univariate nor multivariate Cox regression showed any significance for the independent impact of M3R on overall survival.

3. Discussion

3.1. Key Findings

We aimed to examine the potential of M3R expression as a prognostic factor for survivability in human CRC patients, as its expression and inhibition have shown therapeutic potential in animal and in vitro trials [24]. We found that high M3R expression correlated with increased survivability, significantly with lower tumor grade and non-mucinous subtype, associating with a more favorable outcome as compared to low M3R expression, which was significantly correlated with decreased survivability, higher tumor grade and mucinous subtype.

3.2. Correlation with Previous Literature

These findings are surprising and stand in contrast to the previously reported in vitro and in vivo effects of M3R expression and inhibition [20,26–30]. Other examples of a strong inverse correlation between tumor grade and receptor expression are described in the literature, for example, numerous studies concerning breast cancer tumor grade and hormone receptor intensity [31–34], and in astrocytomas, estrogen receptor expression was positive only in low-grade and nil in high-grade astrocytomas [35]. A progressive decrease in progesterone receptor and estrogen receptor 1 mRNA expression was observed from endometrioid endometrial cancers to more aggressive serous tumors as defined by grade level [36]. Pacini et al. examined the expression of muscarinic acetylcholine receptor subtypes M1, M2 and M3 in transitional cell carcinoma of the bladder and found that M1R and M3R were significantly upregulated only in low-grade samples [37]. The correlation between tumor grade and M3R expression in CRCs warrants further investigation.

Aiming to discover further potential treatment approaches, we investigated the role of MR3 expression in the CRC tumor immune microenvironment by immunohistochemical analysis for a selection of promising immunomarkers: CD8, FOXP3, IL17, TIA-1, CD16 and OX40. Each of these have previously been shown to play a role in CRC progression by fellow researchers [16,38–43] and members of our group [11,13,14,44]. Immune cell density of the examined CRC specimens showed that low M3R expression was significantly associated with a higher density of CD8- and TIA-1-positive immune cells. A possible link between increased density of CD8-positive cells in CRC tumors and their level of differentiation has been shown [45]. Sun-Young Lee et al. found that CD8+ T cell infiltration in the tumor stroma was more prominent in moderately and poorly differentiated adenocarcinoma than in adenoma and well-differentiated adenocarcinoma [46]. Similar associations were found in breast cancer, where tumor-infiltrating CD8-positive T cells significantly increased with stage progression [45]. In our study, a higher density of CD8-positive cells was significantly associated with low M3R expression. There is also increasing evidence that a higher density of CD8- and TIA-1-positive immune cells in CRC tumors is a prognostic factor for increased survival [46]. These findings highlight the incomplete picture of interactions between tumor grade, immune cell density, M3R expression and survival.

The overexpression of M3R has been shown in the HT-29 human colorectal adenocarcinoma cell line through subtype-specific muscarinic antagonists and X-ray microanalysis measurement of intracellular ion concentration [21,47]. Prior research has shown that surgical CRC samples may exhibit increased M3R expression by up to 128-fold in 10 out of 18 specimens as compared to an adjacent normal colon [26]. The possible effects of M3R activation in CRC have been studied in vitro using H508 human colon cancer cells, suggesting that muscarinic receptor agonists stimulate cell proliferation, migration and invasion by several post-M3R signaling pathways, one example being acetylcholine-stimulated calcium-dependent phosphorylation of p44/42 mitogen-activated protein kinase (MAPK) [26,27]. Raufman et al. used an animal model employing Apc$^{min/+}$ mice to compare Chrm3$^{+/+}$ mice (capable of M3R expression) to Chrm3$^{-/-}$ mice (not capable of M3R expression) and showed a 70% reduction in the number of tumors and an 81% reduction in tumor volume in the group that was not capable of M3R expression [28].

These in vitro and animal trials are part of an emerging body of evidence pointing to M3R expression rate as a biomarker for increased proliferation and invasiveness of CRC, as recently shown by Hering et al. [24].

Apart from CRC, M3R has clearly been shown to play a role in lung cancer [48–50]. Additionally, muscarinic agonists have been reported to have the ability to stimulate growth for melanoma, pancreatic, breast, ovarian, prostate and brain cancers [50–52]. Thus, these cancer types need to be considered in the context of our study and results in the future.

3.3. Implications

Our findings after examining MR3 expression in surgical samples of more than 600 human CRC patients suggest that while in in vitro and animal model studies, there is considerable potential for M3R inhibition, this may not be the case for clinical treatments. This may either be due to variables that are not present in a laboratory setting or to differences in laboratory variables such as the type of the investigated molecule (e.g., micro-RNA or protein), the type of antibody used, or differences in staining techniques and scoring systems.

CRC cells with high M3R expression could have traits that increase overall survival that are unrelated to tumor proliferation and invasion. An animal trial using Chrm3$^{-/-}$ mice showed that genetic ablation of M3R affected mucus production by decreasing mucin 2 gene expression, thereby facilitating prolonged bacterial adherence and delaying clearance of C. rodentium [53]. CRCs with a low expression rate of M3R could therefore have higher tendencies for bacterial infection. Muscarinic receptor activation on colon epithelial cells has been shown to protect against cytokine-induced barrier dysfunction by inhibiting IL-1β-induced production of chemokines and rearrangement of tight-junction proteins, while this protective effect of acetylcholine was antagonized by atropine [54]. This effect may lead to a stronger inflammatory response and higher inflammation rates in CRCs with low M3R expression.

Cheng et al. used immunohistochemistry to identify the expression of choline acetyltransferase (ChAT), a critical enzyme for acetylcholine synthesis, in surgical specimens of normal colons and colon cancer and found that normal colon enterocytes showed limited to no ChAT staining, whereas one-half of the colon cancer specimens displayed moderate to strong staining, and the other half exhibited weak staining [22]. Despite the small sample size, this suggests a higher rate of ACh production in colon cancer cells. The correlation between high and low M3R expression and ACh production capability of CRC cells in surgical specimens should be investigated.

Experiments have shown a relationship between the M3R expression rate and M3R inhibition or activation in different cell types. Witt-Enderby et al. found that in rabbit bronchi, M2R and M3R were significantly upregulated compared to the control after a 4-week inhibition by atropine [55]. A similar observation was made in rat forebrains by Wall et al., where a 14-day administration of atropine resulted in a 69% increase in the density of M3R [56]. Fukamauchi et al. studied the administration of carbachol, a cholinergic agonist, to cerebellar granule cells and described a time-dependent loss of M3R mRNAs as a result of stimulation [57]. Further experiments showed a decrease of 59.3% in M3R gene transcription in nuclei from cells treated with carbachol and a 230% increase in M3R gene transcription in nuclei from cells treated with atropine [57].

While the retrospective nature of this study is a limitation, our data contribute to the development of targeted, prospective studies in the future. Additionally, the investigated cohort includes CRC patients who underwent surgery between 1985 and 1998, a period in which neoadjuvant therapy regimens had not yet been widely established. Thus, while our results may not represent the efficacy of current clinical treatments fully, they are more likely to portray CRC immunobiology accurately due to the absence of the effect of antineoplastic agents.

We found that CRC tissues with a high M3R expression were significantly more likely to be of the non-mucinous histologic subtype as compared to the mucinous subtype than specimens with a low M3R expression (Table 2). Patients with a mucinous adenocarcinoma (MAC), which we found to be correlated with low M3R expression, were reported to be younger by Kanemitsu et al., have greater disease severity and metastatic spread and a significantly shorter 5-year survival rate than patients with a non-mucinous subtype CRC. The association of low M3R expression with the MAC subtype could be one reason for the decreased survival in the low-M3R group, which requires further investigation.

3.4. Future Perspective and Possibilites

Our findings add an important perspective for future trials to an abundant and currently rapidly increasing number of in vitro genetic and proteomic findings in CRC. In an era of high-throughput screening, next-generation sequencing and proteome-specific therapeutic agents leading to personalized cancer therapies, the inclusion of the tumor (immune) microenvironment is paramount when translating molecular findings into suitable therapies and biomarkers. Thus, we believe that our findings should be investigated in advanced cancer models. Delle Cave et al. already reviewed promising 3D in vitro cancer models for pancreatic cancer [58]. Using such a model to screen for M3R expression and associated tumor cell and microenvironment interactions mechanistically would ultimately generate new treatment options. The first preclinical 3D models for CRC have been proposed [59], but many more are needed. Additionally, M3R signaling could be investigated by using nanoparticles in vitro and in vivo, which have been shown to deliver small molecules specifically to CRC cells [60]. The structure–activity relationships of muscarinic receptor subtypes and the therapeutic effects of novel M3R-specific ligands or modulators also need to be explored [29,30,61]. Tolayat et al. reported that M3R deletion increased proliferation in intestinal stem cells and that M3R expression fine-tuned the cellular response to acetylcholine stimulation, ensuring intestinal tissue homeostasis [20]. In connection with our findings, this warrants further investigation. More established immune markers need to be investigated, such as interferon-gamma, CTLA-4 and CD28, to further characterize the tumor immune microenvironment. Further mechanisms to be explored in order to examine the role of M3R signaling in CRC could include micro-RNAs, members of the CHRM3-dependent oncogenetic pathways and potentially synthetically lethal combinations with M3R signaling members [17,18,62–64]. Future trials may incorporate proteomic screening [65], multiplex immunofluorescence [66] and screening of The Cancer Genome Atlas (TCGA; https://www.cancer.gov/tcga, accessed on 24 April 2023) for the impact of M3R expression on survival in both healthy and CRC patients. Appropriate gene and protein microarrays, bioinformatics and artificial-intelligence-based screening models could also be implemented in future investigations of M3R expression [15,19,67,68].

4. Materials and Methods

4.1. Tissue Microarray (TMA) Construction

A tissue microarray (TMA) was constructed at the Department of Pathology, University Hospital Basel, from each tissue sample from 754 unselected, non-consecutive patients with primary CRC following approval by the Regional Ethical Committee (EKBB, Ethikkommission beider Basel, Switzerland). Formalin-fixed, paraffin-embedded tissue blocks were prepared according to standard procedures. Tissue cylinders with a diameter of 0.6 mm were punched from morphologically representative areas of each donor block and brought into one recipient paraffin block (30 × 25 mm) using a TMA-Grand Master® automated tissue arrayer (3DHisteck, Sysmex AG, Horgen, Switzerland). Each punch was made from the center of the tumor so that each TMA spot consisted of at least 50% tumor cells. The detailed construction technique was previously described by our group [44,69,70].

4.2. Clinicopathological Features

Clinicopathological data for the 754 included CRC patients were collected retrospectively in a non-stratified and non-matched manner. Annotation included patient age, pT/pN stage, grade, histologic subtype, tumor location, diameter, vascular invasion, border configuration, presence of peritumoral lymphocytic inflammation at the invasive tumor front and overall survival. After microscopy and storage using a ZEISS Axio Scan.Z1 slide scanner, tumor border configuration and peritumoral lymphocytic inflammation were evaluated using the original H&E slides of the resection specimens corresponding to each tissue microarray punch [67]. Available follow-up data for the testing and validation cohort had a mean event-free follow-up time of 115 and 36 months, respectively.

4.3. Immunohistochemistry

Immunohistochemical staining was performed using an anti-M3R primary antibody (1:100, AHP1355, Biorad Laboratories, Neuberg, Germany) on a Benchmark immunohistochemistry staining system (Leica Biosystems, Muttenz, Switzerland) with bond polymer refine detection solution (Leica Biosystems) for 3, 3′-diaminobenzidine. Antigen retrieval was performed using citrate solution at pH 6 for 30 min at 95 °C. M3R staining intensity was scored from 0 (no reaction) to 3 (strong reaction) for each TME punch. Low expression of M3R was defined as scores of 0 and 1, and high expression was defined as scores of 2 and 3. Scoring was performed by two trained research fellows (M.S. and M.A.), and data were independently validated by an additional investigator (B.W.). Expression of M3R was scored according to the staining intensity.

4.4. Statistical Analysis

M3R-positive cells were counted on each of the 635 CRC TMA cores. After having proven an association between M3R-positive cells and overall survival (OS) by univariate Cox regression, an optimal threshold was estimated by regression tree analysis. The obtained threshold was found to be almost equal to the 25th-percentile value. Therefore, continuous values were dichotomized, subdividing the collective as CRC with low or high M3R expression. Chi-Square or Fisher's exact tests were used to determine the association of M3R expression and clinicopathological discrete features, and Wilcoxon's signed-rank sum test was used for comparison with continuous values. Survival curves were depicted according to the Kaplan–Meier method and compared with the log-rank test results. Only tests for normal and non-normal distribution were used (Mann–Whitney U). Age and tumor size were evaluated using the Kruskal–Wallis test. Normally distributed data were presented with mean ± SD, and non-normally distributed data were presented with median (range).

The immune cells CD8, FOXP3, IL17, TIA-1, CD16 and OX40 have previously been evaluated for CRC, and CRC cases have been classified accordingly by our group and others [1–11], generating the data used in the present study. The assumption of proportional hazards was verified for all markers by analyzing the correlation of Schoenfeld residuals and the ranks of individual failure times. Any missing clinicopathological information was assumed to be missing at random.

M3R expression data were entered into multivariate Cox regression analysis, and hazard ratios (HRs) and 95% confidence intervals (CIs) were used to determine prognostic effects on survival time. For the immune cell biomarkers, the hazard ratio was calculated per immune cell, subsequently indicating that, e.g., 10 additional immune cells in a sample would generate an HR of $0.99^{10} = 0.9$ or, in the case of 20 more cells, $0.99^{20} = 0.82$.

Additionally, the independent impact of M3R on overall survival was investigated by univariate and multivariate Cox regression.

All *p*-values were two-sided and considered significant when $p < 0.05$. Analyses were performed using STATA 13 (StataCorp, College Station, TX, USA).

5. Conclusions

While our knowledge of CRC is increasing, new questions are also constantly arising, which must be investigated scientifically to improve treatments [37]. Our data offer several new insights that may help to navigate future investigations. This study is highly relevant, as it points out an important, unexpected difference in the prognostic and therapeutic role of M3R expression in CRC between laboratory and clinical settings. Evidently, there are in vivo factors influencing the expression and activation of M3R and its effect on survivability that need to be explored to reveal the broader picture and further utilize M3R expression for therapeutic advances in the treatment of CRC.

Author Contributions: Conceptualization, N.A.H. and B.W.; methodology, R.D. and I.P.; software, M.A.; validation, M.A.S., L.A.L. and J.C.L.; formal analysis, R.D., L.A.L. and M.A.S.; investigation, M.A.S. and M.A.; resources, B.W. and N.A.H.; data curation, L.A.L. and R.D.; writing—original draft preparation, L.A.L. and M.A.S.; writing—review and editing, B.W., J.C.L., I.P., M.A.S. and L.A.L.; visualization, R.D. and M.A.S.; supervision, N.A.H.; project administration, B.W. All authors have read and agreed to the published version of the manuscript.

Funding: This research received no external funding.

Institutional Review Board Statement: The study was conducted in accordance with the Declaration of Helsinki and approved by the ethics committee of the University of Basel (EKBB, Ethikkommission beider Basel, protocol code EK120/13, 30 April 2013).

Informed Consent Statement: Written informed consent was obtained from all subjects involved in the study.

Data Availability Statement: The data presented in this study are available on request from the corresponding author. The data are not publicly available due to patient data protection and the decision of the regional ethical committee at the time of study approval.

Conflicts of Interest: The authors declare no conflict of interest.

References

1. Sung, H.; Ferlay, J.; Siegel, R.L.; Laversanne, M.; Soerjomataram, I.; Jemal, A.; Bray, F. Global Cancer Statistics 2020: GLOBOCAN Estimates of Incidence and Mortality Worldwide for 36 Cancers in 185 Countries. *CA Cancer J. Clin.* **2021**, *71*, 209–249. [CrossRef] [PubMed]
2. Siegel, R.L.; Fedewa, S.A.; Anderson, W.F.; Miller, K.D.; Ma, J.; Rosenberg, P.S.; Jemal, A. Colorectal Cancer Incidence Patterns in the United States, 1974-2013. *J. Natl. Cancer Inst.* **2017**, *109*, djw322. [CrossRef] [PubMed]
3. Molenaar, R.J.; Radivoyevitch, T.; Wilmink, J.W. RE: Colorectal Cancer Incidence Patterns in the United States, 1974-2013. *J. Natl. Cancer Inst.* **2017**, *109*. [CrossRef] [PubMed]
4. Yeo, H.; Betel, D.; Abelson, J.S.; Zheng, X.E.; Yantiss, R.; Shah, M.A. Early-onset Colorectal Cancer is Distinct From Traditional Colorectal Cancer. *Clin. Color. Cancer* **2017**, *16*, 293–299.e6. [CrossRef]
5. Brenner, H.; Kloor, M.; Pox, C.P. Colorectal cancer. *Lancet* **2014**, *383*, 1490–1502. [CrossRef]
6. Zlobec, I.; Lugli, A. Prognostic and predictive factors in colorectal cancer. *Postgrad. Med. J.* **2008**, *84*, 403–411. [CrossRef]
7. Pagès, F.; Galon, J.; Dieu-Nosjean, M.C.; Tartour, E.; Sautès-Fridman, C.; Fridman, W.H. Immune infiltration in human tumors: A prognostic factor that should not be ignored. *Oncogene* **2010**, *29*, 1093–1102. [CrossRef]
8. Lin, J.S.; Piper, M.A.; Perdue, L.A.; Rutter, C.M.; Webber, E.M.; O'Connor, E.; Smith, N.; Whitlock, E.P. Screening for Colorectal Cancer: Updated Evidence Report and Systematic Review for the US Preventive Services Task Force. *JAMA* **2016**, *315*, 2576–2594. [CrossRef]
9. Berg, K.B.; Schaeffer, D.F. SATB2 as an Immunohistochemical Marker for Colorectal Adenocarcinoma: A Concise Review of Benefits and Pitfalls. *Arch. Pathol. Lab. Med.* **2017**, *141*, 1428–1433. [CrossRef]
10. Weixler, B.; Renetseder, F.; Facile, I.; Tosti, N.; Cremonesi, E.; Tampakis, A.; Delko, T.; Eppenberger-Castori, S.; Tzankov, A.; Iezzi, G.; et al. Phosphorylated CXCR4 expression has a positive prognostic impact in colorectal cancer. *Cell. Oncol.* **2017**, *40*, 609–619. [CrossRef]

11. Frey, D.M.; Droeser, R.A.; Viehl, C.T.; Zlobec, I.; Lugli, A.; Zingg, U.; Oertli, D.; Kettelhack, C.; Terracciano, L.; Tornillo, L. High frequency of tumor-infiltrating FOXP3(+) regulatory T cells predicts improved survival in mismatch repair-proficient colorectal cancer patients. *Int. J. Cancer* **2010**, *126*, 2635–2643. [CrossRef]
12. Tosti, N.; Cremonesi, E.; Governa, V.; Basso, C.; Kancherla, V.; Coto-Llerena, M.; Amicarella, F.; Weixler, B.; Däster, S.; Sconocchia, G.; et al. Infiltration by IL22-Producing T Cells Promotes Neutrophil Recruitment and Predicts Favorable Clinical Outcome in Human Colorectal Cancer. *Cancer Immunol. Res.* **2020**, *8*, 1452–1462. [CrossRef]
13. Haak, F.; Obrecht, I.; Tosti, N.; Weixler, B.; Mechera, R.; Däster, S.; von Strauss, M.; Delko, T.; Spagnoli, G.C.; Terracciano, L.; et al. Tumor Infiltration by OX40+ Cells Enhances the Prognostic Significance of CD16+ Cell Infiltration in Colorectal Cancer. *Cancer Control* **2020**, *27*, 903383. [CrossRef]
14. Däster, S.; Eppenberger-Castori, S.; Hirt, C.; Soysal, S.D.; Delko, T.; Nebiker, C.A.; Weixler, B.; Amicarella, F.; Iezzi, G.; Governa, V.; et al. Absence of myeloperoxidase and CD8 positive cells in colorectal cancer infiltrates identifies patients with severe prognosis. *Oncoimmunology* **2015**, *4*, e1050574. [CrossRef]
15. Yue, Y.; Zhang, Q.; Sun, Z. CX3CR1 Acts as a Protective Biomarker in the Tumor Microenvironment of Colorectal Cancer. *Front. Immunol.* **2021**, *12*, 758040. [CrossRef]
16. Yan, L.H.; Liu, X.L.; Mo, S.S.; Zhang, D.; Mo, X.W.; Tang, W.Z. OX40 as a novel target for the reversal of immune escape in colorectal cancer. *Am. J. Transl. Res.* **2021**, *13*, 923–934.
17. Chang, P.Y.; Chen, C.C.; Chang, Y.S.; Tsai, W.S.; You, J.F.; Lin, G.P.; Chen, T.W.; Chen, J.S.; Chan, E.C. MicroRNA-223 and microRNA-92a in stool and plasma samples act as complementary biomarkers to increase colorectal cancer detection. *Oncotarget* **2016**, *7*, 10663–10675. [CrossRef]
18. Toiyama, Y.; Okugawa, Y.; Fleshman, J.; Richard Boland, C.; Goel, A. MicroRNAs as potential liquid biopsy biomarkers in colorectal cancer: A systematic review. *Biochim. Biophys. Acta BBA Rev. Cancer* **2018**, *1870*, 274–282. [CrossRef]
19. Liu, L.; Huang, Y.; Li, Y.; Wang, Q.; Hao, Y.; Liu, L.; Yao, X.; Yao, X.; Wei, Y.; Sun, X.; et al. FJX1 as a candidate diagnostic and prognostic serum biomarker for colorectal cancer. *Clin. Transl. Oncol.* **2022**, *24*, 1964–1974. [CrossRef]
20. Tolaymat, M.; Larabee, S.M.; Hu, S.; Xie, G.; Raufman, J.P. The Role of M3 Muscarinic Receptor Ligand-Induced Kinase Signaling in Colon Cancer Progression. *Cancers* **2019**, *11*, 308. [CrossRef]
21. Kopp, R.; Lambrecht, G.; Mutschler, E.; Moser, U.; Tacke, R.; Pfeiffer, A. Human HT-29 colon carcinoma cells contain muscarinic M3 receptors coupled to phosphoinositide metabolism. *Eur. J. Pharmacol.* **1989**, *172*, 397–405. [CrossRef] [PubMed]
22. Cheng, K.; Samimi, R.; Xie, G.; Shant, J.; Drachenberg, C.; Wade, M.; Davis, R.J.; Nomikos, G.; Raufman, J.P. Acetylcholine release by human colon cancer cells mediates autocrine stimulation of cell proliferation. *Am. J. Physiol.-Gastrointest. Liver Physiol.* **2008**, *295*, G591–G597. [CrossRef] [PubMed]
23. Raufman, J.P.; Cheng, K.; Saxena, N.; Chahdi, A.; Belo, A.; Khurana, S.; Xie, G. Muscarinic receptor agonists stimulate matrix metalloproteinase 1-dependent invasion of human colon cancer cells. *Biochem. Biophys. Res. Commun.* **2011**, *415*, 319–324. [CrossRef] [PubMed]
24. Hering, N.A.; Liu, V.; Kim, R.; Weixler, B.; Droeser, R.A.; Arndt, M.; Pozios, I.; Beyer, K.; Kreis, M.E.; Seeliger, H. Blockage of Cholinergic Signaling via Muscarinic Acetylcholine Receptor 3 Inhibits Tumor Growth in Human Colorectal Adenocarcinoma. *Cancers* **2021**, *13*, 3220. [CrossRef]
25. McShane, L.M.; Altman, D.G.; Sauerbrei, W.; Taube, S.E.; Gion, M.; Clark, G.M. REporting recommendations for tumour MARKer prognostic studies (REMARK). *Br. J. Cancer* **2005**, *93*, 387–391. [CrossRef]
26. Cheng, K.; Shang, A.C.; Drachenberg, C.B.; Zhan, M.; Raufman, J.P. Differential expression of M3 muscarinic receptors in progressive colon neoplasia and metastasis. *Oncotarget* **2017**, *8*, 21106–21114. [CrossRef]
27. Cheng, K.; Zimniak, P.; Raufman, J.P. Transactivation of the epidermal growth factor receptor mediates cholinergic agonist-induced proliferation of H508 human colon cancer cells. *Cancer Res.* **2003**, *63*, 6744–6750. [CrossRef]
28. Raufman, J.P.; Shant, J.; Xie, G.; Cheng, K.; Gao, X.M.; Shiu, B.; Shah, N.; Drachenberg, C.B.; Heath, J.; Wess, J.; et al. Muscarinic receptor subtype-3 gene ablation and scopolamine butylbromide treatment attenuate small intestinal neoplasia in Apcmin/+ mice. *Carcinogenesis* **2011**, *32*, 1396–1402. [CrossRef]
29. Xie, G.; Raufman, J.P. Muscarinic receptor signaling and colon cancer progression. *J. Cancer Metastasis Treat.* **2016**, *2*, 195–200. [CrossRef]
30. Schledwitz, A.; Sundel, M.H.; Alizadeh, M.; Hu, S.; Xie, G.; Raufman, J.P. Differential Actions of Muscarinic Receptor Subtypes in Gastric, Pancreatic, and Colon Cancer. *Int. J. Mol. Sci.* **2021**, *22*, 13153. [CrossRef]
31. Gupta, D.; Gupta, V.; Marwah, N.; Gill, M.; Gupta, S.; Gupta, G.; Jain, P.; Sen, R. Correlation of Hormone Receptor Expression with Histologic Parameters in Benign and Malignant Breast Tumors. *Iran. J. Pathol.* **2015**, *10*, 23–34.
32. Barnes, N.L.; Boland, G.P.; Davenport, A.; Knox, W.F.; Bundred, N.J. Relationship between hormone receptor status and tumour size, grade and comedo necrosis in ductal carcinoma in situ. *Br. J. Surg.* **2005**, *92*, 429–434. [CrossRef]
33. Mudduwa, L.K. Quick score of hormone receptor status of breast carcinoma: Correlation with the other clinicopathological prognostic parameters. *Indian J. Pathol. Microbiol.* **2009**, *52*, 159–163. [CrossRef]
34. Fisher, E.R.; Redmond, C.K.; Liu, H.; Rockette, H.; Fisher, B. Correlation of estrogen receptor and pathologic characteristics of invasive breast cancer. *Cancer* **1980**, *45*, 349–353. [CrossRef]
35. Tavares, C.B.; Gomes-Braga, F.; Sousa, E.B.; Borges, U.S.; Escórcio-Dourado, C.S.; Silva-Sampaio, J.P.D.; Silva, B.B.D. Evaluation of estrogen receptor expression in low-grade and high-grade astrocytomas. *Rev. Assoc. Med. Bras.* **2018**, *64*, 1129–1133. [CrossRef]

36. Kavlashvili, T.; Jia, Y.; Dai, D.; Meng, X.; Thiel, K.W.; Leslie, K.K.; Yang, S. Inverse Relationship between Progesterone Receptor and Myc in Endometrial Cancer. *PLoS ONE* **2016**, *11*, e0148912. [CrossRef]
37. Pacini, L.; De Falco, E.; Di Bari, M.; Coccia, A.; Siciliano, C.; Ponti, D.; Pastore, A.L.; Petrozza, V.; Carbone, A.; Tata, A.M.; et al. M2muscarinic receptors inhibit cell proliferation and migration in urothelial bladder cancer cells. *Cancer Biol. Ther.* **2014**, *15*, 1489–1498. [CrossRef]
38. Schmitt, M.; Greten, F.R. The inflammatory pathogenesis of colorectal cancer. *Nat. Rev. Immunol.* **2021**, *21*, 653–667. [CrossRef]
39. Jiang, W.; He, Y.; He, W.; Wu, G.; Zhou, X.; Sheng, Q.; Zhong, W.; Lu, Y.; Ding, Y.; Lu, Q.; et al. Exhausted CD8+T Cells in the Tumor Immune Microenvironment: New Pathways to Therapy. *Front. Immunol.* **2020**, *11*, 622509. [CrossRef]
40. Sun, X.; Feng, Z.; Wang, Y.; Qu, Y.; Gai, Y. Expression of Foxp3 and its prognostic significance in colorectal cancer. *Int. J. Immunopathol. Pharmacol.* **2017**, *30*, 201–206. [CrossRef]
41. Liu, C.; Liu, R.; Wang, B.; Lian, J.; Yao, Y.; Sun, H.; Zhang, C.; Fang, L.; Guan, X.; Shi, J.; et al. Blocking IL-17A enhances tumor response to anti-PD-1 immunotherapy in microsatellite stable colorectal cancer. *J. ImmunoTherapy Cancer* **2021**, *9*, e001895. [CrossRef] [PubMed]
42. Hurtado, C.G.; Wan, F.; Housseau, F.; Sears, C.L. Roles for Interleukin 17 and Adaptive Immunity in Pathogenesis of Colorectal Cancer. *Gastroenterology* **2018**, *155*, 1706–1715. [CrossRef] [PubMed]
43. Krijgsman, D.; de Vries, N.L.; Skovbo, A.; Andersen, M.N.; Swets, M.; Bastiaannet, E.; Vahrmeijer, A.L.; van de Velde, C.J.H.; Heemskerk, M.H.M.; Hokland, M.; et al. Characterization of circulating T-, NK-, and NKT cell subsets in patients with colorectal cancer: The peripheral blood immune cell profile. *Cancer Immunol. Immunother.* **2019**, *68*, 1011–1024. [CrossRef] [PubMed]
44. Lalos, A.; Tülek, A.; Tosti, N.; Mechera, R.; Wilhelm, A.; Soysal, S.; Daester, S.; Kancherla, V.; Weixler, B.; Spagnoli, G.C.; et al. Prognostic significance of CD8+ T-cells density in stage III colorectal cancer depends on SDF-1 expression. *Sci. Rep.* **2021**, *11*, 775. [CrossRef] [PubMed]
45. Sheu, B.C.; Kuo, W.H.; Chen, R.J.; Huang, S.C.; Chang, K.J.; Chow, S.N. Clinical significance of tumor-infiltrating lymphocytes in neoplastic progression and lymph node metastasis of human breast cancer. *Breast* **2008**, *17*, 604–610. [CrossRef]
46. Oberg, A.; Samii, S.; Stenling, R.; Lindmark, G. Different occurrence of CD8+, CD45R0+, and CD68+ immune cells in regional lymph node metastases from colorectal cancer as potential prognostic predictors. *Int. J. Color. Dis.* **2002**, *17*, 25–29. [CrossRef]
47. Zhang, W.; Roomans, G.M. Evidence for muscarinic 3 receptor mediated ion transport in HT29 cells studied by X-ray microanalysis. *Cell. Organelles Struct.* **1997**, *22*, 379–385. [CrossRef]
48. Wu, J.; Zhou, J.; Yao, L.; Lang, Y.; Liang, Y.; Chen, L.; Zhang, J.; Wang, F.; Wang, Y.; Chen, H.; et al. High expression of M3 muscarinic acetylcholine receptor is a novel biomarker of poor prognostic in patients with non-small cell lung cancer. *Tumour Biol.* **2013**, *34*, 3939–3944. [CrossRef]
49. Lin, G.; Sun, L.; Wang, R.; Guo, Y.; Xie, C. Overexpression of muscarinic receptor 3 promotes metastasis and predicts poor prognosis in non-small-cell lung cancer. *J. Thorac. Oncol.* **2014**, *9*, 170–178. [CrossRef]
50. Spindel, E.R. Muscarinic receptor agonists and antagonists: Effects on cancer. In *Muscarinic Receptors*; Handbook of Experimental Pharmacology; Springer: Berlin/Heidelberg, Germany, 2012; Volume 208, pp. 451–468.
51. Chen, J.; Cheuk, I.W.Y.; Shin, V.Y.; Kwong, A. Acetylcholine receptors: Key players in cancer development. *Surg. Oncol.* **2019**, *31*, 46–53. [CrossRef]
52. Russo, P.; Del Bufalo, A.; Milic, M.; Salinaro, G.; Fini, M.; Cesario, A. Cholinergic receptors as target for cancer therapy in a systems medicine perspective. *Curr. Mol. Med.* **2014**, *14*, 1126–1138. [CrossRef]
53. McLean, L.P.; Smith, A.; Cheung, L.; Sun, R.; Grinchuk, V.; Vanuytsel, T.; Desai, N.; Urban, J.F., Jr.; Zhao, A.; Raufman, J.P.; et al. Type 3 Muscarinic Receptors Contribute to Clearance of Citrobacter rodentium. *Inflamm. Bowel Dis.* **2015**, *21*, 1860–1871. [CrossRef]
54. Dhawan, S.; Hiemstra, I.H.; Verseijden, C.; Hilbers, F.W.; Te Velde, A.A.; Willemsen, L.E.; Stap, J.; den Haan, J.M.; de Jonge, W.J. Cholinergic receptor activation on epithelia protects against cytokine-induced barrier dysfunction. *Acta Physiol.* **2015**, *213*, 846–859. [CrossRef]
55. Witt-Enderby, P.A.; Yamamura, H.I.; Halonen, M.; Lai, J.; Palmer, J.D.; Bloom, J.W. Regulation of airway muscarinic cholinergic receptor subtypes by chronic anticholinergic treatment. *Mol. Pharmacol.* **1995**, *47*, 485–490.
56. Wall, S.J.; Yasuda, R.P.; Li, M.; Ciesla, W.; Wolfe, B.B. Differential regulation of subtypes m1-m5 of muscarinic receptors in forebrain by chronic atropine administration. *J. Pharmacol. Exp. Ther.* **1992**, *262*, 584–588.
57. Fukamauchi, F.; Saunders, P.A.; Hough, C.; Chuang, D.M. Agonist-induced down-regulation and antagonist-induced up-regulation of m2- and m3-muscarinic acetylcholine receptor mRNA and protein in cultured cerebellar granule cells. *Mol. Pharmacol.* **1993**, *44*, 940–949.
58. Delle Cave, D.; Rizzo, R.; Sainz, B., Jr.; Gigli, G.; Del Mercato, L.L.; Lonardo, E. The Revolutionary Roads to Study Cell-Cell Interactions in 3D In Vitro Pancreatic Cancer Models. *Cancers* **2021**, *13*, 930. [CrossRef]
59. Sensi, F.; D'Angelo, E.; D'Aronco, S.; Molinaro, R.; Agostini, M. Preclinical three-dimensional colorectal cancer model: The next generation of in vitro drug efficacy evaluation. *J. Cell. Physiol.* **2018**, *234*, 181–191. [CrossRef]
60. Managò, S.; Tramontano, C.; Delle Cave, D.; Chianese, G.; Zito, G.; De Stefano, L.; Terracciano, M.; Lonardo, E.; De Luca, A.C.; Rea, I. SERS Quantification of Galunisertib Delivery in Colorectal Cancer Cells by Plasmonic-Assisted Diatomite Nanoparticles. *Small* **2021**, *17*, e2101711. [CrossRef]

61. Okimoto, R.; Ino, K.; Ishizu, K.; Takamatsu, H.; Sakamoto, K.; Yuyama, H.; Fuji, H.; Someya, A.; Ohtake, A.; Ishigami, T.; et al. Potentiation of Muscarinic M(3) Receptor Activation through a New Allosteric Site with a Novel Positive Allosteric Modulator ASP8302. *J. Pharmacol. Exp. Ther.* **2021**, *379*, 64–73. [CrossRef]
62. Aktan, Ç.; Tekin, F.; Oruç, N.; Özütemiz, Ö. CHRM3-Associated miRNAs May Play a Role in Bile Acid-Induced Proliferation of H508 Colon Cancer Cells. *Turk. J. Gastroenterol.* **2023**, *34*, 298–307. [CrossRef] [PubMed]
63. Invrea, F.; Punzi, S.; Petti, C.; Minelli, R.; Peoples, M.D.; Bristow, C.A.; Vurchio, V.; Corrado, A.; Bragoni, A.; Marchiò, C.; et al. Synthetic Lethality Screening Highlights Colorectal Cancer Vulnerability to Concomitant Blockade of NEDD8 and EGFR Pathways. *Cancers* **2021**, *13*, 3805. [CrossRef] [PubMed]
64. Picco, G.; Cattaneo, C.M.; van Vliet, E.J.; Crisafulli, G.; Rospo, G.; Consonni, S.; Vieira, S.F.; Rodríguez, I.S.; Cancelliere, C.; Banerjee, R.; et al. Werner Helicase Is a Synthetic-Lethal Vulnerability in Mismatch Repair-Deficient Colorectal Cancer Refractory to Targeted Therapies, Chemotherapy, and Immunotherapy. *Cancer Discov.* **2021**, *11*, 1923–1937. [CrossRef] [PubMed]
65. Barpanda, A.; Tuckley, C.; Ray, A.; Banerjee, A.; Duttagupta, S.P.; Kantharia, C.; Srivastava, S. A protein microarray-based serum proteomic investigation reveals distinct autoantibody signature in colorectal cancer. *Proteom. Clin. Appl.* **2023**, *17*, e2200062. [CrossRef]
66. Viratham Pulsawatdi, A.; Craig, S.G.; Bingham, V.; McCombe, K.; Humphries, M.P.; Senevirathne, S.; Richman, S.D.; Quirke, P.; Campo, L.; Domingo, E.; et al. A robust multiplex immunofluorescence and digital pathology workflow for the characterisation of the tumour immune microenvironment. *Mol. Oncol.* **2020**, *14*, 2384–2402. [CrossRef]
67. Chen, J.; Wang, Z.; Shen, X.; Cui, X.; Guo, Y. Identification of novel biomarkers and small molecule drugs in human colorectal cancer by microarray and bioinformatics analysis. *Mol. Genet. Genom. Med.* **2019**, *7*, e00713. [CrossRef]
68. Yin, Z.; Yao, C.; Zhang, L.; Qi, S. Application of artificial intelligence in diagnosis and treatment of colorectal cancer: A novel Prospect. *Front. Med.* **2023**, *10*, 1128084. [CrossRef]
69. Sauter, G.; Simon, R.; Hillan, K. Tissue microarrays in drug discovery. *Nat. Rev. Drug Discov.* **2003**, *2*, 962–972. [CrossRef]
70. Däster, S.; Eppenberger-Castori, S.; Mele, V.; Schäfer, H.M.; Schmid, L.; Weixler, B.; Soysal, S.D.; Droeser, R.A.; Spagnoli, G.C.; Kettelhack, C.; et al. Low Expression of Programmed Death 1 (PD-1), PD-1 Ligand 1 (PD-L1), and Low CD8+ T Lymphocyte Infiltration Identify a Subgroup of Patients with Gastric and Esophageal Adenocarcinoma with Severe Prognosis. *Front. Med.* **2020**, *7*, 144. [CrossRef]

Disclaimer/Publisher's Note: The statements, opinions and data contained in all publications are solely those of the individual author(s) and contributor(s) and not of MDPI and/or the editor(s). MDPI and/or the editor(s) disclaim responsibility for any injury to people or property resulting from any ideas, methods, instructions or products referred to in the content.

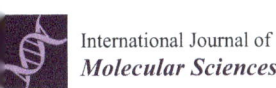

Article

KRAS, NRAS, BRAF, HER2 and MSI Status in a Large Consecutive Series of Colorectal Carcinomas

Aleksandr S. Martianov [1,2], Natalia V. Mitiushkina [1], Anastasia N. Ershova [2], Darya E. Martynenko [1], Mikhail G. Bubnov [1], Priscilla Amankwah [2], Grigory A. Yanus [1,2], Svetlana N. Aleksakhina [1], Vladislav I. Tiurin [1], Aigul R. Venina [1], Aleksandra A. Anuskina [1], Yuliy A. Gorgul [1], Anna D. Shestakova [1], Mikhail A. Maidin [1], Alexey M. Belyaev [1], Liliya S. Baboshkina [1], Aglaya G. Iyevleva [1] and Evgeny N. Imyanitov [1,2,*]

1 Department of Tumor Growth Biology, N.N. Petrov Institute of Oncology, 197758 St. Petersburg, Russia
2 Department of Medical Genetics, St.-Petersburg Pediatric Medical University, 194100 St. Petersburg, Russia
* Correspondence: evgeny@imyanitov.spb.ru; Tel.: +7-812-4399528

Abstract: This study aimed to analyze clinical and regional factors influencing the distribution of actionable genetic alterations in a large consecutive series of colorectal carcinomas (CRCs). *KRAS*, *NRAS* and *BRAF* mutations, *HER2* amplification and overexpression, and microsatellite instability (MSI) were tested in 8355 CRC samples. *KRAS* mutations were detected in 4137/8355 (49.5%) CRCs, with 3913 belonging to 10 common substitutions affecting codons 12/13/61/146, 174 being represented by 21 rare hot-spot variants, and 35 located outside the "hot" codons. *KRAS* Q61K substitution, which leads to the aberrant splicing of the gene, was accompanied by the second function-rescuing mutation in all 19 tumors analyzed. *NRAS* mutations were detected in 389/8355 (4.7%) CRCs (379 hot-spot and 10 non-hot-spot substitutions). *BRAF* mutations were identified in 556/8355 (6.7%) CRCs (codon 600: 510; codons 594–596: 38; codons 597–602: 8). The frequency of HER2 activation and MSI was 99/8008 (1.2%) and 432/8355 (5.2%), respectively. Some of the above events demonstrated differences in distribution according to patients' age and gender. In contrast to other genetic alterations, *BRAF* mutation frequencies were subject to geographic variation, with a relatively low incidence in areas with an apparently warmer climate (83/1726 (4.8%) in Southern Russia and North Caucasus vs. 473/6629 (7.1%) in other regions of Russia, $p = 0.0007$). The simultaneous presence of two drug targets, *BRAF* mutation and MSI, was observed in 117/8355 cases (1.4%). Combined alterations of two driver genes were detected in 28/8355 (0.3%) tumors (*KRAS/NRAS*: 8; *KRAS/BRAF*: 4; *KRAS/HER2*: 12; *NRAS/HER2*: 4). This study demonstrates that a substantial portion of *RAS* alterations is represented by atypical mutations, *KRAS* Q61K substitution is always accompanied by the second gene-rescuing mutation, *BRAF* mutation frequency is a subject to geographical variations, and a small fraction of CRCs has simultaneous alterations in more than one driver gene.

Keywords: *KRAS*; *NRAS*; *BRAF*; microsatellite instability; *HER2*; colorectal cancer

1. Introduction

Colorectal cancer (CRC) affects approximately 1.9 million people per year, thus holding the third position in cancer morbidity worldwide [1]. Molecular genetic testing has become an essential component of CRC management. Patients with metastatic CRC usually receive *KRAS*, *NRAS*, *BRAF*, microsatellite instability (MSI) and *HER2* testing [2,3]. *KRAS/NRAS* analysis is complicated because of a wide spectrum of activating mutations affecting these genes [4]. While tumors with wild-type *RAS* genes are highly sensitive to anti-EGFR therapy, erroneous administration of cetuximab or panitumumab to patients with *RAS*-mutated CRC may facilitate tumor growth [5,6]. CRCs carrying amino acid substitutions in codon 600 have a particularly poor prognosis and are potentially responsive to the combination of BRAF inhibitors and anti-EGFR antibodies [7]. *HER2*-driven CRCs can be managed by

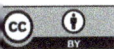

various antagonists of HER2 kinase [8]. Microsatellite instability occurs in CRCs caused by Lynch syndrome, as well as in a subset of sporadic cancers. The identification of MSI in CRC tissue may call for germline DNA testing. In addition, microsatellite unstable tumors are sensitive to immune checkpoint inhibitors. MSI analysis is employed not only for the management of metastatic tumors but also for patients with early-stage CRC [9,10].

The frequencies of genetic alterations observed in CRC patients vary across studies. It is very likely that technical bias contributes to these variations. *RAS* testing was initially limited to *KRAS* exon 2 and 3 hotspot mutations, and was supplemented by so-called "extended" *RAS* analysis (hotspot substitutions in *KRAS* exon 4 and *NRAS* exons 2, 3 and 4) only a few years ago [4,11]. Reliable analysis of *KRAS/NRAS* status still presents a challenge, as several available commercial assays limit the detection of *RAS* mutations to a number of relatively common events, thus missing a substantial portion of clinically relevant genetic alterations. Sanger sequencing and pyrosequencing are capable of detecting the entire spectrum of mutations. However, these sequencing methods are not efficient in tumor samples containing a low proportion of tumor cells. Next-generation sequencing (NGS) is certainly the method of choice. However, its use is still limited due to high cost and the need to accumulate multiple samples for a single run [4,6,11,12].

We have developed an inexpensive CRC diagnostic pipeline, which is capable of detecting both "typical" and "atypical" mutations in *KRAS*, *NRAS* and *BRAF* genes, even in samples with a low proportion of tumor cells, includes *HER2* and MSI testing, and is characterized by low cost. This uniform methodology was applied to 8355 consecutive CRC samples obtained from various parts of Russia. This study provides interesting insights into region-specific variations in mutation frequencies, ratios between "common" and "rare" genetic alterations, and the co-occurrence of multiple driver mutations.

2. Results

KRAS mutations were identified in 4137/8355 (49.5%) CRCs (Supplementary Table S1). A total of 3913/4137 (94.6%) mutations affected hot-spots and had a frequency above 1% among *KRAS*-mutated CRCs (G12D: 1193 (28.8%), G12V: 874 (21.1%), G13D: 727 (17.6%), G12C: 276 (6.7%), A146T: 235 (5.7%), G12A: 206 (5.0%), G12S: 200 (4.8%), Q61H: 108 (2.6%), A146V: 51 (1.2%), G12R: 43 (1.0%)). A total of 174/4137 (4.2%) CRCs carried 21 rare variants affecting the hot-spots; amino acid substitutions (Q61L: 35 (0.9%), G13C: 24 (0.6%), Q61R: 24 (0.6%), A59T: 21 (0.5%), Q61K: 21 (0.5%), G13R: 10 (0.2%), A146P: 6 (0.2%), A59E: 6 (0.2%), A59G: 6 (0.2%), G12F: 5 (0.1%), Q61P: 4 (0.1%), G13S: 2 (0.05%); G12L, G13V, Q61D: 1 (0.02%) each) or non-missense variants (G13dup: 2 (0.05%); A59del, G12Rfs*22, G12Sfs*22, G13_V14delinsDI, G60_Q61delinsE: 1 (0.02%) each) were present. A total of 35/4137 (0.9%) CRCs had mutations located outside the "hot" codons (V14I: 6 (0.2%), A18D: 5 (0.1%), L19F: 5 (0.1%), Q22K: 5 (0.1%), G60D: 4 (0.1%); A66X, E62K, E63del, G10_A11dup, G10dup, G10R, G10V, K147E, L19_T20delinsFS, T58I: 1 (0.02%) each), with most of them resulting in the activation of KRAS protein [4]. In addition, 12/4137 (0.3%) tumors carried two mutations, and one CRC had three distinct *KRAS* mutations. *KRAS* mutations were more common in females (52.0% vs. 47.0%, $p < 0.0001$) and in patients aged above 50 years (50.2% vs. 45.3%, $p = 0.002$) (Supplementary Table S2, Figures 1 and 2). The distribution of *KRAS* mutation frequencies was relatively even across different geographic regions (Supplementary Table S3, Figure 3).

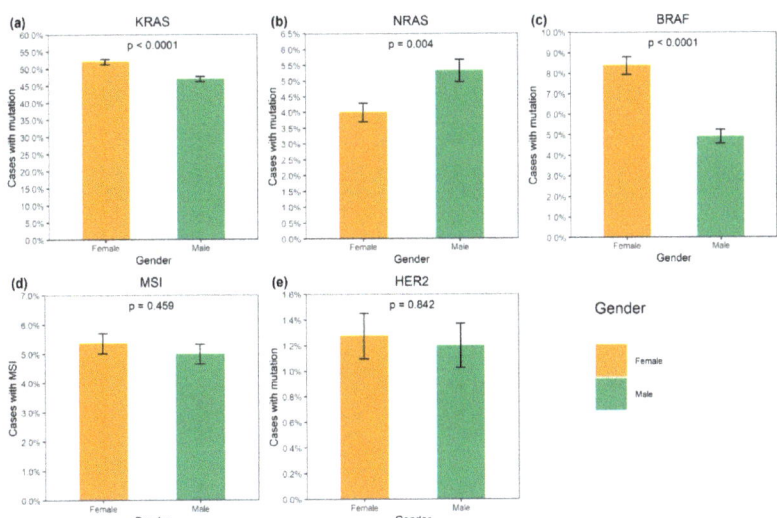

Figure 1. Association of genetic alterations with gender. (**a**) *KRAS* mutation, (**b**) *NRAS* mutation, (**c**) *BRAF* mutation, (**d**) MSI, (**e**) *HER2* amplification.

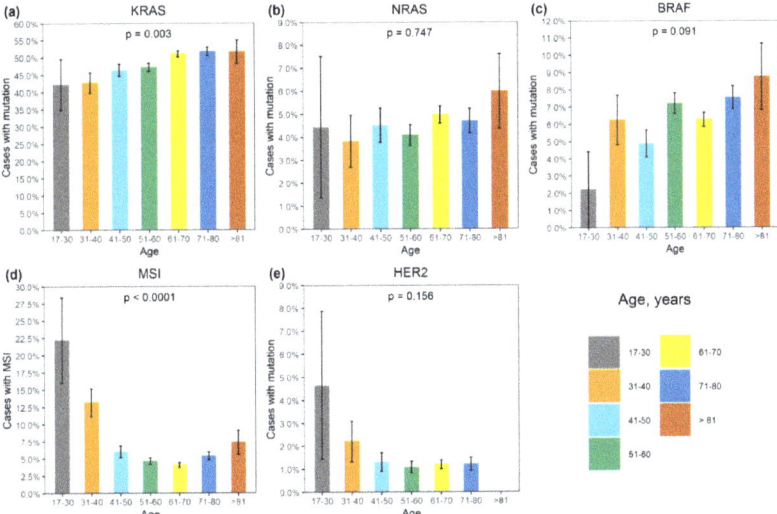

Figure 2. Association of genetic alterations with age. (**a**) *KRAS* mutation, (**b**) *NRAS* mutation, (**c**) *BRAF* mutation, (**d**) MSI, (**e**) *HER2* amplification.

A recent study revealed that *KRAS* Q61K mutation is not activating per se as it leads to the aberrant splicing and disruption of the gene function [13]. Instead, Kobayashi et al. [13] have shown that when occurring in tumors, *KRAS* Q61K is almost always accompanied by another mutation (usually a G60G silent mutation affecting codon 60), which restores the normal processing of the *KRAS* RNA transcript. *KRAS* Q61K substitution was observed in 21 CRCs in our data set, with 19 specimens available for pyrosequencing analysis. Strikingly, all 19 analyzed tumors indeed carried a second *KRAS* alteration, with GQ60_61GK function-restoring mutation being the most prevalent (17/19, 89.5%; c.180_181delinsAA: 15; c.180_181delinsCA: 2).

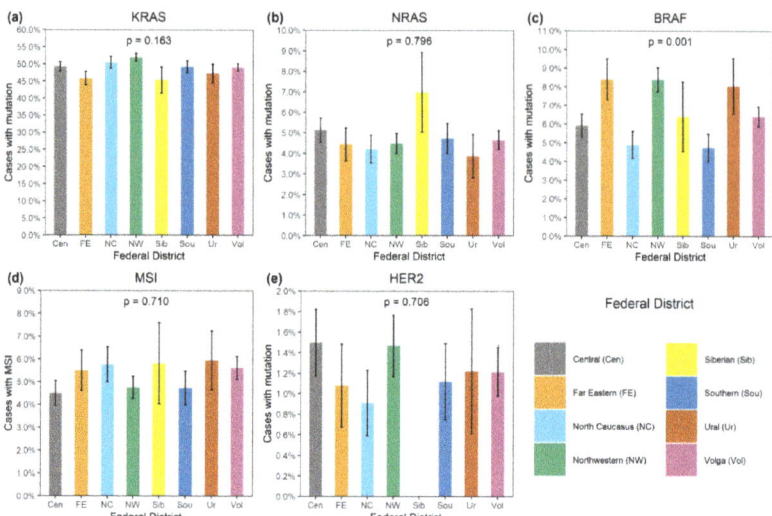

Figure 3. Distribution of genetic alterations in patients from various regions of Russia. (**a**) *KRAS* mutation, (**b**) *NRAS* mutation, (**c**) *BRAF* mutation, (**d**) MSI, (**e**) *HER2* amplification.

NRAS mutations were detected in 389/8355 (4.7%) CRCs. Several hot-spot mutations were relatively common (Q61K: 95 (24.4%), G12D: 67 (17.2%), Q61R: 59 (15.2%), Q61L: 38 (9.8%), G13R: 21 (5.4%), Q61H: 19 (4.9%), G12V: 18 (4.6%), G13D: 18 (4.6%), G12C: 14 (3.6%), G12S: 12 (3.1%), G12A: 7 (1.8%), G13V: 6 (1.5%)). There were 10/389 (2.6%) CRCs carrying missense mutations located outside hot spots (G60E: 2 (0.5%); A11T, A18T, A59T, A66V, E62K, E63D, G15E, Y64C: 1 (0.3%) each). *NRAS* mutations were slightly more prevalent in males (5.3% vs. 4.0%, $p = 0.004$). Their occurrence was not affected by the age at diagnosis or geographic region (Supplementary Tables S2 and S3; Figures 1–3).

BRAF mutations were identified in 556/8355 (6.7%) CRCs. Of these, 510/556 (91.7%) were kinase-activating codon 600 substitutions (509 V600E and 1 V600K). A total of 38/556 (6.8%) CRCs carried mutations affecting codons 594, 595 or 596, which result in the down-regulation of BRAF kinase activity but increased ERK signaling via bypass mechanisms [14,15]. There were also rare instances of *BRAF*-activating mutations affecting codons 597 ($n = 2$), 599 ($n = 2$), 601 ($n = 3$) and 602 ($n = 1$). *BRAF* mutations were almost twice more common in females than in males (8.4% vs. 4.9%, $p < 0.0001$) and tended to have different frequencies in different age groups (17–30 years old: 1/45 (2.2%), 31–40: 18/288 (6.3%), 41–50: 39/796 (4.9%), 51–60: 139/1925 (7.2%), 61–70: 217/3458 (6.3%), 71–80: 122/1613 (7.6%), >81: 19/217 (8.7%)) (Supplementary Table S2, Figures 1 and 2). In contrast to *RAS* mutations, *BRAF* mutation frequencies were subject to geographic variation, with a relatively low occurrence in areas with an apparently warmer climate (4.8% in Southern Russia and North Caucasus vs. 7.1% in other regions of Russia, $p = 0.0007$) (Supplementary Table S3, Figures 3 and 4).

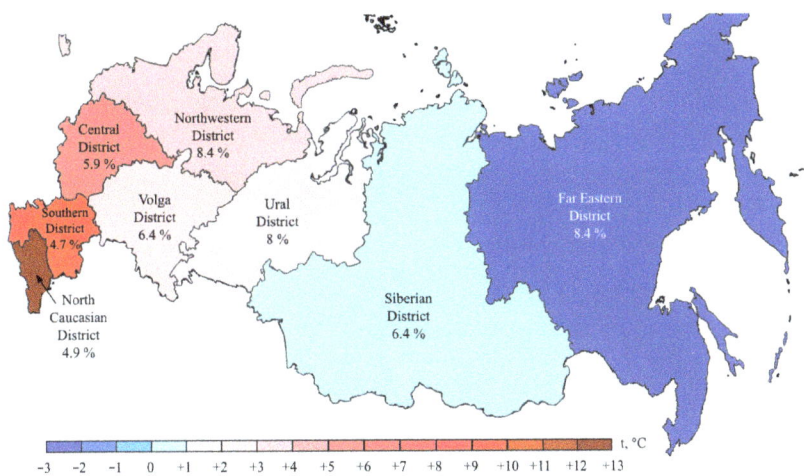

Figure 4. *BRAF* mutation frequencies in CRC patients from various region of Russia. The color bar represents an average annual temperature.

MSI was detected in 432/8355 (5.2%) CRCs. There was a striking increase in MSI frequency in patients below 40 years of age (48/333, 14.4%), which is almost certainly related to the high proportion of Lynch syndrome in younger individuals [2]. Patients aged 51–70 years demonstrated relatively low MSI occurrence (318/6996, 4.5%). A trend towards elevated MSI incidence in older age groups (71–80: 87/1613 (5.4%); >81: 16/217 (7.4%), $p < 0.0001$) was observed (Supplementary Table S2, Figure 2). The frequency of detection of MSI was 317/6324 (5.0%) when using a single marker BAT26, and 115/2031 (5.7%) with the pentaplex panel. Out of 115 CRCs with MSI detected by the pentaplex panel, only 4 did not show the instability for the BAT26 marker.

BRAF mutations were detected in 117/432 (27.1%) microsatellite-unstable CRCs. Double MSI/*BRAF*-positive tumors were significantly more common in women than in men (92/4151, 2.2% vs. 25/4204, 0.6%, $p < 0.0001$) and in elderly individuals (0.09% in patients below 50 years, 1.5% in 51–80 years age group and 3.7% in individuals older than 80 years, $p < 0.0001$).

Approximately one third of MSI-positive cases contained *KRAS* alterations (138/432, 31.9%). The simultaneous occurrence of MSI and *KRAS* mutations decreased with age (4.3% in patients below 50 years, 1.2% in 51–80 years age group and 0.9% in individuals older than 80 years, $p < 0.0001$).

HER2 activation by gene amplification and overexpression was detected in 99/8008 CRCs (1.2%) (Supplementary Tables S2 and S3). No significant correlation with clinical characteristics of the disease was observed, although the statistical analysis was compromised by the low frequency of this event.

A small fraction of CRCs contained combinations of mutations in distinct driver genes (*KRAS* and *NRAS* mutations: 8 (0.1%), *KRAS* and *BRAF* mutations: 4 (0.05%), *KRAS* mutation and *HER2* amplification/overexpression 12 (0.15%), *NRAS* mutation and *HER2* amplification/overexpression: 4 (0.05%)) (Supplementary Table S4). The total frequency of combined driver events was 26/8355 (0.3%).

3. Discussion

This study describes a large series of consecutive CRCs, which were collected in various regions of Russia and genetically tested using a low-cost, but nevertheless comprehensive, methodology capable of evaluating the entire spectrum of medically relevant alterations (hot-spot and rare mutations in *KRAS*, *NRAS* and *BRAF* oncogenes; *HER2* amplification/overexpression; MSI). Strikingly, the observed frequency of *RAS* mutations is on the upper limit of inter-study variations, suggesting that the combination of HRM, allele-specific PCR and pyrosequencing is reliable for detection of both "typical" and "atypical" mutations [11,16–18]. For example, the occurrence of *KRAS* alterations in the current study (49.5%) was higher than that reported at cBioPortal, a resource hosting genomic data from large cancer sequencing consortiums and individual studies (44.7%) (Supplementary Table S5) [19,20]. Our study underscores that clinical CRC *RAS* testing should not be limited to allele-specific PCR, as a substantial portion of *RAS* mutations is destined to be missed by this approach [4,6,21]. This is an important finding, given that the anti-EGFR therapeutic antibodies cetuximab and panitumumab are contraindicated for *RAS*-mutated CRCs and may even boost tumor progression in this category of patients [5,6].

KRAS Q61K is a rare genetic event. A recent study led to a surprising finding suggesting that Q61K substitution inactivates the *KRAS* gene if present alone, but is almost always accompanied by the second function-rescuing mutation in naturally occurring tumors [13]. The large size of our data set permitted us to analyze a substantial number of CRCs carrying *KRAS* Q61K substitution, and we provide, apparently, the first independent confirmation of the report of Kobayashi et al. [13].

There are hundreds of reports describing the distribution of *KRAS* and *NRAS* mutations in CRC patients. Although patients' race, age, gender and other factors appear to have some impact, it seems that the differences in the observed frequencies are significantly more attributed to the variations in the methodology of the mutation testing than to genuine clinical or biological reasons [11,18,22]. Indeed, our study confirmed the mild influence of age and gender on the probability of detecting *RAS* activation [11,16,19,20] (Supplementary Tables S2 and S6), while the pattern of *RAS* mutations was relatively uniform across various regions of Russia, suggesting a limited impact of lifestyle, environmental or other external factors.

In contrast, this investigation revealed strong regional differences in the distribution of *BRAF* mutations, suggesting that this event is more characteristic of areas with a relatively cold climate. This is an interesting observation, with either diet, lifestyle or other climate-related factors assuming a role in determining the probability of developing *BRAF*-mutated CRC disease. Previous studies revealed race-specific differences in the distribution of *BRAF* mutations, i.e., an increased prevalence of this event in CRC patients of European vs. African or Asian descent [18,23]. Some investigations reported ethnic variations with regard to the frequency of *BRAF* alterations in CRC observed within the subjects of the same race [24]. In our study, a low rate of *BRAF* oncogene involvement was detected in patients from the North Caucasus and Southern Russia (Figure 4). While the population of the North Caucasus is represented by White non-Slavic people, the ethnic composition of the Southern Russia is identical to other regions of this country. There is also some evidence for a moderate contribution of smoking or dietary factors in determining the probability of development of *BRAF*-mutated CRC [25–27].

The comparison of data obtained for *HER2* activation and MSI with other studies is a complicated task. *HER2* overexpression is usually analyzed using immunohistochemical staining [28,29]. We have incorporated the determination of *HER2* status into the molecular genetic pipeline using the analysis of *HER2* extra copies as a primary test and the quantitation of the *HER2* RNA transcript as a confirmation of the functional relevance of *HER2* amplification. This approach, although promising, still needs to be rigorously validated against clinically accepted methodologies of *HER2* CRC testing. MSI frequencies are significantly influenced by several factors. MSI is a relatively common occurrence in the early-onset CRC; however, its incidence may depend on a population-specific incidence of Lynch-syndrome-associated germ-line pathogenic variants. Furthermore, MSI is particularly characteristic of very elderly subjects, so the age distribution of a given CRC patient series is a strong confounding factor [2].

The driver mutations affecting *KRAS*, *NRAS*, *BRAF* and *HER2* genes are generally mutually exclusive. This study along with similar reports and cBioPortal data describes rare instances of combined alterations of the above genes [19,20,30,31] (Supplementary Table S5).

It is of question whether this phenomenon reflects intratumoral genetic heterogeneity, i.e., the situation where distinct cell clones carry distinct genetic alterations, or true instances of the co-occurrence of several driver events in the same cell. The combination of HER2 amplification/overexpression with RAS mutations seems to be particularly common, being detected in 16/99 (16%) HER2-associated tumors. The responsiveness of these CRCs to HER2-targeted therapy needs to be evaluated in clinical studies.

In conclusion, this investigation produced several findings of potential importance. Atypical KRAS and NRAS mutations represent a substantial portion of RAS alterations which need to be considered in clinical testing. KRAS Q61K substitution is a gene-inactivating event if occurring alone, but it is always accompanied by the second function-rescuing mutation in naturally occurring CRCs. The frequency of BRAF but not other CRC-specific genetic aberrations may be a subject of climate-related variations. There are rare instances of CRCs carrying simultaneous alterations in several genes involved in MAPK signaling cascade. The analysis of biological mechanisms underlying the latter two observations deserves further consideration.

4. Materials and Methods

This study included 8355 consecutive CRCs, which were referred for molecular genetic analysis to the N.N. Petrov Institute of Oncology (St.-Petersburg, Russia) within years 2021–2022. Formalin-fixed paraffin-embedded (FFPE) CRC samples were subjected to microscope-guided manual tumor cell dissection, and nucleic acids (DNA and RNA) were extracted from the tumor cells using Trizol reagent as described previously [32]. In brief, tissue sections were washed with 70% ethanol, air-dried and then incubated overnight in 200 µL of lysis buffer (10 mM Tris–HCl (pH 8.0), 0.1 mM EDTA (pH 8.0), 2% SDS, 20 mg/mL proteinase K) at 65 °C. After sample cooling at room temperature, 200 µL Trizol and 90 µL chloroform–isoamyl alcohol mix (24:1) were added, samples were shaken rigorously and centrifuged at full speed (15,000× g) for 15 min at 0 °C. The supernatant was transferred into new tubes, to which 1 µL of glycogen (20 mg/mL) and 1 volume (300 µL) of cold isopropanol were added. The samples were vortexed and left overnight at −20 °C. The tubes were then centrifuged at 15,000× g for 30 min. Isopropanol was removed, and the precipitate was rinsed once in 70% ethanol for 10 min. After thorough removal of ethanol, the precipitate was dried at 50 °C, and then dissolved in 100 µL of sterile water at 50 °C for 5 min. RNA was enzymatically converted into cDNA only in samples positive for HER2 gene amplification [33]. The reaction setup included two steps. First, 10 µL of nucleic acid sample was mixed with 1 µL dNTP mix (25 µmol each) and 2 µL of hexaprimers (0.25 µmol) in a total volume of 15 µL and incubated for 3 min at 70 °C, 3 min at 65 °C and 1 min at 60 °C in order to denature RNA and anneal primers. After sample cooling on ice, 4 µL 5^X RT buffer (Amgen, Thousand Oaks, CA, USA), 0.3 µL M-Mulv reverse transcriptase (Amgen, Thousand Oaks, CA, USA), 0.2 µL and RiboLock RNase Inhibitor (Thermo Scientific, Waltham, MA, USA) were added. The total volume of the reverse transcription (RT) reaction was 20 µL. Reaction conditions were 20 °C for 5 min, 38 °C for 30 min and 95 °C for 5 min. After the completion of cDNA synthesis, 80 µL of water was added to the sample. cDNA quality was checked by the Cycle threshold (Ct) of the housekeeping gene SDHA obtained in qPCR. Samples with SDHA(Ct) < 34 cycles were considered suitable for further analysis of HER2 expression.

Testing for KRAS, NRAS and BRAF mutations was performed by a combination of high-resolution melting (HRM) analysis, allele-specific PCR (AS-PCR), digital droplet PCR and pyrosequencing. First, the presence of KRAS (exons 2, 3, and 4), NRAS (exons 2, 3, and 4), and BRAF (exon 15) alterations was determined by HRM of PCR products. Cases showing abnormal melting patterns were further tested for hot-spot variants by the corresponding AS-PCR assays (KRAS exon 2: codons 12, 13; exon 3: codons 59, 61; exon 4: codon 146; NRAS exon 2: codons 12, 13; exon 3: codon 61; BRAF exon 15: codon 600). Tumor samples with equivocal results were additionally analyzed by digital droplet PCR. Cases with abnormal HRM curves negative for relevant hot-spot variants were subjected to pyrosequencing. The list of the primers, assay conditions and utilized equipment is given in Supplementary Table S7.

HER2 gene amplification was determined by a quantitative real-time PCR assay (Supplementary Table S7). Tumor samples with extra copies of HER2 DNA were subsequently tested for HER2 mRNA overexpression. The thresholds for HER2 DNA amplification and RNA overexpression were determined by comparing the IHC/FISH-validated HER2-positive and negative control samples. These thresholds were dCt < 0 and dCt < −1.9 for DNA amplification and RNA overexpression, respectively, where $dCt = Ct_{HER2} - Ct_{reference}$.

Microsatellite instability (MSI) status was evaluated by fragment analysis of either a single marker (BAT26; 6324 samples) or five mononucleotide markers (BAT25, BAT26, NR21, NR22 and NR24; 2031 samples) using the GenomeLab GeXP Genetic Analysis System (Beckman Coulter, Brea, CA, USA) (Supplementary Table S7). For pentaplex panel, tumors with two or more shifts were classified as MSI-positive.

Mutation frequencies and their associations with clinical parameters were analyzed using a Chi-square test with Yates correction or Fisher's exact test. Statistical comparisons were performed using R software (version 3.2.1, http://www.r-project.org (accessed on 16 February 16 2023)). The level of statistical significance was set at $\alpha = 0.05$.

Supplementary Materials: The following supporting information can be downloaded at: https://www.mdpi.com/article/10.3390/ijms24054868/s1.

Author Contributions: Conceptualization, A.S.M., E.N.I.; methodology, A.S.M., N.V.M., M.G.B., G.A.Y., S.N.A.; investigation, A.N.E., D.E.M., M.G.B., P.A., V.I.T., A.R.V., A.A.A., A.D.S., M.A.M., L.S.B.; data curation, A.S.M., Y.A.G., A.G.I.; writing—original draft preparation, A.S.M., S.N.A., A.G.I.; writing—review and editing, E.N.I.; visualization, A.S.M., Y.A.G.; supervision, A.M.B., E.N.I.; funding acquisition G.A.Y. All authors have read and agreed to the published version of the manuscript.

Funding: This research has been supported by the Russian Science Foundation, grant number 18-75-10070.

Institutional Review Board Statement: The study was conducted in accordance with the Declaration of Helsinki and approved by the Ethics Committee of N.N. Petrov Institute of Oncology.

Informed Consent Statement: Informed consent was obtained from all subjects involved in the study.

Data Availability Statement: The data that support the findings of this study are available from the corresponding author upon reasonable request.

Conflicts of Interest: The authors declare no conflict of interest.

References

1. Sung, H.; Ferlay, J.; Siegel, R.L.; Laversanne, M.; Soerjomataram, I.; Jemal, A.; Bray, F. Global Cancer Statistics 2020: GLOBOCAN Estimates of Incidence and Mortality Worldwide for 36 Cancers in 185 Countries. *CA Cancer J. Clin.* **2021**, *71*, 209–249. [CrossRef] [PubMed]
2. Imyanitov, E.; Kuligina, E. Molecular testing for colorectal cancer: Clinical applications. *World. J. Gastrointest. Oncol.* **2021**, *13*, 1288–1301. [CrossRef]
3. Crutcher, M.; Waldman, S. Biomarkers in the development of individualized treatment regimens for colorectal cancer. *Front. Med.* **2022**, *9*, 1062423. [CrossRef] [PubMed]
4. Loree, J.M.; Wang, Y.; Syed, M.A.; Sorokin, A.V.; Coker, O.; Xiu, J.; Weinberg, B.A.; Vanderwalde, A.M.; Tesfaye, A.; Raymond, V.M.; et al. Clinical and Functional Characterization of Atypical KRAS/NRAS Mutations in Metastatic Colorectal Cancer. *Clin. Cancer Res.* **2021**, *27*, 4587–4598. [CrossRef] [PubMed]
5. Douillard, J.Y.; Oliner, K.S.; Siena, S.; Tabernero, J.; Burkes, R.; Barugel, M.; Humblet, Y.; Bodoky, G.; Cunningham, D.; Jassem, J.; et al. Panitumumab-FOLFOX4 treatment and RAS mutations in colorectal cancer. *N. Engl. J. Med.* **2013**, *369*, 1023–1034. [CrossRef] [PubMed]
6. Van Krieken, J.H.; Rouleau, E.; Ligtenberg, M.J.; Normanno, N.; Patterson, S.D.; Jung, A. RAS testing in metastatic colorectal cancer: Advances in Europe. *Virchows Arch.* **2016**, *468*, 383–396. [CrossRef] [PubMed]
7. Grassi, E.; Corbelli, J.; Papiani, G.; Barbera, M.A.; Gazzaneo, F.; Tamberi, S. Current Therapeutic Strategies in BRAF-Mutant Metastatic Colorectal Cancer. *Front. Oncol.* **2021**, *11*, 601722. [CrossRef]

18. Yoshikawa, A.; Nakamura, Y. Molecular Basis of HER2-Targeted Therapy for HER2-Positive Colorectal Cancer. *Cancers* 2022, *15*, 183. [CrossRef]
19. Buchler, T. Microsatellite Instability and Metastatic Colorectal Cancer—A Clinical Perspective. *Front. Oncol.* 2022, *12*, 888181. [CrossRef]
20. Taieb, J.; Svrcek, M.; Cohen, R.; Basile, D.; Tougeron, D.; Phelip, J.M. Deficient mismatch repair/microsatellite unstable colorectal cancer: Diagnosis, prognosis and treatment. *Eur. J. Cancer* 2022, *175*, 136–157. [CrossRef]
21. Levin-Sparenberg, E.; Bylsma, L.C.; Lowe, K.; Sangare, L.; Fryzek, J.P.; Alexander, D.D. A Systematic Literature Review and Meta-Analysis Describing the Prevalence of KRAS, NRAS, and BRAF Gene Mutations in Metastatic Colorectal Cancer. *Gastroenterol. Res.* 2020, *13*, 184–198. [CrossRef] [PubMed]
22. Belardinilli, F.; Capalbo, C.; Malapelle, U.; Pisapia, P.; Raimondo, D.; Milanetti, E.; Yasaman, M.; Liccardi, C.; Paci, P.; Sibilio, P.; et al. Clinical Multigene Panel Sequencing Identifies Distinct Mutational Association Patterns in Metastatic Colorectal Cancer. *Front. Oncol.* 2020, *10*, 560. [CrossRef] [PubMed]
23. Kobayashi, Y.; Chhoeu, C.; Li, J.; Price, K.S.; Kiedrowski, L.A.; Hutchins, J.L.; Hardin, A.I.; Wei, Z.; Hong, F.; Bahcall, M.; et al. Silent mutations reveal therapeutic vulnerability in RAS Q61 cancers. *Nature* 2022, *603*, 335–342. [CrossRef] [PubMed]
24. Yao, Z.; Yaeger, R.; Rodrik-Outmezguine, V.S.; Tao, A.; Torres, N.M.; Chang, M.T.; Drosten, M.; Zhao, H.; Cecchi, F.; Hembrough, T.; et al. Tumours with class 3 BRAF mutants are sensitive to the inhibition of activated RAS. *Nature* 2017, *548*, 234–238. [CrossRef]
25. Owsley, J.; Stein, M.K.; Porter, J.; In, G.K.; Salem, M.; O'Day, S.; Elliott, A.; Poorman, K.; Gibney, G.; VanderWalde, A. Prevalence of class I-III BRAF mutations among 114,662 cancer patients in a large genomic database. *Exp. Biol. Med.* 2021, *246*, 31–39. [CrossRef]
26. Peeters, M.; Kafatos, G.; Taylor, A.; Gastanaga, V.M.; Oliner, K.S.; Hechmati, G.; Terwey, J.H.; van Krieken, J.H. Prevalence of RAS mutations and individual variation patterns among patients with metastatic colorectal cancer: A pooled analysis of randomised controlled trials. *Eur. J. Cancer* 2015, *51*, 1704–1713. [CrossRef]
27. Kafatos, G.; Banks, V.; Burdon, P.; Neasham, D.; Anger, C.; Manuguid, F.; Lowe, K.A.; Cheung, P.; Taieb, J.; van Krieken, J.H. Biomarker testing and mutation prevalence in metastatic colorectal cancer patients in five European countries using a large oncology database. *Future Oncol.* 2021, *17*, 1483–1494. [CrossRef]
28. Myer, P.A.; Lee, J.K.; Madison, R.W.; Pradhan, K.; Newberg, J.Y.; Isasi, C.R.; Klempner, S.J.; Frampton, G.M.; Ross, J.S.; Venstrom, J.M.; et al. The Genomics of Colorectal Cancer in Populations with African and European Ancestry. *Cancer Discov.* 2022, *12*, 1282–1293. [CrossRef]
29. Cerami, E.; Gao, J.; Dogrusoz, U.; Gross, B.E.; Sumer, S.O.; Aksoy, B.A.; Jacobsen, A.; Byrne, C.J.; Heuer, M.L.; Larsson, E.; et al. The cBio cancer genomics portal: An open platform for exploring multidimensional cancer genomics data. *Cancer Discov.* 2012, *2*, 401–404. [CrossRef]
30. Gao, J.; Aksoy, B.A.; Dogrusoz, U.; Dresdner, G.; Gross, B.; Sumer, S.O.; Sun, Y.; Jacobsen, A.; Sinha, R.; Larsson, E.; et al. Integrative analysis of complex cancer genomics and clinical profiles using the cBioPortal. *Sci. Signal.* 2013, *6*, pl1. [CrossRef]
31. Pietrantonio, F.; Yaeger, R.; Schrock, A.B.; Randon, G.; Romero-Cordoba, S.; Rossini, D.; Fucà, G.; Ross, J.S.; Kotani, D.; Madison, R.; et al. Atypical RAS Mutations in Metastatic Colorectal Cancer. *JCO Precis. Oncol.* 2019, *3*, 1–11. [CrossRef] [PubMed]
32. Turpin, A.; Genin, M.; Hebbar, M.; Occelli, F.; Lanier, C.; Vasseur, F.; Descarpentries, C.; Pannier, D.; Ploquin, A. Spatial heterogeneity of KRAS mutations in colorectal cancers in northern France. *Cancer Manag. Res.* 2019, *11*, 8337–8344. [CrossRef] [PubMed]
33. Yoon, H.H.; Shi, Q.; Alberts, S.R.; Goldberg, R.M.; Thibodeau, S.N.; Sargent, D.J.; Sinicrope, F.A. Alliance for Clinical Trials in Oncology. Racial Differences in BRAF/KRAS Mutation Rates and Survival in Stage III Colon Cancer Patients. *J. Natl. Cancer Inst.* 2015, *107*, djv186. [CrossRef] [PubMed]
34. English, D.R.; Young, J.P.; Simpson, J.A.; Jenkins, M.A.; Southey, M.C.; Walsh, M.D.; Buchanan, D.D.; Barker, M.A.; Haydon, A.M.; Royce, S.G.; et al. Ethnicity and risk for colorectal cancers showing somatic BRAF V600E mutation or CpG island methylator phenotype. *Cancer Epidemiol. Biomark. Prev.* 2008, *17*, 1774–1780. [CrossRef] [PubMed]
35. Rozek, L.S.; Herron, C.M.; Greenson, J.K.; Moreno, V.; Capella, G.; Rennert, G.; Gruber, S.B. Smoking, gender, and ethnicity predict somatic BRAF mutations in colorectal cancer. *Cancer Epidemiol. Biomark. Prev.* 2010, *19*, 838–843. [CrossRef] [PubMed]
36. Mehta, R.S.; Song, M.; Nishihara, R.; Drew, D.A.; Wu, K.; Qian, Z.R.; Fung, T.T.; Hamada, T.; Masugi, Y.; da Silva, A.; et al. Dietary Patterns and Risk of Colorectal Cancer: Analysis by Tumor Location and Molecular Subtypes. *Gastroenterology* 2017, *152*, 1944–1953.e1. [CrossRef] [PubMed]
37. Wang, L.; He, X.; Ugai, T.; Haruki, K.; Lo, C.H.; Hang, D.; Akimoto, N.; Fujiyoshi, K.; Wang, M.; Fuchs, C.S.; et al. Risk Factors and Incidence of Colorectal Cancer According to Major Molecular Subtypes. *JNCI Cancer Spectr.* 2020, *5*, pkaa089. [CrossRef]
38. Roy-Chowdhuri, S.; Davies, K.D.; Ritterhouse, L.L.; Snow, A.N. ERBB2 (HER2) Alterations in Colorectal Cancer. *J. Mol. Diagn.* 2022, *24*, 1064–1066. [CrossRef]
39. Sun, Q.; Li, Q.; Gao, F.; Wu, H.; Fu, Y.; Yang, J.; Fan, X.; Cui, X.; Pu, X. HER2 overexpression/amplification status in colorectal cancer: A comparison between immunohistochemistry and fluorescence in situ hybridization using five different immunohistochemical scoring criteria. *J. Cancer Res. Clin. Oncol.* 2022. ahead of print. [CrossRef]
40. Afrăsânie, V.A.; Gafton, B.; Marinca, M.V.; Alexa-Stratulat, T.; Miron, L.; Rusu, C.; Ivanov, A.V.; Balan, G.G.; Croitoru, A.E. The Coexistence of RAS and BRAF Mutations in Metastatic Colorectal Cancer: A Case Report and Systematic Literature Review. *J. Gastrointestin. Liver Dis.* 2020, *29*, 251–256. [CrossRef]

31. Uchida, S.; Kojima, T.; Sugino, T. Frequency and Clinicopathological Characteristics of Patients With KRAS/BRAF Double-Mutant Colorectal Cancer: An In Silico Study. *Pathol. Oncol. Res.* **2022**, *28*, 1610206. [CrossRef] [PubMed]
32. Yanus, G.A.; Belyaeva, A.V.; Ivantsov, A.O.; Kuligina, E.S.; Suspitsin, E.N.; Mitiushkina, N.V.; Aleksakhina, S.N.; Iyevleva, A.G.; Zaitseva, O.A.; Yatsuk, O.S.; et al. Pattern of clinically relevant mutations in consecutive series of Russian colorectal cancer patients. *Med. Oncol.* **2013**, *30*, 686. [CrossRef] [PubMed]
33. Mitiushkina, N.V.; Romanko, A.A.; Preobrazhenskaya, E.V.; Tiurin, V.I.; Ermachenkova, T.I.; Martianov, A.S.; Mulkidjan, R.S.; Sokolova, T.N.; Kholmatov, M.M.; Bizin, I.V.; et al. Comprehensive evaluation of the test for 5′-/3′-end mRNA unbalanced expression as a screening tool for ALK and ROS1 fusions in lung cancer. *Cancer Med.* **2022**, *17*, 3226–3237. [CrossRef] [PubMed]

Disclaimer/Publisher's Note: The statements, opinions and data contained in all publications are solely those of the individual author(s) and contributor(s) and not of MDPI and/or the editor(s). MDPI and/or the editor(s) disclaim responsibility for any injury to people or property resulting from any ideas, methods, instructions or products referred to in the content.

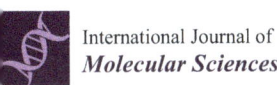

Sleep Fragmentation Accelerates Carcinogenesis in a Chemical-Induced Colon Cancer Model

Da-Been Lee [1,2], Seo-Yeon An [3], Sang-Shin Pyo [2,4], Jinkwan Kim [2,4], Suhng-Wook Kim [1,5,*] and Dae-Wui Yoon [2,4,*]

1. Department of Health and Safety Convergence Science, Graduate School, Korea University, Seoul 02841, Republic of Korea
2. Sleep Medicine Institute, Jungwon University, Goesan-gun 20204, Chungcheongbuk-do, Republic of Korea
3. Next&Bio Inc., Techno Complex Building 6F, Korea University, Seoul 02841, Republic of Korea
4. Department of Biomedical Laboratory Science, Jungwon University, Goesan-gun 20204, Chungcheongbuk-do, Republic of Korea
5. BK21 FOUR R&E Center for Learning Health Systems, Korea University, Seoul 02841, Republic of Korea
* Correspondence: swkimkorea@korea.ac.kr (S.-W.K.); ydw@jwu.ac.kr (D.-W.Y.); Tel.: +82-2-3290-5686 (S.-W.K.); +82-43-830-8863 (D.-W.Y.)

Abstract: Aims of this study were to test whether sleep fragmentation (SF) increased carcinogenesis and to investigate the possible mechanisms of carcinogenesis in a chemical-induced colon cancer model. In this study, eight-week-old C57BL/6 mice were divided into Home cage (HC) and SF groups. After the azoxymethane (AOM) injection, the mice in the SF group were subjected to SF for 77 days. SF was accomplished in a sleep fragmentation chamber. In the second protocol, mice were divided into 2% dextran sodium sulfate (DSS)-treated, HC, and SF groups and were exposed to the HC or SF procedures. Immunohistochemical and immunofluorescent stainings were conducted to determine the level of 8-OHdG and reactive oxygen species (ROS), respectively. Quantitative real-time polymerase chain reaction was used to assess the relative expression of inflammatory and ROS-generating genes. The number of tumors and average tumor size were significantly higher in the SF group than in the HC group. The intensity (%) of the 8-OHdG stained area was significantly higher in the SF group than in the HC group. The fluorescence intensity of ROS was significantly higher in the SF group than the HC group. SF accelerated cancer development in a murine AOM/DSS-induced model of colon cancer, and the increased carcinogenesis was associated with ROS- and oxidative stress-induced DNA damage.

Keywords: carcinogenesis; colon cancer; reactive oxygen species; sleep fragmentation

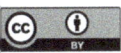

1. Introduction

In recent years, evidence about the significant association between sleep disorders and cancer has accumulated. Many studies have demonstrated that various types of sleep disorders, such as circadian rhythm sleep-wake disorders, insomnia, hypersomnia, and sleep-related breathing disorders, are risk factors for cancer. However, systematic reviews and meta-analyses of the association between sleep duration and cancer risk have shown that the increase in cancer risk due to altered sleep duration is limited to specific ethnicities and differs by cancer type [1], suggesting that different sleep problems might have different effects on cancer risk.

Sleep fragmentation (SF) is frequently found in patients with obstructive sleep apnea (OSA), periodic limb movements, insomnia, and chronic pain. It can also be induced by environmental factors such as light, noise, and inappropriate temperature or humidity during sleep. The influence of SF, which can be defined as frequent disruption of sleep architecture despite the optimal duration of sleep [2], on cancer incidence or adverse prognosis has been investigated relatively little, possibly due to limitations on human study. However, experimental studies using mice showed that fragmented sleep accelerates tumor growth and progression through the recruitment of tumor-associated macrophages and the reduction of nicotinamide adenine dinucleotide phosphate (NADPH) oxidase type 2 activity [3,4]. Those studies investigated the effects of SF on tumors inoculated in mice, but the effects of SF on carcinogenesis remain unexamined. For this study, we hypothesized that chronic SF can accelerate tumor development as well as tumor growth. To test our hypothesis, we used chemical-induced colon carcinogenesis models with azoxymethane (AOM) and dextran sodium sulfate (DSS). We chose this colon cancer model using a carcinogen and a colitis-inducing substance for two main reasons. First, previous human studies reported that OSA, a common sleep-breathing disorder that causes SF, is significantly associated with colorectal neoplasia [5]. Second, it takes too long to observe spontaneous carcinogenesis in an animal model of sleep disturbance without genetic modification or the administration of a carcinogen. Even intermittent hypoxia (IH), a more severe model than SF that also mimics OSA, took more than 3 months to induce spontaneous carcinogenesis in old mice (15 months).

In this study, we used two different experimental protocols. In the first protocol, we explored the effect of SF on chemical-induced colon carcinogenesis and its possible mechanisms using macroscopic examinations of colon tumors and histological and molecular analyses. In the second protocol, we conducted an additional experiment to test the possible mechanisms hypothesized from the results of the first protocol.

2. Results

2.1. Comparison of Tumor Number and Size between the HC and SF Groups

In Experiment 1, we compared the tumor number and size between the HC and SF groups after sacrificing the mice. The total number of tumors was significantly higher in the SF group than in the HC group (Figure 1A,B). We classified tumor size as <2 mm or >2 mm. The number of tumors larger and smaller than 2 mm was both significantly higher in the SF group than in the HC group (Figure 1C,D). The tumors were also larger in the SF group than in the HC group (Figure 1E). Inflammation is known to shorten colon length, so we measured colon length to assess whether SF exacerbated the inflammatory status of the colon in the AOM/DSS-treated mice. The colon length did not differ significantly between the HC and SF groups (8.9 ± 1.7 vs. 9.2 ± 2.0) (Figure 1F,G).

2.2. Histological Assessments of Colon

The AOM/DSS colon carcinogenesis model is based on the induction of colitis. Therefore, we first hypothesized that the increased carcinogenesis caused by SF was due to the exacerbation of colitis. In the H & E stain results, however, we found no significant difference in the inflammation score between the HC and SF groups (1.3 ± 0.2 vs. 1.5 ± 0.3) (Figure 2A,B). Next, we performed IHC staining to assess the level of 8-OHdG, a well-known oxidative stress-induced DNA damage marker, because a previous study reported that sleep deprivation specifically increased ROS in the colon [6]. ROS is also an important cause of carcinogenesis [7,8]. Spearman's correlation analysis also showed a significant positive correlation between 8-OHdG intensity and the number of tumors in Figure 2C ($r = 0.731$; p-value $= 0.0004$). The intensity of the 8-OHdG stained area (%) was higher in the SF group than in the HC group (Figure 2D,E). These IHC and correlation analysis results imply that the increased tumor development caused by SF was associated with elevated 8-OHdG levels in the colon.

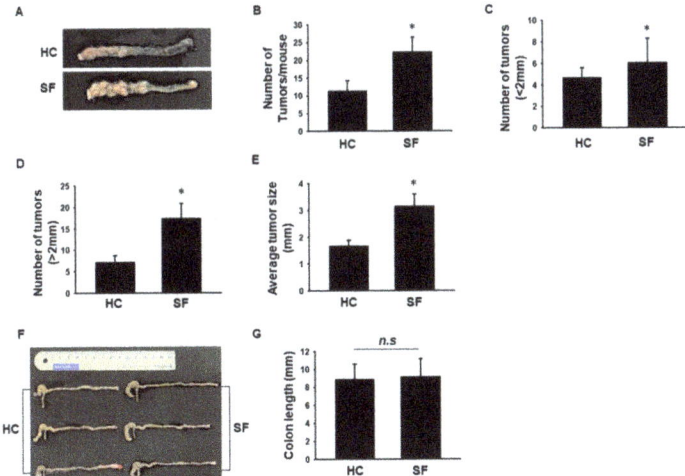

Figure 1. Tumor growth in mice in the home cage control (HC) and sleep fragmentation (SF) groups. (**A**). Macroscopic view of colon tumors that developed in the mice of the HC and SF groups. (**B**). Comparison of the number of tumors. (**C**). Comparison of the number of tumors < 2 mm. (**D**). Comparison of the number of tumors > 2 mm. (**E**). Average tumor size in the HC and SF groups. (**F**). Representative images of mouse colons from the HC and SF groups. (**G**) Comparison of colon lengths between the HC and SF groups. Data are presented as the mean ± S.E.M. * $p < 0.05$ compared with the HC group, as determined by the Mann-Whitney U test. n.s. non-significant.

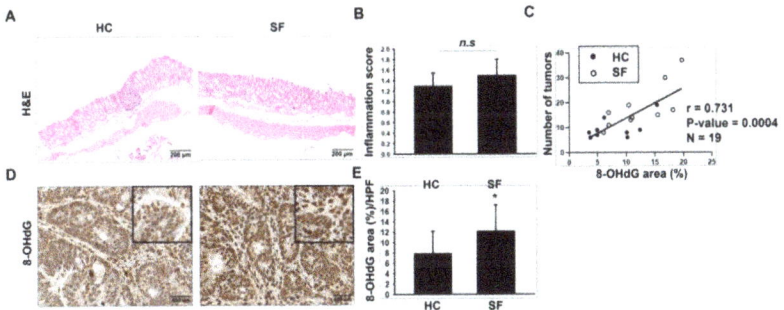

Figure 2. Results of H & E staining and immunohistochemical staining for 8-OHdG. (**A**) Representative H & E-stained images of colon tissue and (**B**) comparison of inflammation scores. (**C**) Spearman's correlation analysis between number of tumors and 8-OHdG area (%). (**D**) Representative immunohistochemical-stained images for 8-hydroxyl-2′-deoxyguanosine (8-OHdG) in the colons of mice from the HC and SF groups and (**E**) quantification of the stained area (%). Data are presented as the mean ± S.E.M. * $p < 0.05$ compared with the HC group, as determined by the Mann-Whitney U test. n.s. non-significant.

2.3. ROS Measurements in Colon Tissue

To evaluate whether SF itself can elevate oxidative stress in the colon, we designed an SF experiment without AOM/DSS treatment (Experiment 2). The confocal microscope analysis showed that the fluorescence intensities of ROS in the colon were significantly higher in the SF group than in the HC group (Figure 3A,B).

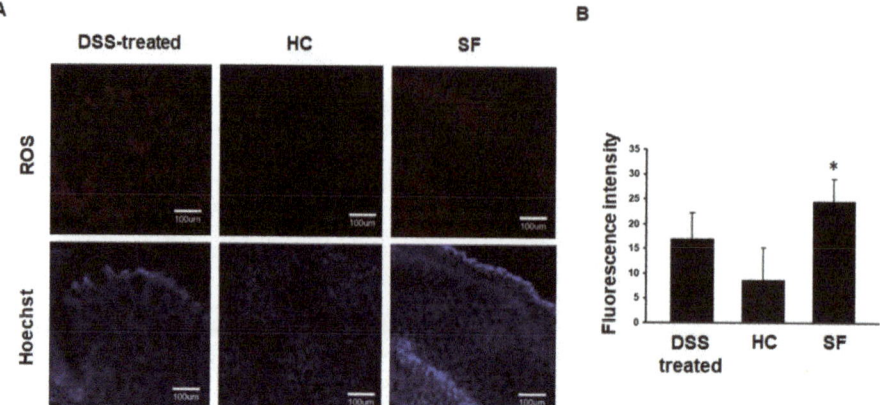

Figure 3. Confocal microscopic images showing ROS in colon tissue from mice in the DSS-treated, HC, and SF groups. (**A**). Representative confocal images of ROS in the colons of mice in the 2% DSS-treated (n = 3), HC (n = 5), and SF (n = 5) groups. (**B**). Comparison of fluorescence intensity showing ROS in colon tissues across the groups. Data are presented as the mean ± S.E.M. * $p < 0.05$ compared with the HC group, as determined by the Mann-Whitney U test.

2.4. Gene Expression Analysis

Next, we conducted qRT-PCR to assess the gene expression associated with ROS generation and inflammation in the colon (Experiment 2). The level of *NOX1*, a colonic epithelium-specific ROS-generating enzyme, tended to increase in the SF group, but the difference from the HC group did not reach statistical significance (Figure 4), possibly due to our small sample size. The level of *NOX2*, a macrophage-specific ROS-generating enzyme, did not differ between the groups. No significant differences between the HC and SF groups were found in proinflammatory cytokine (*IL-1β* and *IL-6*) levels, supporting the results of Experiment 1 that SF increased oxidative stress in the colon without exacerbating inflammation.

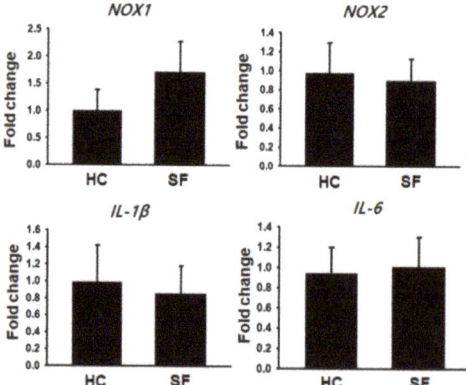

Figure 4. Expression of genes related to ROS generation and inflammation in tumor tissues from mice in the HC and SF groups. Comparison of relative NOX1, NOX2, IL-1β, and IL-6 mRNA expression levels in tumors from mice in the HC and SF groups. Data are presented as the mean ± S.E.M3.

3. Discussion

This chemical-induced carcinogenesis study has shown that chronic SF increases colon carcinogenesis in mice. Tumor size was also larger in the colons of SF mice than in the control mice. Elevated ROS and the resulting oxidative DNA damage were associated with

SF-induced carcinogenesis. To our knowledge, no previous studies have examined the direct effect of SF on carcinogenesis; therefore, our results support the previous finding that OSA is associated with an increased risk of colon cancer and further suggest that SF alone might contribute to cancer development even in the absence of confounding conditions such as sleep duration or IH.

Epidemiology studies about the association between sleep disorders and cancer have already shown that chronically altered sleep cycles [9] or short sleep duration [10] increase colorectal cancer risk. Sleep quality is also an important factor in cancer risk. The English Longitudinal Study of Ageing examined the association between sleep quality and incident cancer risk and found that poor sleep quality, as assessed by questionnaire, was associated with an increase in the long-term incident cancer risk (HR 1.586, 95% CI 1.149–2.189) [11]. Increased production of glucocorticoids, activation of the sympathetic nervous system, and exacerbated inflammation have been suggested as possible mechanisms linking sleep disorders and cancer pathogenesis [12,13], but the causal relationship between them is still ambiguous due to a lack of appropriate experimental models and design limitations in human studies.

SF is a common feature of many types of sleep disorders, and it is particularly characteristic of patients with OSA, in whom the cessation of breathing causes arousal during sleep, which opens the airway but interferes with sleep continuation. These arousals can occur several to dozens of times per hour during sleep.

Most human and animal studies that have investigated the influence of SF on body systems have focused on cognitive function, the cardiovascular system, or metabolism. They have reported a significant causal effect of SF or cross-sectional relationships between SF and poor cognitive function [14], endothelial dysfunction [15], atherosclerosis [16], and insulin resistance [17]. To the best of our knowledge, only two previous animal studies examined the effect of SF on tumors. Hakim et al. used mice deficient in TLR4 or its downstream molecules MYD88 or TRIF [3]. After the engraftment of tumor cells, the mice were subjected to SF for 28 days and examined for tumor growth and invasiveness. SF accelerated tumor growth and increased tumor invasiveness to adjacent tissue through changes in the microenvironment that facilitated cancer progression. The other study that examined the effect of SF on tumors also reported increased tumor growth in mice subjected to SF and that increased tumor growth was mediated by phagocytic Nox2 activity within the tumor [4]. In those two studies, however, tumor cells were implanted into mice before SF. Therefore, those studies cannot confirm the carcinogenic effect of SF.

We found elevated ROS in the colon tissue of mice subjected only to SF. Although it is difficult to say that the increased ROS found in the AOM/DSS experiments was the direct or sole cause of SF-induced colon carcinogenesis because we did not perform an intensive mechanistic study using pharmacological inhibition or genetic manipulation experiments, it is well known that ROS-induced genomic instability, such as 8-OHdG accumulation, is an important cause of carcinogenesis [18,19].

Many studies have reported altered or increased oxidative stress in different organs during sleep disturbance. In rodents, antioxidant defense responses to sleep loss were decreased in the liver [20], and ROS were elevated in hepatocytes by REM sleep deprivation [21], implying that the liver is susceptible to sleep loss. Sleep loss also alters antioxidant responses in the brain [22,23]. However, it is not known whether the increased oxidative stress caused by sleep disturbances is a cause or a result of other damage.

ROS accumulation in the gut is a critical factor in death caused by sleep deprivation (SD). Vaccaro et al. showed that SD induced ROS accumulation, oxidative stress, and DNA damage only in the guts of flies and mice [6]. Elevated oxidative stress shortened the lifespans of both animals, and gut-specific expression of antioxidant enzymes through genetic manipulation extended the survival of both. These findings indicate that the detrimental effects of SD are not equally distributed to all organs and are concentrated in the gut in terms of oxidative stress. Although the sleep disturbance model used in Vaccaro's study differed slightly from our model (SF vs. SD), our results support Vaccaro's findings and further suggest a possible role of SF in colon carcinogenesis.

4. Materials and Methods

4.1. Experimental Design

Thirty-seven male, 8-week-old C57BL/6 mice (DBL Co., Ltd., Eumseong, Republic of Korea) were used in this study, which consisted of two different protocols (Figure 5A,B). The first protocol (Experiment 1) examined the effect of SF on colon carcinogenesis. The mice in Experiment 1 were randomly divided into two groups: home cage control (HC; n = 12) and SF (n = 12). Mice in both groups received one intraperitoneal injection of AOM (10 mg/kg; Sigma-Aldrich, St. Louis, MO, USA). Then, the mice in the HC and SF groups were exposed to normal conditions and the SF protocol, respectively, for 77 days. 2% DSS (MP Biomedicals, Santa Ana, CA, USA) was given in the drinking water on Days 7–14, Days 28–35, and Days 49–56. The mice were sacrificed on Day 77, and tissue samples were harvested for further analysis. The second protocol (Experiment 2) tested our hypothesis that SF alone can elevate reactive oxygen species (ROS). Mice in the HC (n = 5) and SF groups (n = 5) were maintained in normal conditions and the SF chamber for 4 weeks without any administration of AOM or DSS. The 2% DSS group (n = 3) was given 2% DSS in their drinking water between 3 and 4 weeks as a positive control of the ROS measurements. Both experimental protocols were approved by the Jungwon University Institutional Animal Use and Care Committee and are in close agreement with the NIH Guide on the Care and Use of Animals.

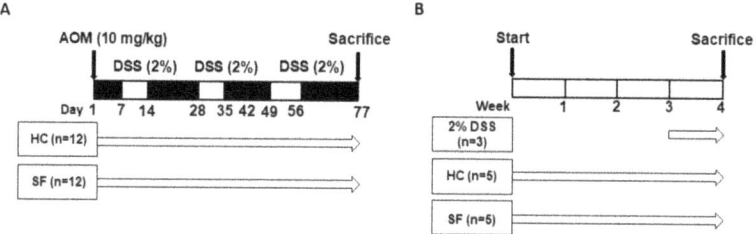

Figure 5. Schematic representation of the experimental protocols. (**A**). Schematic design of Experiment 1. A single intraperitoneal injection of 10 mg/kg azoxymethane (AOM) was given to mice in both the control and sleep fragmentation (SF) groups. Subsequently, mice in the control group were maintained in a normal cage until the end of the experiment (77 days). Mice in the SF group were subjected to SF, which was accomplished by a sweeping bar activated every 2 min (30/h). Dextran sodium sulfate (DSS) was given in the drinking water on Days 7–14, 28–35, and 49–56. (**B**). Schematic design of Experiment 2. Mice in the control and SF groups were maintained in normal cages and SF chambers, respectively, for 4 weeks. 2% DSS was given to other mice in their drinking water at 3–4 weeks as a positive control.

4.2. Sleep Fragmentation

To induce SF, we used a commercially available SF chamber (Model 80391; Lafayette Instrument, Lafayette, IN, USA). The chamber has a sweeping bar inside that moves from one end to the other. When it touches the mice, they awaken from sleep. To mimic the arousal frequency shown in patients with severe sleep apnea (30 awakenings/h), the sweeping bar was set to move once every 2 min. Although we did not perform simultaneous electroencephalography monitoring to evaluate whether SF was appropriately induced, several studies using the same chamber have already validated this SF model [24,25].

4.3. Histological Evaluation

Colon tissue was harvested on Day 77 and washed with cold phosphate-buffered saline (PBS). To compare the colon length between the HC and SF groups, colons from the cecum to the rectum were placed on a plate with a black background and photographed with a digital camera. After taking those colon images, the cecum was removed, and the remaining colon was opened longitudinally along the main axis to expose the internal tumors. After taking a picture of the inside of each colon, the colons were divided into their distal parts and middle parts for histological analysis and quantitative real-time polymerase chain reaction experiments, respectively. Tumor number and size were evaluated by two independent investigators and expressed as the mean value of the two measurements. To obtain reproducible results, the number of tumors was counted by dividing them into those that were 2 mm or larger and those that were 2 mm or smaller [26]. Hematoxylin and eosin (H & E) staining was performed for general histological assessments and colonic inflammation score calculation. After H & E staining, five random areas of the colon per tissue slide were used to calculate the colonic inflammation score. Colonic inflammation was classified into five grades (Grade 0 to Grade 4) based on the criteria of Cooper et al. [27,28].

4.4. Immunofluorescent ROS Staining

Immunofluorescent staining of colon tissue from mice in the HC and SF groups in Experiment 2 was conducted to measure ROS using a protocol from a previous study [6]. Distal colons excised from the mice were immediately placed on dry ice and embedded in the O.C.T. compound (Tissue-Tek). 30-μm thick sections were obtained using a cryomicrotome. The sections were air-dried and then incubated with 10 μM dihydroethidium (Sigma-Aldrich, St. Louis, MO, USA) at 37 °C for 30 min. After being washed with PBS, the sections were incubated with 1 μg/mL Hoechst 33342 (Thermo Fisher, Waltham, MA, USA) at room temperature for 10 min. Then, the sections were mounted with Fluoroshield (Sigma-Aldrich, St. Louis, MO, USA). The red fluorescence of each image was obtained by excitation at 610 nm and collected at 600–780 nm using confocal microscopy (LSM 700, Carl Zeiss, Jena, Germany).

4.5. Immunohistochemical 8-OHdG Staining

For immunohistochemistry (IHC), excised colon tissue was fixed with 10% neutral-buffered formalin, embedded in paraffin, and cut into 4-μm slices using a rotary microtome. For antigen retrieval, tissue slides were autoclaved with HIER citrate buffer (pH 6.0; Zytomed Systems, Berlin, Germany). IHC for 8-OHdG staining was conducted using a commercial mouse and rabbit-specific HRP/DAB detection kit (Abcam, Cambridge, UK). After being incubated with 3% hydrogen peroxide in methanol for 10 min, the sections were treated with a blocking solution for 1 h at room temperature to remove nonspecific background reactions. Following treatment with blocking solution, the sections were incubated with anti-8-OHdG/8-oxo-dG monoclonal antibody (1:200; JalCA, Nikken SEIL CO, Shizuoka, Japan) for 1 h at 4 °C. After washing the samples with TBST four times, a biotinylated goat anti-polyvalent was applied to the tissues and incubated for 10 min at 4 °C. After being treated with streptavidin peroxidase for 10 min, the sections were developed with 3,3′-diaminobenzidine solution. As a counterstain, hematoxylin QS (Vector Laboratories, Inc., Burlingame, CA, USA) was applied to the tissues for 1 min, and then the sections were dehydrated, cleared, and mounted for microscopic examination. The stained slides were scanned with a Pannoramic SCAN II slide scanner (3d Histech, Budapest, Hungary). Then, 4–5 high-power field images (400 X) per slide were randomly acquired. The intensity (%) of the stained area in each image was blindly analyzed using ImageJ (NIH, Bethesda, MD, USA).

4.6. Quantitative Real-Time Polymerase Chain Reaction (qRT-PCR)

Total RNA was extracted from the colon tissue using an RNeasy mini kit (Qiagen, Germantown, MD, USA). One microgram of total RNA was used for cDNA synthesis and reverse transcribed using a Tetro cDNA synthesis kit (Bioline, London, UK). qRT-PCR was performed using a StepOne Plus™ real-time PCR system (Applied Biosystems, Waltham, MA, USA). TaqMan real-time PCR master mixes were used for TaqMan assay–based real-time PCR. The following TaqMan primer and probes were purchased from Applied Biosystems: NADPH oxidase 2 (NOX2) assay# Mm01287743_m1, NOX1 assay# Mm00549170_m1, interleukin (IL)-1β assay# Mm00434228_m1, IL-6 assay# Mm00446190_m1, and β-actin assay# Mm02619580_g1. All reactions were performed in duplicate. The 2ΔΔ method was used for the relative comparison of genes between the HC and SF groups. β-actin was used as a housekeeping gene for normalization.

4.7. Statistical Analysis

Data are expressed as the mean ± standard error of the mean (S.E.M). Differences in the means were evaluated using the non-parametric Kruskal-Wallis test. Mann-Whitney U-tests were used for the post hoc analyses and comparisons of variables between two independent groups. Spearman's rank correlation coefficients were calculated to evaluate correlations between the intensity of 8-OHdG stained areas (%) and the number of tumors. All statistical analyses were performed using IBM SPSS version 21.0 (SPSS; Chicago, IL, USA), and a p-value < 0.05 was considered to be statistically significant.

5. Conclusions

We found that SF has carcinogenic effects in the murine AOM/DSS colon cancer model. Moreover, elevated oxidative stress-induced DNA damage correlated with an increase in carcinogenesis. Our findings suggest that SF is a risk factor for colon cancer and that preventing ROS accumulation is important for preventing the development of SF-induced colon cancer. Further studies are needed to elucidate whether SF can induce carcinogenesis in other visceral organs and determine the exact mechanism by which SF promotes carcinogenesis.

Author Contributions: Conceptualization, S.-W.K. and D.-W.Y.; methodology, D.-B.L., S.-Y.A. and S.-S.P.; formal analysis, D.-B.L., J.K. and D.-W.Y.; writing, D.-B.L. and D.-W.Y.; supervision, S.-W.K. and D.-W.Y.; funding acquisition, D.-W.Y. All authors have read and agreed to the published version of the manuscript.

Funding: This study was supported by the Jungwon University Research Grant (2020-016). The funders have no role in the study.

Institutional Review Board Statement: All animals used in the study were treated in accordance with the NIH Guide for the Care and Use of Laboratory Animals and the whole procedure was approved by the Animal Ethics Committee of Jungwon University.

Informed Consent Statement: Not applicable.

Data Availability Statement: The data presented in this study are available on request from the corresponding author.

Conflicts of Interest: The authors declare no conflict of interest.

References

1. Chen, Y.; Tan, F.; Wei, L.; Li, X.; Lyu, Z.; Feng, X.; Wen, Y.; Guo, L.; He, J.; Dai, M.; et al. Sleep duration and the risk of cancer: A systematic review and meta-analysis including dose-response relationship. *BMC Cancer* **2018**, *18*, 1149. [CrossRef] [PubMed]
2. Bhagavan, S.M.; Sahota, P.K. Sleep Fragmentation and Atherosclerosis: Is There a Relationship? *Mo. Med.* **2021**, *118*, 272–276. [PubMed]
3. Hakim, F.; Wang, Y.; Zhang, S.X.; Zheng, J.; Yolcu, E.S.; Carreras, A.; Khalyfa, A.; Shirwan, H.; Almendros, I.; Gozal, D. Fragmented sleep accelerates tumor growth and progression through recruitment of tumor-associated macrophages and TLR4 signaling. *Cancer Res.* **2014**, *74*, 1329–1337. [CrossRef] [PubMed]
4. Zheng, J.; Almendros, I.; Wang, Y.; Zhang, S.X.; Carreras, A.; Qiao, Z.; Gozal, D. Reduced NADPH oxidase type 2 activity mediates sleep fragmentation-induced effects on TC1 tumors in mice. *Oncoimmunology* **2015**, *4*, e976057. [CrossRef]
5. Lee, S.; Kim, B.G.; Kim, J.W.; Lee, K.L.; Koo, D.L.; Nam, H.; Im, J.P.; Kim, J.S.; Koh, S.J. Obstructive sleep apnea is associated with an increased risk of colorectal neoplasia. *Gastrointest. Endosc.* **2017**, *85*, 568–573.e1. [CrossRef]
6. Vaccaro, A.; Kaplan Dor, Y.; Nambara, K.; Pollina, E.A.; Lin, C.; Greenberg, M.E.; Rogulja, D. Sleep Loss Can Cause Death through Accumulation of Reactive Oxygen Species in the Gut. *Cell* **2020**, *181*, 1307–1328.e15. [CrossRef]
7. Afanas'ev, I. Reactive oxygen species signaling in cancer: Comparison with aging. *Aging Dis.* **2011**, *2*, 219–230.

8. Pan, J.S.; Hong, M.Z.; Ren, J.L. Reactive oxygen species: A double-edged sword in oncogenesis. *World J. Gastroenterol.* **2009**, *15*, 1702–1707. [CrossRef]
9. Schernhammer, E.S.; Laden, F.; Speizer, F.E.; Willett, W.C.; Hunter, D.J.; Kawachi, I.; Fuchs, C.S.; Colditz, G.A. Night-shift work and risk of colorectal cancer in the nurses' health study. *J. Natl. Cancer Inst.* **2003**, *95*, 825–828. [CrossRef]
10. Thompson, C.L.; Larkin, E.K.; Patel, S.; Berger, N.A.; Redline, S.; Li, L. Short duration of sleep increases risk of colorectal adenoma. *Cancer* **2011**, *117*, 841–847. [CrossRef]
11. Song, C.; Zhang, R.; Wang, C.; Fu, R.; Song, W.; Dou, K.; Wang, S. Sleep quality and risk of cancer: Findings from the English longitudinal study of aging. *Sleep* **2021**, *44*, zsaa192. [CrossRef] [PubMed]
12. Mogavero, M.P.; DelRosso, L.M.; Fanfulla, F.; Bruni, O.; Ferri, R. Sleep disorders and cancer: State of the art and future perspectives. *Sleep Med. Rev.* **2021**, *56*, 101409. [CrossRef] [PubMed]
13. Walker, W.H., 2nd; Borniger, J.C. Molecular Mechanisms of Cancer-Induced Sleep Disruption. *Int. J. Mol. Sci.* **2019**, *20*, 2780. [CrossRef] [PubMed]
14. Kaneshwaran, K.; Olah, M.; Tasaki, S.; Yu, L.; Bradshaw, E.M.; Schneider, J.A.; Buchman, A.S.; Bennett, D.A.; De Jager, P.L.; Lim, A.S.P. Sleep fragmentation, microglial aging, and cognitive impairment in adults with and without Alzheimer's dementia. *Sci. Adv.* **2019**, *5*, eaax7331. [CrossRef]
15. Carreras, A.; Zhang, S.X.; Peris, E.; Qiao, Z.; Gileles-Hillel, A.; Li, R.C.; Wang, Y.; Gozal, D. Chronic sleep fragmentation induces endothelial dysfunction and structural vascular changes in mice. *Sleep* **2014**, *37*, 1817–1824. [CrossRef]
16. McAlpine, C.S.; Kiss, M.G.; Rattik, S.; He, S.; Vassalli, A.; Valet, C.; Anzai, A.; Chan, C.T.; Mindur, J.E.; Kahles, F.; et al. Sleep modulates haematopoiesis and protects against atherosclerosis. *Nature* **2019**, *566*, 383–387. [CrossRef] [PubMed]
17. Zhang, S.X.; Khalyfa, A.; Wang, Y.; Carreras, A.; Hakim, F.; Neel, B.A.; Brady, M.J.; Qiao, Z.; Hirotsu, C.; Gozal, D. Sleep fragmentation promotes NADPH oxidase 2-mediated adipose tissue inflammation leading to insulin resistance in mice. *Int. J. Obes.* **2014**, *38*, 619–624. [CrossRef]
18. Nishida, N.; Arizumi, T.; Takita, M.; Kitai, S.; Yada, N.; Hagiwara, S.; Inoue, T.; Minami, Y.; Ueshima, K.; Sakurai, T.; et al. Reactive oxygen species induce epigenetic instability through the formation of 8-hydroxydeoxyguanosine in human hepatocarcinogenesis. *Dig. Dis.* **2013**, *31*, 459–466. [CrossRef]
19. Shibutani, S.; Takeshita, M.; Grollman, A.P. Insertion of specific bases during DNA synthesis past the oxidation-damaged base 8-oxodG. *Nature* **1991**, *349*, 431–434. [CrossRef]
20. Everson, C.A.; Laatsch, C.D.; Hogg, N. Antioxidant defense responses to sleep loss and sleep recovery. *Am. J. Physiol. Regul. Integr. Comp. Physiol.* **2005**, *288*, R374–R383. [CrossRef]
21. Pandey, A.; Kar, S.K. Rapid Eye Movement sleep deprivation of rat generates ROS in the hepatocytes and makes them more susceptible to oxidative stress. *Sleep Sci.* **2018**, *11*, 245–253. [CrossRef] [PubMed]
22. Alzoubi, K.H.; Khabour, O.F.; Rashid, B.A.; Damaj, I.M.; Salah, H.A. The neuroprotective effect of vitamin E on chronic sleep deprivation-induced memory impairment: The role of oxidative stress. *Behav. Brain Res.* **2012**, *226*, 205–210. [CrossRef] [PubMed]
23. Kanazawa, L.K.S.; Vecchia, D.D.; Wendler, E.M.; Hocayen, P.A.S.; Dos Reis Lívero, F.A.; Stipp, M.C.; Barcaro, I.M.R.; Acco, A.; Andreatini, R. Quercetin reduces manic-like behavior and brain oxidative stress induced by paradoxical sleep deprivation in mice. *Free Radic. Biol. Med.* **2016**, *99*, 79–86. [CrossRef] [PubMed]
24. Nair, D.; Zhang, S.X.; Ramesh, V.; Hakim, F.; Kaushal, N.; Wang, Y.; Gozal, D. Sleep fragmentation induces cognitive deficits via nicotinamide adenine dinucleotide phosphate oxidase-dependent pathways in mouse. *Am. J. Respir. Crit. Care Med.* **2011**, *184*, 1305–1312. [CrossRef] [PubMed]
25. Ramesh, V.; Nair, D.; Zhang, S.X.; Hakim, F.; Kaushal, N.; Kayali, F.; Wang, Y.; Li, R.C.; Carreras, A.; Gozal, D. Disrupted sleep without sleep curtailment induces sleepiness and cognitive dysfunction via the tumor necrosis factor-α pathway. *J. Neuroinflammation* **2012**, *9*, 91. [CrossRef]
26. Thaker, A.I.; Shaker, A.; Rao, M.S.; Ciorba, M.A. Modeling colitis-associated cancer with azoxymethane (AOM) and dextran sulfate sodium (DSS). *J. Vis. Exp.* **2012**, *67*, 4100.
27. Cooper, H.S.; Murthy, S.N.; Shah, R.S.; Sedergran, D.J. Clinicopathologic study of dextran sulfate sodium experimental murine colitis. *Lab Investig.* **1993**, *69*, 238–249.
28. Suzuki, R.; Kohno, H.; Sugie, S.; Nakagama, H.; Tanaka, T. Strain differences in the susceptibility to azoxymethane and dextran sodium sulfate-induced colon carcinogenesis in mice. *Carcinogenesis* **2006**, *27*, 162–169. [CrossRef]

Disclaimer/Publisher's Note: The statements, opinions and data contained in all publications are solely those of the individual author(s) and contributor(s) and not of MDPI and/or the editor(s). MDPI and/or the editor(s) disclaim responsibility for any injury to people or property resulting from any ideas, methods, instructions or products referred to in the content.

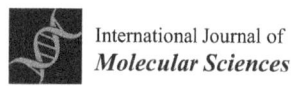

Article

Development of a Novel Anti-CD44 Variant 6 Monoclonal Antibody C$_{44}$Mab-9 for Multiple Applications against Colorectal Carcinomas

Ryo Ejima [1,†], Hiroyuki Suzuki [1,*,†], Tomohiro Tanaka [1], Teizo Asano [2], Mika K. Kaneko [2] and Yukinari Kato [1,2,*]

[1] Department of Molecular Pharmacology, Tohoku University Graduate School of Medicine, 2-1 Seiryo-machi, Aoba-ku, Sendai 980-8575, Japan
[2] Department of Antibody Drug Development, Tohoku University Graduate School of Medicine, 2-1 Seiryo-machi, Aoba-ku, Sendai 980-8575, Japan
* Correspondence: hiroyuki.suzuki.b4@tohoku.ac.jp (H.S.); yukinari.kato.e6@tohoku.ac.jp (Y.K.); Tel.: +81-22-717-8207 (H.S. & Y.K.)
† These authors contributed equally to this work.

Abstract: CD44 is a cell surface glycoprotein, and its isoforms are produced by the alternative splicing with the standard and variant exons. The CD44 variant exon-containing isoforms (CD44v) are overexpressed in carcinomas. CD44v6 is one of the CD44v, and its overexpression predicts poor prognosis in colorectal cancer (CRC) patients. CD44v6 plays critical roles in CRC adhesion, proliferation, stemness, invasiveness, and chemoresistance. Therefore, CD44v6 is a promising target for cancer diagnosis and therapy for CRC. In this study, we established anti-CD44 monoclonal antibodies (mAbs) by immunizing mice with CD44v3-10-overexpressed Chinese hamster ovary (CHO)-K1 cells. We then characterized them using enzyme-linked immunosorbent assay, flow cytometry, western blotting, and immunohistochemistry. One of the established clones (C$_{44}$Mab-9; IgG$_1$, kappa) reacted with a peptide of the variant 6-encoded region, indicating that C$_{44}$Mab-9 recognizes CD44v6. Furthermore, C$_{44}$Mab-9 reacted with CHO/CD44v3-10 cells or CRC cell lines (COLO201 and COLO205) by flow cytometry. The apparent dissociation constant (K_D) of C$_{44}$Mab-9 for CHO/CD44v3-10, COLO201, and COLO205 was 8.1×10^{-9} M, 1.7×10^{-8} M, and 2.3×10^{-8} M, respectively. C$_{44}$Mab-9 detected the CD44v3-10 in western blotting, and partially stained the formalin-fixed paraffin-embedded CRC tissues in immunohistochemistry. Collectively, C$_{44}$Mab-9 is useful for detecting CD44v6 in various applications.

Keywords: CD44; CD44v6; monoclonal antibody; colorectal cancer

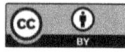

1. Introduction

Colorectal cancer (CRC) has become the second cancer type for the estimated deaths in men and women combined in the United States, 2023 [1]. The development of CRC is classically explained by Fearon and Vogelstein model; the sequential genetic changes including *APC* (adenomatous polyposis coli), *KRAS*, *DCC* (deleted in colorectal cancer, chromosome 18q), and *TP53* lead to CRC progression [2]. However, CRC exhibits heterogeneous outcomes and drug responses. Therefore, the large-scale data analysis by an international consortium classified the CRC into four consensus molecular subtypes, including the microsatellite instability immune, the canonical, the metabolic, and the mesenchymal types [3]. In addition, various marker proteins have been investigated for the prediction of prognosis and drug responses of CRC [4,5]. Among them, recent studies suggest that CD44 plays a critical role in tumor progression through its cancer-initiating and metastasis-promoting properties [6].

CD44 is a polymorphic integral membrane protein, which binds to hyaluronic acid (HA), and contributes to cell-matrix adhesion, cell proliferation, migration, and tumor metastasis [7]. When the CD44 is transcribed, its pre-messenger RNA can be received alternative splicing and maturated into mRNAs that encode various CD44 isoforms [8]. The mRNA assembles with ten standard exons and the sixth variant exon encodes CD44v6, which plays critical roles in cell proliferation, migration, survival, and angiogenesis [9,10]. Functionally, CD44v6 can interact with HA via the standard exons-encoded region [11]. Furthermore, the v6-encoded region functions as a co-receptor of various receptors for epidermal growth factor, hepatocyte growth factor, C-X-C motif chemokine 12, and osteopontin [12]. Therefore, the receptor tyrosine kinase or G protein-coupled receptor signaling pathways are potentiated in the presence of CD44v6 [13]. These functions are essential for homeostasis or regeneration in normal tissues. Importantly, CD44v6 overexpression plays a critical role in CRC progression. For instance, CD44v6 is involved in colorectal carcinoma invasiveness, colonization, and metastasis [14]. Therefore, CD44v6 is a promising target for cancer diagnosis and therapy.

The clinical significance of CD44v6 in CRC deserves consideration. Anti-CD44v6 therapies mainly include the blocking of the v6-encoded region by monoclonal antibody (mAb) [12]. First, humanized anti-CD44v6 mAbs (BIWA-4 and BIWA-8) labeled with ^{186}Re exhibited therapeutic efficacy in head and neck squamous cell carcinoma (SCC) xenograft-bearing mice [15]. Furthermore, the humanized anti-CD44v6 mAb, bivatuzumab-mertansine (anti-tubulin agent) conjugate, was evaluated in clinical trials [16]. However, the clinical trials were discontinued due to severe skin toxicity, including a case of lethal epidermal necrolysis [17]. The efficient accumulation of mertansine was most likely responsible for the high toxicity [17,18]. Therefore, the development of anti-CD44v6 mAbs with more potent and fewer side effects is desired.

We established the novel anti-CD44 mAbs, C_{44}Mab-5 (IgG$_1$, kappa) [19] and C_{44}Mab-46 (IgG$_1$, kappa) [20] by Cell-Based Immunization and Screening (CBIS) method and immunization of CD44v3-10 ectodomain, respectively. Both C_{44}Mab-5 and C_{44}Mab-46 recognize the first five standard exons-encoding sequences [21–23]. Therefore, they can recognize both CD44s and CD44v (pan-CD44). Furthermore, C_{44}Mab-5 and C_{44}Mab-46 exhibited high reactivity for flow cytometry and immunohistochemical analysis in oral [19] and esophageal [20] SCCs. C_{44}Mab-5 reacted with oral cancer cells such as Ca9-22, HO-1-u-1, SAS, HSC-2, HSC-3, and HSC-4 using flow cytometry [19]. Moreover, immunohistochemical analysis revealed that C_{44}Mab-5 detected 166/182 (91.2%) of oral cancers [19]. In contrast, C_{44}Mab-46 reacted with esophageal squamous cell carcinoma (ESCC) cell lines (KYSE70 and KYSE770) using flow cytometry [20]. In immunohistochemical analyses using C_{44}Mab−46 against ESCC tissue microarrays, C_{44}Mab−46 stained 63 of 67 (94.0%) cases of ESCC [20].

We also examined the antitumor effects of C_{44}Mab-5 in mouse xenograft models [24]. We converted the mouse IgG$_1$ subclass antibody (C_{44}Mab-5) into an IgG$_{2a}$ subclass antibody (5-mG$_{2a}$), and further produced a defucosylated version (5-mG$_{2a}$-f) using FUT8-deficient ExpiCHO-S (BINDS-09) cells. In vitro analysis demonstrated that 5-mG$_{2a}$-f showed moderate antibody-dependent cellular cytotoxicity (ADCC) and complement-dependent cytotoxicity activities against HSC-2 and SAS oral cancer cells. In vivo analysis revealed that 5-mG$_{2a}$-f significantly reduced tumor growth in HSC-2 and SAS xenografts in comparison to control mouse IgG, even after injection seven days post-tumor inoculation. These results suggested that treatment with 5-mG$_{2a}$-f may represent a useful therapy for patients with CD44-expressing oral cancers.

For epitope mapping of C_{44}Mab-5, we employed the RIEDL tag system ("RIEDL" peptide and LpMab-7 mAb) [23]. We inserted the "RIEDL" peptide into the CD44 protein from the 21st to 41st amino acids. The transfectants produced were stained by LpMab-7 and C_{44}Mab-5 in flow cytometry. C_{44}Mab-5 did not react with the 30th-36th amino acids of the deletion mutant of CD44. Further, the reaction of C_{44}Mab-5 to RIEDL tag-inserted CD44 from the 25th to 36th amino acids was lost, although LpMab-7 detected most of the RIEDL tag-inserted CD44 from the 21st to 41st amino acids. These results indicated that the epitope of C_{44}Mab-5 for CD44 was determined to be the peptide from the 25th to 36th amino acids of CD44 using the RIEDL insertion for epitope mapping (REMAP) method.

In this study, we developed a novel anti-CD44v6 mAb, C_{44}Mab-9 (IgG$_1$, kappa) by CBIS method, and evaluated its applications, including flow cytometry, western blotting, and immunohistochemical analyses.

2. Results

2.1. Establishment of Anti-CD44v6 mAb, C_{44}Mab-9

We employed the CBIS method to develop anti-CD44 mAbs. In the CBIS method, we prepared a stable transfectant as an immunogen. Then, we performed the high throughput hybridoma screening using flow cytometry (Figure 1). In this study, mice were immunized with CHO/CD44v3-10 cells. Hybridomas were seeded into 96-well plates, and CHO/CD44v3-10-positive and CHO-K1-negative wells were selected. After limiting dilution, anti-CD44 mAb-producing clones were finally established. We next performed an enzyme-linked immunosorbent assay (ELISA) to determine the epitope of each mAb. Among them, C_{44}Mab-9 (IgG$_1$, kappa) was shown to recognize the only CD44p351–370 peptide (EETATQKEQWFGNRWHEGYR), which is corresponding to variant 6-encoded sequence (Table 1).

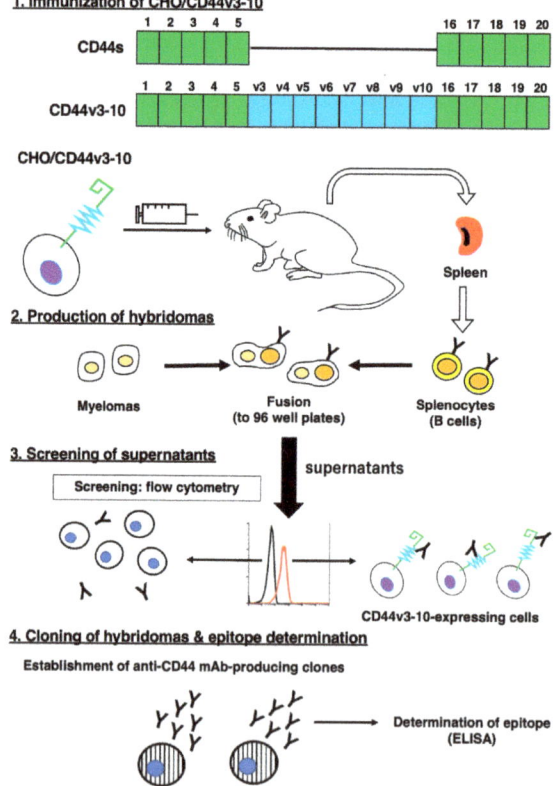

Figure 1. A schematic illustration of ant-human CD44 mAbs production. A BALB/c mouse was intraperitoneally immunized with CHO/CD44v3-10 cells. Hybridomas were produced by the fusion of the splenocytes and P3U1 cells. Then, the screening was performed by flow cytometry using parental CHO-K1 and CHO/CD44v3-10 cells. After cloning and additional screening, a clone C_{44}Mab-9 (IgG$_1$, kappa) was established. Finally, the binding epitopes were determined by enzyme-linked immunosorbent assay (ELISA) using peptides that cover the extracellular domain of CD44v3-10.

Table 1. The determination of the binding epitope of C$_{44}$Mab-9 by ELISA.

Peptide	Coding Exon *	Sequence	C$_{44}$Mab-9
CD44p21–40	2	QIDLNITCRFAGVFHVEKNG	–
CD44p31–50	2	AGVFHVEKNGRYSISRTEAA	–
CD44p41–60	2	RYSISRTEAADLCKAFNSTL	–
CD44p51–70	2	DLCKAFNSTLPTMAQMEKAL	–
CD44p61–80	2/3	PTMAQMEKALSIGFETCRYG	–
CD44p71–90	2/3	SIGFETCRYGFIEGHVVIPR	–
CD44p81–100	3	FIEGHVVIPRIHPNSICAAN	–
CD44p91–110	3	IHPNSICAANNTGVYILTSN	–
CD44p101–120	3	NTGVYILTSNTSQYDTYCFN	–
CD44p111–130	3/4	TSQYDTYCFNASAPPEEDCT	–
CD44p121–140	3/4	ASAPPEEDCTSVTDLPNAFD	–
CD44p131–150	4/5	SVTDLPNAFDGPITITIVNR	–
CD44p141–160	4/5	GPITITIVNRDGTRYVQKGE	–
CD44p151–170	5	DGTRYVQKGEYRTNPEDIYP	–
CD44p161–180	5	YRTNPEDIYPSNPTDDDVSS	–
CD44p171–190	5	SNPTDDDVSSGSSSERSSTS	–
CD44p181–200	5	GSSSERSSTSGGYIFYTFST	–
CD44p191–210	5	GGYIFYTFSTVHPIPDEDSP	–
CD44p201–220	5	VHPIPDEDSPWITDSTDRIP	–
CD44p211–230	5/v3	WITDSTDRIPATSTSSNTIS	–
CD44p221–240	5/v3	ATSTSSNTISAGWEPNEENE	–
CD44p231–250	v3	AGWEPNEENEDERDRHLSFS	–
CD44p241–260	v3	DERDRHLSFSGSGIDDDEDF	–
CD44p251–270	v3/v4	GSGIDDDEDFISSTISTTPR	–
CD44p261–280	v3/v4	ISSTISTTPRAFDHTKQNQD	–
CD44p271–290	v4	AFDHTKQNQDWTQWNPSHSN	–
CD44p281–300	v4	WTQWNPSHSNPEVLLQTTTR	–
CD44p291–310	v4/v5	PEVLLQTTTRMTDVDRNGTT	–
CD44p301–320	v4/v5	MTDVDRNGTTAYEGNWNPEA	–
CD44p311–330	v5	AYEGNWNPEAHPPLIHHEHH	–
CD44p321–340	v5	HPPLIHHEHHEEEETPHSTS	–
CD44p331–350	v5/v6	EEEETPHSTSTIQATPSSTT	–
CD44p341–360	v5/v6	TIQATPSSTTEETATQKEQW	–
CD44p351–370	v6	EETATQKEQWFGNRWHEGYR	+

Table 1. Cont.

Peptide	Coding Exon *	Sequence	C_{44}Mab-9
CD44p361–380	v6	FGNRWHEGYRQTPREDSHST	−
CD44p371–390	v6/v7	QTPREDSHSTTGTAAASAHT	−
CD44p381–400	v6/v7	TGTAAASAHTSHPMQGRTTP	−
CD44p391–410	v7	SHPMQGRTTPSPEDSSWTDF	−
CD44p401–420	v7	SPEDSSWTDFFNPISHPMGR	−
CD44p411–430	v7/v8	FNPISHPMGRGHQAGRRMDM	−
CD44p421–440	v7/v8	GHQAGRRMDMDSSHSTTLQP	−
CD44p431–450	v8	DSSHSTTLQPTANPNTGLVE	−
CD44p441–460	v8	TANPNTGLVEDLDRTGPLSM	−
CD44p451–470	v8/v9	DLDRTGPLSMTTQQSNSQSF	−
CD44p461–480	v8/v9	TTQQSNSQSFSTSHEGLEED	−
CD44p471–490	v9	STSHEGLEEDKDHPTTSTLT	−
CD44p481–500	v9/v10	KDHPTTSTLTSSNRNDVTGG	−
CD44p491–510	v9/v10	SSNRNDVTGGRRDPNHSEGS	−
CD44p501–520	v10	RRDPNHSEGSTTLLEGYTSH	−
CD44p511–530	v10	TTLLEGYTSHYPHTKESRTF	−
CD44p521–540	v10	YPHTKESRTFIPVTSAKTGS	−
CD44p531–550	v10	IPVTSAKTGSFGVTAVTVGD	−
CD44p541–560	v10	FGVTAVTVGDSNSNVNRSLS	−
CD44p551–570	v10/16	SNSNVNRSLSGDQDTFHPSG	−
CD44p561–580	v10/16	GDQDTFHPSGGSHTTHGSES	−
CD44p571–590	16/17	GSHTTHGSESDGHSHGSQEG	−
CD44p581–600	16/17	DGHSHGSQEGGANTTSGPIR	−
CD44p591–606	17	GANTTSGPIRTPQIPEAAAA	−

+, OD655 ≥ 0.3; −, OD655 < 0.1. * The CD44 exons are illustrated in Figure 1.

2.2. Flow Cytometric Analysis of C_{44}Mab-9 to CD44-Expressing Cells

We next confirmed the reactivity of C_{44}Mab-9 against CHO/CD44v3-10 and CHO/CD44s cells by flow cytometry. As shown in Figure 2A, C_{44}Mab-9 recognized CHO/CD44v3-10 cells in a dose-dependent manner, but neither CHO/CD44s (Figure 2B) nor CHO-K1 (Figure 2C) cells. The CHO/CD44s cells were recognized by a pan-CD44 mAb, C_{44}Mab-46 [20] (Supplemental Figure S1). Furthermore, C_{44}Mab-9 also recognized endogenous CD44v6 in CRC cell lines as it reacted with both COLO201 (Figure 2D) and COLO205 (Figure 2E) in a dose-dependent manner.

Next, we determined the binding affinity of C_{44}Mab-9 with CHO/CD44v3-10, COLO201, and COLO205 using flow cytometry. The dissociation constant (K_D) of C_{44}Mab-9 for CHO/CD44v3-10, COLO201, and COLO205 was 8.1×10^{-9} M, 1.7×10^{-8} M, and 2.3×10^{-8} M, respectively, indicating that C_{44}Mab-9 possesses a moderate affinity for CD44v3-10 or endogenous CD44v6-expressing cells (Figure 3).

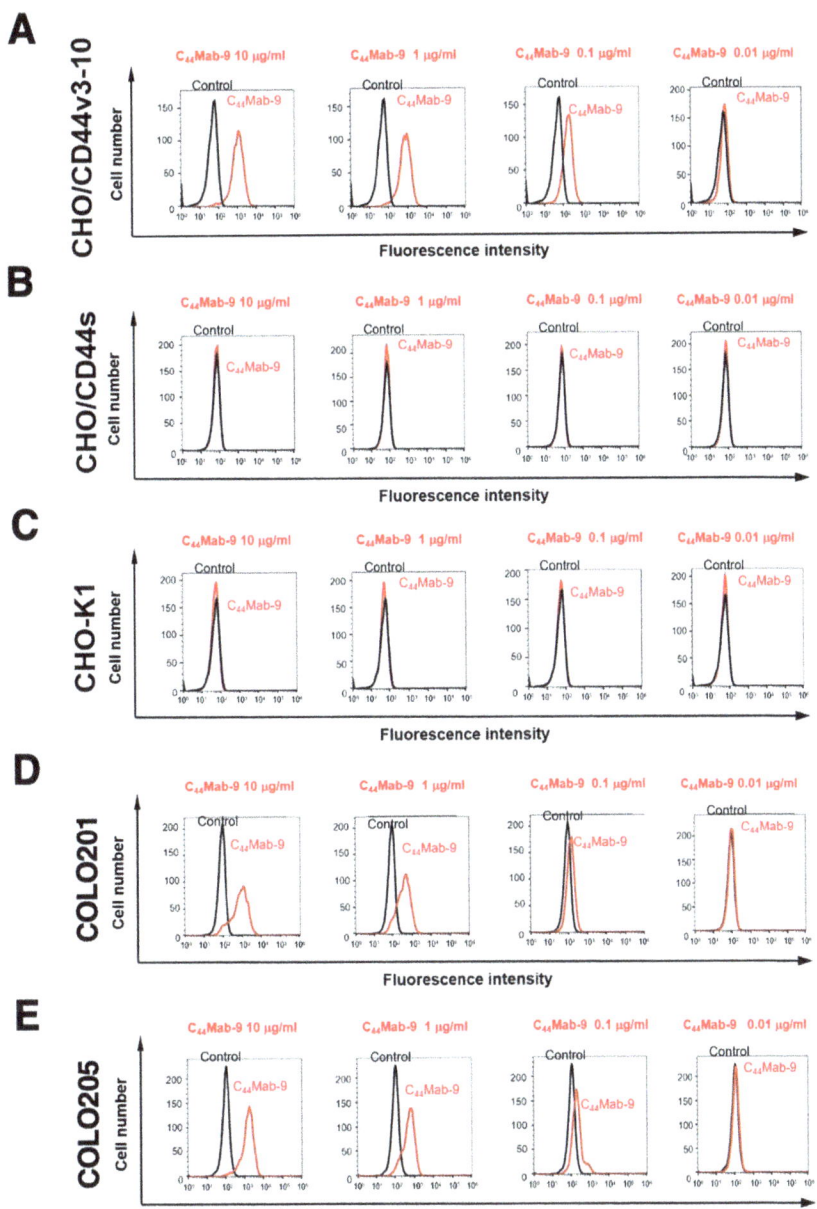

Figure 2. Flow cytometry to CD44-expressing cells using C$_{44}$Mab-9. CHO/CD44v3-10 (**A**), CHO/CD44s (**B**), CHO-K1 (**C**), COLO201 (**D**), and COLO205 (**E**) were treated with 0.01–10 µg/mL of C$_{44}$Mab-9, followed by treatment with Alexa Fluor 488-conjugated anti-mouse IgG (Red line). The black line represents the negative control (blocking buffer).

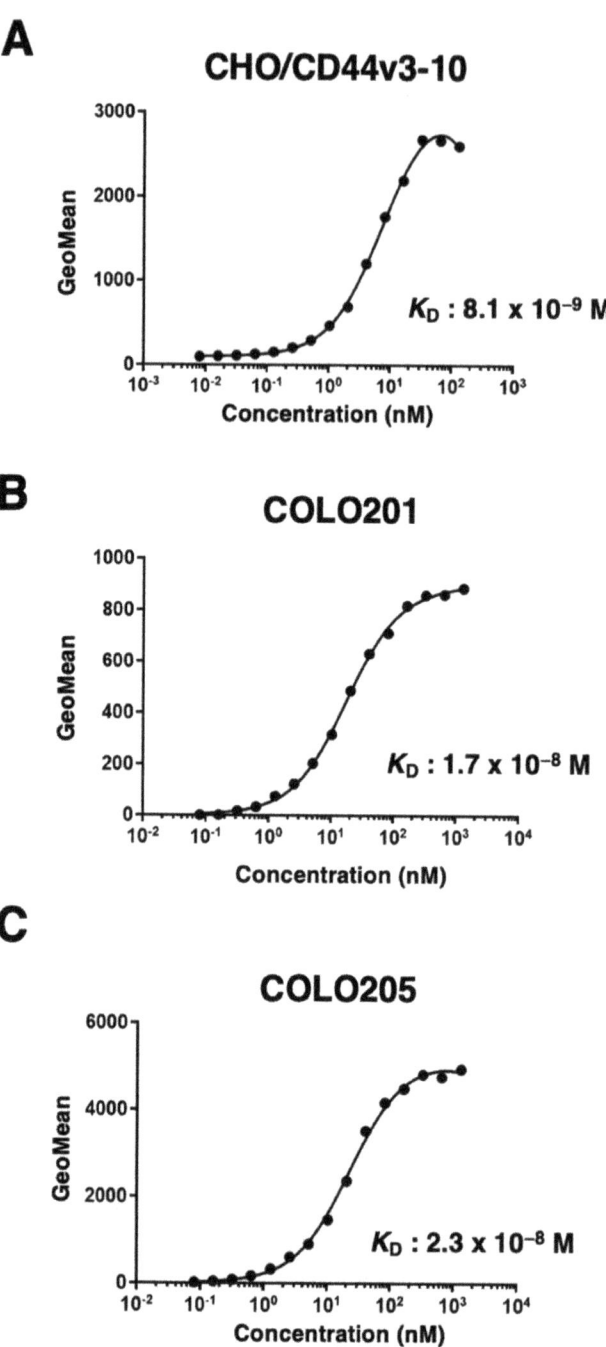

Figure 3. The determination of the binding affinity of C_{44}Mab-9 to CD44-expressing cells. CHO/CD44v3-10 (**A**), COLO201 (**B**), and COLO205 (**C**) cells were suspended in 100 μL of serially diluted C_{44}Mab-9 at indicated concentrations. Then, cells were treated with Alexa Fluor 488-conjugated anti-mouse IgG. Fluorescence data were subsequently collected, followed by the calculation of the apparent dissociation constant (K_D) by GraphPad PRISM 8.

2.3. Western Blot Analysis

We next performed western blot analysis to assess the sensitivity of C_{44}Mab-9. Total cell lysates of CHO-K1, CHO/CD44s, and CHO/CD44v3-10 were analyzed. As shown in Figure 4, C_{44}Mab-9 detected CD44v3-10 as a more than 180-kDa band. However, C_{44}Mab-9 did not detect any bands from lysates of CHO-K1 and CHO/CD44s cells. An anti-pan-CD44 mAb, C_{44}Mab-46, recognized the lysates from both CHO/CD44s (~75 kDa) and CHO/CD44v3-10 (>180 kDa). These results indicated that C_{44}Mab-9 specifically detects exogenous CD44v3-10.

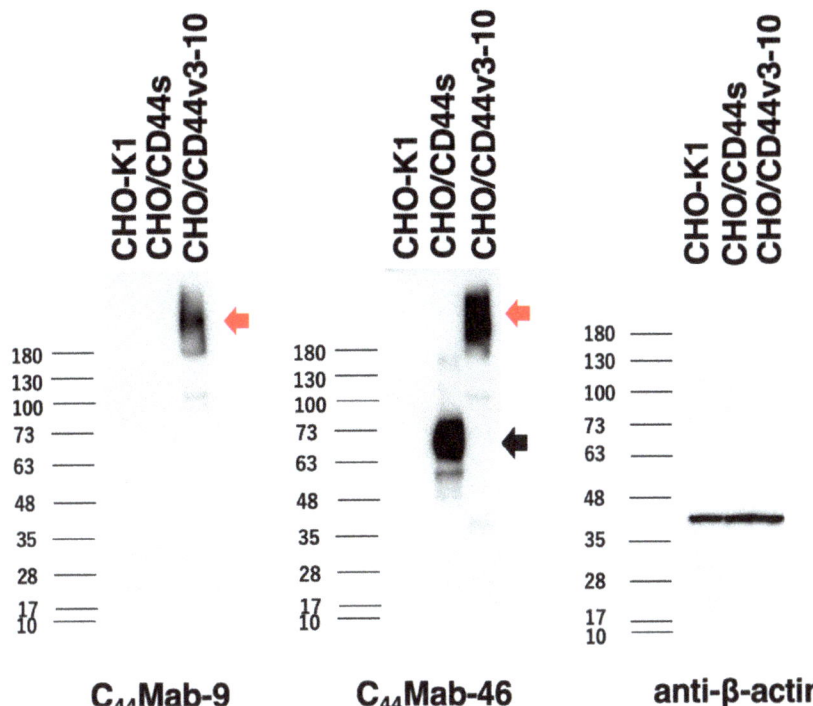

Figure 4. Western blotting by C_{44}Mab-9. The cell lysates of CHO-K1, CHO/CD44s, and CHO/CD44v3-10 (10 μg of protein) were electrophoresed and transferred onto polyvinylidene difluoride (PVDF) membranes. The membranes were incubated with 10 μg/mL of C_{44}Mab-9, 10 μg/mL of C_{44}Mab-46, and 1 μg/mL of anti-β-actin mAb, followed by incubation with peroxidase-conjugated anti-mouse immunoglobulins. The black arrow indicates the CD44s (~75 kDa). The red arrows indicate the CD44v3-10 (>180 kDa).

2.4. Immunohistochemical Analysis Using C_{44}Mab-9 against Tumor Tissues

We next examined whether C_{44}Mab-9 could be used for immunohistochemical analyses using formalin-fixed paraffin-embedded (FFPE) sections. Since previous anti-CD44v6 mAbs could detect CD44v6 in SCC tissues at a high frequency, we first stained an oral SCC tissue. As shown in Figure 5A, C_{44}Mab-9 exhibited clear membranous staining, and could clearly distinguish tumor cells from stromal tissues. In contrast, C_{44}Mab-46 stained both (Figure 5B). We next investigated CRC sections. C_{44}Mab-9 showed membranous staining in CRC cells, but not stromal tissues (Figure 5C). In contrast, C_{44}Mab-46 also stained both (Figure 5D). These results indicated that C_{44}Mab-9 is useful for immunohistochemical analysis of FFPE tumor sections.

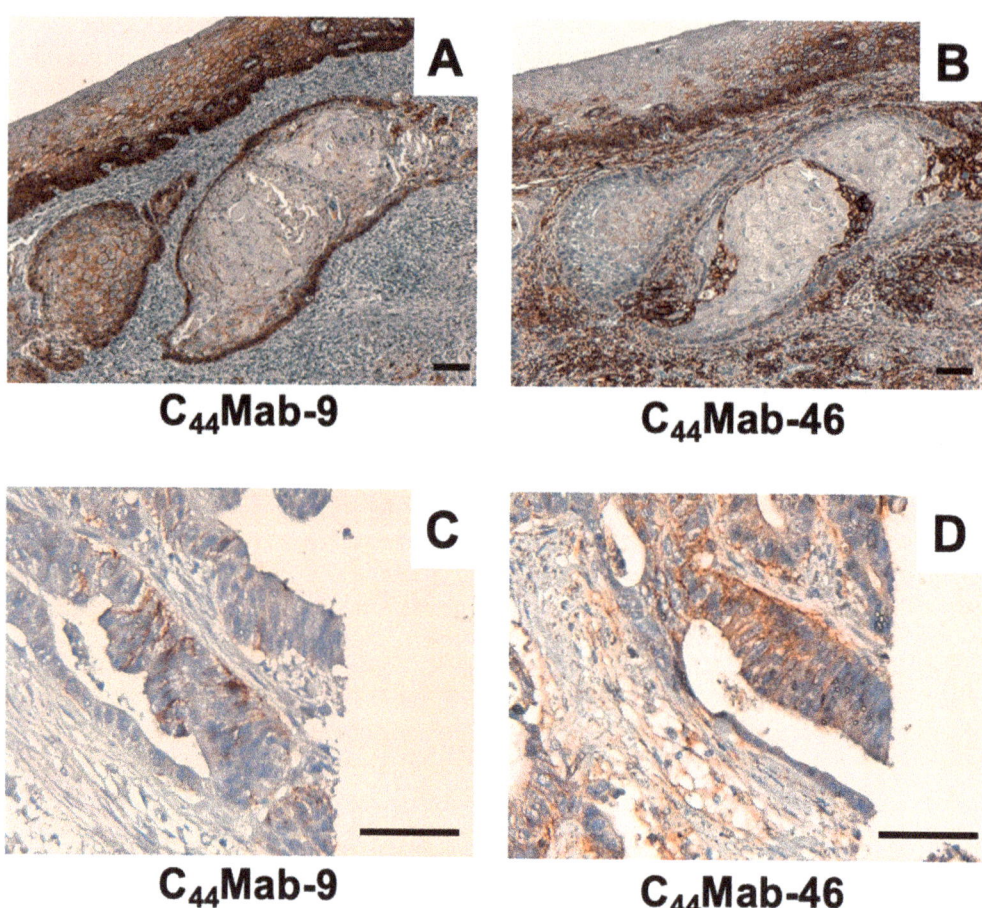

Figure 5. Immunohistochemical analysis using C_{44}Mab-9 and C_{44}Mab-46. (**A,B**) Oral SCC sections were incubated with 1 µg/mL of C_{44}Mab-9 (**A**) and C_{44}Mab-46 (**B**). (**C,D**) CRC sections were incubated with 1 µg/mL of C_{44}Mab-9 (**C**) and C_{44}Mab-46 (**D**), followed by treatment with the Envision+ kit. The color was developed using DAB, and sections were counterstained with hematoxylin. Scale bar = 100 µm.

3. Discussion

In this study, we developed C_{44}Mab-9 using the CBIS method (Figure 1), and determined its epitope as variant 6 encoded region (Table 1). Then, we showed the usefulness of C_{44}Mab-9 for multiple applications, including flow cytometry (Figures 2 and 3), western blotting (Figure 4), and immunohistochemistry (Figure 5).

Anti-CD44v6 mAbs (clones 2F10, VFF4, VFF7, and VFF18) were previously developed, and mainly used for tumor diagnosis and therapy. The 2F10 was established by the immunization of CD44v3-10-Fc protein produced by COS1 cells. The exon specificity of the 2F10 was determined by indirect immunofluorescent staining of COS1 cells transfected with human CD44v cDNAs, including CD44v3-10, CD44v6-10, CD44v7-10, CD44v8-10, and CD44v10 [25]. Therefore, the 2F10 is thought to recognize the peptide or glycopeptide structure of CD44v6. However, the detailed binding epitope of 2F10 has not been determined.

The VFF series mAbs were established by the immunization of bacterial-expressed CD44v3-10 fused with glutathione S-transferase [26,27]. Afterward, VFF4 and VFF 7 were used in the immunohistochemical analysis [28], and VFF18 was humanized as BIWA-

4 [15], and developed to bivatuzumab-mertansine drug conjugate for clinical trials [17,18]. The VFF18 bound only to the fusion proteins, containing a variant 6-encoded region. Furthermore, the VFF18 recognized several synthetic peptides, spanning the variant 6-encoded region in ELISA, and the WFGNRWHEGYR peptide was determined as the epitope [26]. As shown in Table 1, C_{44}Mab-9 also recognized a synthetic peptide (CD44p351–370), which possesses the above sequence. In contrast, a synthetic peptide (CD44p361–380) possesses the FGNRWHEGYR sequence, which is not recognized by C_{44}Mab-9. Therefore, C_{44}Mab-9 and VFF18 recognize CD44v6 with a similar variant 6-encoded region. Detailed epitope mapping for C_{44}Mab-9 is required in the future.

A mutated version of BIWA-4, called BIWA-8, was constructed for improving binding affinity. This was achieved by two amino acid mutations of the light chain without changing the humanized heavy chain [15]. The BIWA-8 was further engineered to chimeric antigen receptors (CARs). The CD44v6 CAR-T exhibited antitumor effects against primary human acute myeloid leukemia and multiple myeloma cells in immunocompromised mice [29]. Furthermore, the CD44v6 CAR-T also showed efficacy in xenograft models of lung and ovarian carcinomas [30], which is expected for a wider development toward solid tumors. However, Greco et al. demonstrated that the N-glycosylation of CD44v6 protects tumor cells from the CD44v6 CAR-T targeting [31]. This phenomenon is probably due to the masking of CD44v6 CAR binding by the N-glycosylation because the original VFF18 was established by bacterial-expressed CD44v3-10 immunization and recognized the peptidic epitope lacking the N-glycosylation [26]. In contrast, C_{44}Mab-9 was established by immunization of CHO/CD44v3-10 cells, but recognizes a synthetic peptide (Table 1). Meanwhile, C_{44}Mab-9 could detect more than 180 kDa, heavily glycosylated CD44v3-10 in western blot analysis (Figure 4). Further studies are required to reveal whether the N-glycosylation affects the recognition by C_{44}Mab-9 for future application to CAR-T therapy.

The clinical significance of CD44v6 expression in patients with CRC using immunohistochemical analysis remains controversial. The elevated expression has been associated with poor prognosis, linked to adverse prognosis [32,33]. However, others have reported that CD44v6 expression is associated with a favorable outcome [34,35]. Various clones of anti-CD44v6 mAbs appeared to influence the outcome of the clinical significance. Among these clinical studies, Saito et al. used VFF18 and showed similar staining patterns of C_{44}Mab-9 (Figure 5). They also found that CD44v6 expression was observed in poorly differentiated CRC without E-cadherin expression. Furthermore, the high CD44v6 expression exhibited a significant inverse correlation with E-cadherin expression and was found to be an independent poor prognostic factor in disease-free survival and overall survival [36]. In the future, we should evaluate the clinical significance of the C_{44}Mab-9-positive CRC with E-cadherin expression.

Large-scale genomic analyses of CRCs defined 4 subtypes: (1) microsatellite instability immune; (2) canonical; (3) metabolic; (4) mesenchymal types [3]. Since the CD44v6 expression was observed in a part of CRC tissues (Figure 5), the relationship to the subtypes should be evaluated. In addition, the mechanism of CD44v6 upregulation including the transcriptional regulation and the v6 inclusion by alternative splicing should be determined. The inclusion of CD44 variant exons was reported to be promoted by the ERK-Sam68 axis [37]. Moreover, CD44v6 forms a ternary complex with MET and HGF, which is essential for the c-MET activation [38]. This positive feedback is a potential mechanism to promote the variant exon inclusion.

CD44v6-positive CRC cells exhibited cancer-initiating cell properties [39]. Cytokines, HGF, C-X-C motif chemokine 12, and osteopontin, secreted from tumor-associated fibroblasts, promote the CD44v6 expression in the cancer-initiating cells, which promotes migration and metastasis of CRC cells [14]. Clinically, circulating-tumor cells (CTCs), which express EpCAM, MET, and CD44, identify a subset with increased metastasis-initiating phenotype [40], suggesting that CD44v6 plays an important role in cancer-initiating cell property cooperating with MET. In addition, CTC culture methods, including two-dimensional (2D) expansion, 3D organoids/spheroids culture, and xenograft formation in mice, have been developed to evaluate the character of CTCs [41]. Therefore, the biological property to affect cell proliferation and invasiveness by C_{44}Mab-9 should be investigated because CD44v6 can potentiate the MET signaling by forming the ternary complex with HGF [38]. Therefore, it would be valuable to examine the effect of C_{44}Mab-9 on CTC proliferation in vitro and metastasis in vivo.

To evaluate the in vivo effect, we previously converted the IgG$_1$ subclass of mAbs into a mouse IgG$_{2a}$, and produced a defucosylated version. These defucosylated IgG$_{2a}$ mAbs exhibited potent ADCC in vitro, and reduced tumor growth in mouse xenograft models [24,42–48]. Therefore, the production of a class-switched and defucosylated version of C_{44}Mab-9 is required to evaluate the antitumor activity in vivo.

4. Materials and Methods

4.1. Cell Lines

Mouse multiple myeloma P3X63Ag8U.1 (P3U1) and CHO-K1 cell lines were obtained from the American Type Culture Collection (ATCC, Manassas, VA, USA). These cells were cultured in Roswell Park Memorial Institute (RPMI)-1640 medium (Nacalai Tesque, Inc., Kyoto, Japan), supplemented with 10% heat-inactivated fetal bovine serum (FBS; Thermo Fisher Scientific, Inc., Waltham, MA, USA), 100 U/mL penicillin, 100 μg/mL streptomycin, and 0.25 μg/mL amphotericin B (Nacalai Tesque, Inc.). Human colorectal cancer cell lines, COLO201 and COLO205, were obtained from ATCC and the Cell Resource Center for Biomedical Research Institute of Development, Aging, and Cancer at Tohoku University, respectively. The COLO201 and COLO205 were cultured in RPMI-1640 medium, supplemented with 10% heat-inactivated FBS, 100 units/mL of penicillin, and 100 μg/mL streptomycin (Nacalai Tesque, Inc.). All the cells were grown in a humidified incubator at 37 °C with 5% CO_2.

CD44s cDNA was amplified using HotStar HiFidelity Polymerase Kit (Qiagen Inc., Hilden, Germany) using LN229 cDNA as a template. CD44v3-10 ORF was obtained from the RIKEN BRC through the National Bio-Resource Project of the MEXT, Japan. CD44s and CD44v3-10 cDNAs were subcloned into pCAG-Ble-ssPA16 vector possessing signal sequence and N-terminal PA16 tag (GLEGGVAMPGAEDDVV) [19,49–52], which is detected by NZ-1 [53–68]. CHO/CD44s and CHO/CD44v3-10 were established by transfecting pCAG-Ble/PA16-CD44s and pCAG-Ble/PA16-CD44v3-10 into CHO-K1 cells using a Neon transfection system (Thermo Fisher Scientific, Inc.).

4.2. Hybridoma Production

The female BALB/c mice (6-weeks old) were purchased from CLEA Japan (Tokyo, Japan). Animals were housed under specific pathogen-free conditions. All animal experiments were also conducted according to relevant guidelines and regulations to minimize animal suffering and distress in the laboratory. The Animal Care and Use Committee of Tohoku University (Permit number: 2019NiA-001) approved animal experiments. The mice were monitored daily for health during the full four-week duration of the experiment. A reduction of more than 25% of the total body weight was defined as a humane endpoint. During sacrifice, the mice were euthanized through cervical dislocation, after which death was verified through respiratory and cardiac arrest. The mice were intraperitoneally immunized with CHO/CD44v3-10 (1 × 10^8 cells) and Imject Alum (Thermo Fisher Scientific Inc.) as an adjuvant, which stimulates a nonspecific immune response for mixed antigens using this formulation of aluminum hydroxide and magnesium hydroxide. After three additional immunizations of CHO/CD44v3-10 (1 × 10^8 cells), a booster injection of CHO/CD44v3-10 was intraperitoneally administered 2 days before harvesting the spleen cells. The splenocytes were fused with P3U1 cells using polyethylene glycol 1500 (PEG1500; Roche Diagnostics, Indianapolis, IN, USA). The supernatants, which are positive for CHO/CD44v3–10 cells and negative for CHO-K1 cells, were selected by the flow cytometry-based high throughput screening using SA3800 Cell Analyzers (Sony Corp., Tokyo, Japan).

4.3. ELISA

Fifty-eight synthesized peptides (Sigma-Aldrich Corp., St. Louis, MO, USA), which cover the CD44v3-10 extracellular domain [21], were immobilized on Nunc Maxisorp 96-well immunoplates (Thermo Fisher Scientific Inc) at a concentration of 1 µg/mL for 30 min at 37 °C. After washing with phosphate-buffered saline (PBS) containing 0.05% (v/v) Tween 20 (PBST; Nacalai Tesque, Inc.) using Microplate Washer, HydroSpeed (Tecan, Zürich, Switzerland), wells were blocked with 1% (w/v) bovine serum albumin (BSA)-containing PBST for 30 min at 37 °C. C_{44}Mab-9 was added to each well, and then incubated with peroxidase-conjugated anti-mouse immunoglobulins (1:2000 diluted; Agilent Technologies Inc., Santa Clara, CA, USA). Enzymatic reactions were performed using 1 Step Ultra TMB (Thermo Fisher Scientific Inc.). The optical density at 655 nm was measured using an iMark microplate reader (Bio-Rad Laboratories, Inc., Berkeley, CA, USA).

4.4. Flow Cytometry

CHO-K1 and CHO/CD44v3-10 were isolated using 0.25% trypsin and 1 mM ethylenediamine tetraacetic acid (EDTA; Nacalai Tesque, Inc.) treatment. COLO201 and COLO205 were isolated by brief pipetting. The cells were treated with primary mAbs or blocking buffer (0.1% bovine serum albumin (BSA; Nacalai Tesque, Inc.) in phosphate-buffered saline [PBS]; control) for 30 min at 4 °C. Subsequently, the cells were incubated in Alexa Fluor 488-conjugated anti-mouse IgG (1:2000; Cell Signaling Technology, Inc.) for 30 min at 4 °C. Fluorescence data were collected using the SA3800 Cell Analyzer and analyzed using SA3800 software ver. 2.05 (Sony Corporation).

4.5. Determination of Dissociation Constant (K_D) by Flow Cytometry

Serially diluted C_{44}Mab-9 was suspended with CHO/CD44v3-10, COLO201, and COLO205 cells. The cells were further treated with Alexa Fluor 488-conjugated anti-mouse IgG (1:200). Fluorescence data were collected using BD FACSLyric and analyzed using BD FACSuite software version 1.3 (BD Biosciences). To determine the dissociation constant (K_D), GraphPad Prism 8 (the fitting binding isotherms to built-in one-site binding models; GraphPad Software, Inc., La Jolla, CA, USA) was used.

4.6. Western Blot Analysis

The cell lysates (10 µg of protein) were separated on 5–20% polyacrylamide gels (FUJIFILM Wako Pure Chemical Corporation, Osaka, Japan) and transferred onto polyvinylidene difluoride (PVDF) membranes (Merck KGaA, Darmstadt, Germany). After blocking (4% skim milk (Nacalai Tesque, Inc.) in PBS with 0.05% Tween 20), the membranes were incubated with 10 µg/mL of C_{44}Mab-9, 10 µg/mL of C_{44}Mab-46 or 1 µg/mL of an anti-β-actin mAb (clone AC-15; Sigma-Aldrich Corp.), and then incubated with peroxidase-conjugated anti-mouse immunoglobulins (diluted 1:1000; Agilent Technologies, Inc., Santa Clara, CA, USA). Finally, the signals were detected with a chemiluminescence reagent, ImmunoStar LD (FUJIFILM Wako Pure Chemical Corporation) using a Sayaca-Imager (DRC Co., Ltd., Tokyo, Japan).

4.7. Immunohistochemical Analysis

The FFPE oral SCC tissue was obtained from Tokyo Medical and Dental University [69]. FFPE sections of colorectal carcinoma tissue array (Catalog number: CO483a) were purchased from US Biomax Inc. (Rockville, MD, USA). The sections were autoclaved in citrate buffer (pH 6.0; Nichirei biosciences, Inc., Tokyo, Japan) for 20 min. After blocking with SuperBlock T20 (Thermo Fisher Scientific, Inc.), the sections were incubated with C_{44}Mab-9 (1 µg/mL) and C_{44}Mab-46 (1 µg/mL) for 1 h at room temperature and then treated with the EnVision+ Kit for mouse (Agilent Technologies, Inc.) for 30 min. The color was developed using 3,3'-diaminobenzidine tetrahydrochloride (DAB; Agilent Technologies Inc.) for 2 min. Hematoxylin (FUJIFILM Wako Pure Chemical Corporation) was used for the counterstaining. Leica DMD108 (Leica Microsystems GmbH, Wetzlar, Germany) was used to examine the sections and obtain images.

Supplementary Materials: The following supporting information can be downloaded at: https://www.mdpi.com/article/10.3390/ijms24044007/s1.

Author Contributions: R.E., T.T. and T.A. performed the experiments. M.K.K. and Y.K. designed the experiments. R.E. and H.S. analyzed the data. R.E., H.S. and Y.K. wrote the manuscript. All authors have read and agreed to the published version of the manuscript.

Funding: This research was supported in part by Japan Agency for Medical Research and Development (AMED) under Grant Numbers: JP22ama121008 (to Y.K.), JP22am0401013 (to Y.K.), JP22bm1004001 (to Y.K.), JP22ck0106730 (to Y.K.), and JP21am0101078 (to Y.K.), and by the Japan Society for the Promotion of Science (JSPS) Grants-in-Aid for Scientific Research (KAKENHI) grant nos. 21K20789 (to T.T.), 22K06995 (to H.S.), 21K15523 (to T.A.), 21K07168 (to M.K.K.), and 22K07224 (to Y.K.).

Institutional Review Board Statement: The animal study protocol was approved by the Animal Care and Use Committee of Tohoku University (Permit number: 2019NiA-001) for studies involving animals.

Data Availability Statement: All related data and methods are presented in this paper. Additional inquiries should be addressed to the corresponding authors.

Acknowledgments: The authors would like to thank Saori Okuno, and Saori Handa (Department of Antibody Drug Development, Tohoku University Graduate School of Medicine) for technical assistance.

Conflicts of Interest: The authors declare no conflict of interest involving this article.

References

1. Siegel, R.L.; Miller, K.D.; Wagle, N.S.; Jemal, A. Cancer statistics, 2023. *CA Cancer J. Clin.* **2023**, *73*, 17–48. [CrossRef] [PubMed]
2. Fearon, E.R.; Vogelstein, B. A genetic model for colorectal tumorigenesis. *Cell* **1990**, *61*, 759–767. [CrossRef] [PubMed]
3. Guinney, J.; Dienstmann, R.; Wang, X.; de Reyniès, A.; Schlicker, A.; Soneson, C.; Marisa, L.; Roepman, P.; Nyamundanda, G.; Angelino, P.; et al. The consensus molecular subtypes of colorectal cancer. *Nat. Med.* **2015**, *21*, 1350–1356. [CrossRef] [PubMed]
4. Puccini, A.; Seeber, A.; Berger, M.D. Biomarkers in Metastatic Colorectal Cancer: Status Quo and Future Perspective. *Cancers* **2022**, *14*, 4828. [CrossRef]
5. Zöller, M. CD44: Can a cancer-initiating cell profit from an abundantly expressed molecule? *Nat. Rev. Cancer* **2011**, *11*, 254–267. [CrossRef]
6. Abbasian, M.; Mousavi, E.; Arab-Bafrani, Z.; Sahebkar, A. The most reliable surface marker for the identification of colorectal cancer stem-like cells: A systematic review and meta-analysis. *J. Cell Physiol.* **2019**, *234*, 8192–8202. [CrossRef]
7. Ponta, H.; Sherman, L.; Herrlich, P.A. CD44: From adhesion molecules to signalling regulators. *Nat. Rev. Mol. Cell Biol.* **2003**, *4*, 33–45. [CrossRef]
8. Yan, Y.; Zuo, X.; Wei, D. Concise Review: Emerging Role of CD44 in Cancer Stem Cells: A Promising Biomarker and Therapeutic Target. *Stem. Cells Transl. Med.* **2015**, *4*, 1033–1043. [CrossRef]
9. Chen, C.; Zhao, S.; Karnad, A.; Freeman, J.W. The biology and role of CD44 in cancer progression: Therapeutic implications. *J. Hematol. Oncol.* **2018**, *11*, 64. [CrossRef]
10. Günthert, U.; Hofmann, M.; Rudy, W.; Reber, S.; Zöller, M.; Haussmann, I.; Matzku, S.; Wenzel, A.; Ponta, H.; Herrlich, P. A new variant of glycoprotein CD44 confers metastatic potential to rat carcinoma cells. *Cell* **1991**, *65*, 13–24. [CrossRef]
11. Slevin, M.; Krupinski, J.; Gaffney, J.; Matou, S.; West, D.; Delisser, H.; Savani, R.C.; Kumar, S. Hyaluronan-mediated angiogenesis in vascular disease: Uncovering RHAMM and CD44 receptor signaling pathways. *Matrix Biol.* **2007**, *26*, 58–68. [CrossRef] [PubMed]
12. Ma, L.; Dong, L.; Chang, P. CD44v6 engages in colorectal cancer progression. *Cell. Death Dis.* **2019**, *10*, 30. [CrossRef] [PubMed]
13. Orian-Rousseau, V.; Morrison, H.; Matzke, A.; Kastilan, T.; Pace, G.; Herrlich, P.; Ponta, H. Hepatocyte growth factor-induced Ras activation requires ERM proteins linked to both CD44v6 and F-actin. *Mol. Biol. Cell.* **2007**, *18*, 76–83. [CrossRef] [PubMed]
14. Todaro, M.; Gaggianesi, M.; Catalano, V.; Benfante, A.; Iovino, F.; Biffoni, M.; Apuzzo, T.; Sperduti, I.; Volpe, S.; Cocorullo, G.; et al. CD44v6 is a marker of constitutive and reprogrammed cancer stem cells driving colon cancer metastasis. *Cell. Stem Cell.* **2014**, *14*, 342–356. [CrossRef] [PubMed]
15. Verel, I.; Heider, K.H.; Siegmund, M.; Ostermann, E.; Patzelt, E.; Sproll, M.; Snow, G.B.; Adolf, G.R.; van Dongen, G.A. Tumor targeting properties of monoclonal antibodies with different affinity for target antigen CD44V6 in nude mice bearing head-and-neck cancer xenografts. *Int. J. Cancer* **2002**, *99*, 396–402. [CrossRef]
16. Orian-Rousseau, V.; Ponta, H. Perspectives of CD44 targeting therapies. *Arch. Toxicol.* **2015**, *89*, 3–14. [CrossRef]

7. Tijink, B.M.; Buter, J.; de Bree, R.; Giaccone, G.; Lang, M.S.; Staab, A.; Leemans, C.R.; van Dongen, G.A. A phase I dose escalation study with anti-CD44v6 bivatuzumab mertansine in patients with incurable squamous cell carcinoma of the head and neck or esophagus. *Clin. Cancer Res.* **2006**, *12*, 6064–6072. [CrossRef]
8. Riechelmann, H.; Sauter, A.; Golze, W.; Hanft, G.; Schroen, C.; Hoermann, K.; Erhardt, T.; Gronau, S. Phase I trial with the CD44v6-targeting immunoconjugate bivatuzumab mertansine in head and neck squamous cell carcinoma. *Oral Oncol.* **2008**, *44*, 823–829. [CrossRef]
9. Yamada, S.; Itai, S.; Nakamura, T.; Yanaka, M.; Kaneko, M.K.; Kato, Y. Detection of high CD44 expression in oral cancers using the novel monoclonal antibody, C(44)Mab-5. *Biochem. Biophys. Rep.* **2018**, *14*, 64–68. [CrossRef]
10. Goto, N.; Suzuki, H.; Tanaka, T.; Asano, T.; Kaneko, M.K.; Kato, Y. Development of a Novel Anti-CD44 Monoclonal Antibody for Multiple Applications against Esophageal Squamous Cell Carcinomas. *Int. J. Mol. Sci.* **2022**, *23*, 5535. [CrossRef]
11. Takei, J.; Asano, T.; Suzuki, H.; Kaneko, M.K.; Kato, Y. Epitope Mapping of the Anti-CD44 Monoclonal Antibody (C44Mab-46) Using Alanine-Scanning Mutagenesis and Surface Plasmon Resonance. *Monoclon. Antib. Immunodiagn. Immunother.* **2021**, *40*, 219–226. [CrossRef] [PubMed]
12. Asano, T.; Kaneko, M.K.; Takei, J.; Tateyama, N.; Kato, Y. Epitope Mapping of the Anti-CD44 Monoclonal Antibody (C44Mab-46) Using the REMAP Method. *Monoclon. Antib. Immunodiagn. Immunother.* **2021**, *40*, 156–161. [CrossRef] [PubMed]
13. Asano, T.; Kaneko, M.K.; Kato, Y. Development of a Novel Epitope Mapping System: RIEDL Insertion for Epitope Mapping Method. *Monoclon. Antib. Immunodiagn. Immunother.* **2021**, *40*, 162–167. [CrossRef]
14. Takei, J.; Kaneko, M.K.; Ohishi, T.; Hosono, H.; Nakamura, T.; Yanaka, M.; Sano, M.; Asano, T.; Sayama, Y.; Kawada, M.; et al. A defucosylated anti-CD44 monoclonal antibody 5-mG2a-f exerts antitumor effects in mouse xenograft models of oral squamous cell carcinoma. *Oncol. Rep.* **2020**, *44*, 1949–1960. [CrossRef]
15. Fox, S.B.; Fawcett, J.; Jackson, D.G.; Collins, I.; Gatter, K.C.; Harris, A.L.; Gearing, A.; Simmons, D.L. Normal human tissues, in addition to some tumors, express multiple different CD44 isoforms. *Cancer Res.* **1994**, *54*, 4539–4546. [PubMed]
16. Heider, K.H.; Sproll, M.; Susani, S.; Patzelt, E.; Beaumier, P.; Ostermann, E.; Ahorn, H.; Adolf, G.R. Characterization of a high-affinity monoclonal antibody specific for CD44v6 as candidate for immunotherapy of squamous cell carcinomas. *Cancer Immunol. Immunother.* **1996**, *43*, 245–253. [CrossRef] [PubMed]
17. Heider, K.H.; Mulder, J.W.; Ostermann, E.; Susani, S.; Patzelt, E.; Pals, S.T.; Adolf, G.R. Splice variants of the cell surface glycoprotein CD44 associated with metastatic tumour cells are expressed in normal tissues of humans and cynomolgus monkeys. *Eur. J. Cancer* **1995**, *31a*, 2385–2391. [CrossRef]
18. Wang, Z.; Tang, Y.; Xie, L.; Huang, A.; Xue, C.; Gu, Z.; Wang, K.; Zong, S. The Prognostic and Clinical Value of CD44 in Colorectal Cancer: A Meta-Analysis. *Front. Oncol.* **2019**, *9*, 309. [CrossRef]
19. Casucci, M.; Nicolis di Robilant, B.; Falcone, L.; Camisa, B.; Norelli, M.; Genovese, P.; Gentner, B.; Gullotta, F.; Ponzoni, M.; Bernardi, M.; et al. CD44v6-targeted T cells mediate potent antitumor effects against acute myeloid leukemia and multiple myeloma. *Blood* **2013**, *122*, 3461–3472. [CrossRef]
20. Porcellini, S.; Asperti, C.; Corna, S.; Cicoria, E.; Valtolina, V.; Stornaiuolo, A.; Valentinis, B.; Bordignon, C.; Traversari, C. CAR T Cells Redirected to CD44v6 Control Tumor Growth in Lung and Ovary Adenocarcinoma Bearing Mice. *Front. Immunol.* **2020**, *11*, 99. [CrossRef] [PubMed]
21. Greco, B.; Malacarne, V.; De Girardi, F.; Scotti, G.M.; Manfredi, F.; Angelino, E.; Sirini, C.; Camisa, B.; Falcone, L.; Moresco, M.A.; et al. Disrupting N-glycan expression on tumor cells boosts chimeric antigen receptor T cell efficacy against solid malignancies. *Sci. Transl. Med.* **2022**, *14*, eabg3072. [CrossRef] [PubMed]
22. Mulder, J.W.; Kruyt, P.M.; Sewnath, M.; Oosting, J.; Seldenrijk, C.A.; Weidema, W.F.; Offerhaus, G.J.; Pals, S.T. Colorectal cancer prognosis and expression of exon-v6-containing CD44 proteins. *Lancet* **1994**, *344*, 1470–1472. [CrossRef]
23. Wielenga, V.J.; Heider, K.H.; Offerhaus, G.J.; Adolf, G.R.; van den Berg, F.M.; Ponta, H.; Herrlich, P.; Pals, S.T. Expression of CD44 variant proteins in human colorectal cancer is related to tumor progression. *Cancer Res.* **1993**, *53*, 4754–4756. [PubMed]
24. Zlobec, I.; Günthert, U.; Tornillo, L.; Iezzi, G.; Baumhoer, D.; Terracciano, L.; Lugli, A. Systematic assessment of the prognostic impact of membranous CD44v6 protein expression in colorectal cancer. *Histopathology* **2009**, *55*, 564–575. [CrossRef]
25. Nanashima, A.; Yamaguchi, H.; Sawai, T.; Yasutake, T.; Tsuji, T.; Jibiki, M.; Yamaguchi, E.; Nakagoe, T.; Ayabe, H. Expression of adhesion molecules in hepatic metastases of colorectal carcinoma: Relationship to primary tumours and prognosis after hepatic resection. *J. Gastroenterol. Hepatol.* **1999**, *14*, 1004–1009. [CrossRef] [PubMed]
26. Saito, S.; Okabe, H.; Watanabe, M.; Ishimoto, T.; Iwatsuki, M.; Baba, Y.; Tanaka, Y.; Kurashige, J.; Miyamoto, Y.; Baba, H. CD44v6 expression is related to mesenchymal phenotype and poor prognosis in patients with colorectal cancer. *Oncol. Rep.* **2013**, *29*, 1570–1578. [CrossRef] [PubMed]
27. Matter, N.; Herrlich, P.; König, H. Signal-dependent regulation of splicing via phosphorylation of Sam68. *Nature* **2002**, *420*, 691–695. [CrossRef]
28. Orian-Rousseau, V.; Chen, L.; Sleeman, J.P.; Herrlich, P.; Ponta, H. CD44 is required for two consecutive steps in HGF/c-Met signaling. *Genes Dev.* **2002**, *16*, 3074–3086. [CrossRef]
29. Wang, Z.; Zhao, K.; Hackert, T.; Zöller, M. CD44/CD44v6 a Reliable Companion in Cancer-Initiating Cell Maintenance and Tumor Progression. *Front. Cell. Dev. Biol.* **2018**, *6*, 97. [CrossRef]

40. Baccelli, I.; Schneeweiss, A.; Riethdorf, S.; Stenzinger, A.; Schillert, A.; Vogel, V.; Klein, C.; Saini, M.; Bäuerle, T.; Wallwiener, M.; et al. Identification of a population of blood circulating tumor cells from breast cancer patients that initiates metastasis in a xenograft assay. *Nat. Biotechnol.* **2013**, *31*, 539–544. [CrossRef]
41. Rupp, B.; Ball, H.; Wuchu, F.; Nagrath, D.; Nagrath, S. Circulating tumor cells in precision medicine: Challenges and opportunities. *Trends Pharmacol. Sci.* **2022**, *43*, 378–391. [CrossRef]
42. Li, G.; Suzuki, H.; Ohishi, T.; Asano, T.; Tanaka, T.; Yanaka, M.; Nakamura, T.; Yoshikawa, T.; Kawada, M.; Kaneko, M.K.; et al. Antitumor activities of a defucosylated anti-EpCAM monoclonal antibody in colorectal carcinoma xenograft models. *Int. J. Mol. Med.* **2023**, *51*, 1–14. [CrossRef]
43. Nanamiya, R.; Takei, J.; Ohishi, T.; Asano, T.; Tanaka, T.; Sano, M.; Nakamura, T.; Yanaka, M.; Handa, S.; Tateyama, N.; et al. Defucosylated Anti-Epidermal Growth Factor Receptor Monoclonal Antibody (134-mG(2a)-f) Exerts Antitumor Activities in Mouse Xenograft Models of Canine Osteosarcoma. *Monoclon. Antib. Immunodiagn. Immunother.* **2022**, *41*, 1–7. [CrossRef]
44. Kawabata, H.; Suzuki, H.; Ohishi, T.; Kawada, M.; Kaneko, M.K.; Kato, Y. A Defucosylated Mouse Anti-CD10 Monoclonal Antibody (31-mG(2a)-f) Exerts Antitumor Activity in a Mouse Xenograft Model of CD10-Overexpressed Tumors. *Monoclon. Antib. Immunodiagn. Immunother.* **2022**, *41*, 59–66. [CrossRef]
45. Kawabata, H.; Ohishi, T.; Suzuki, H.; Asano, T.; Kawada, M.; Suzuki, H.; Kaneko, M.K.; Kato, Y. A Defucosylated Mouse Anti-CD10 Monoclonal Antibody (31-mG(2a)-f) Exerts Antitumor Activity in a Mouse Xenograft Model of Renal Cell Cancers. *Monoclon. Antib. Immunodiagn. Immunother.* **2022**, *41*, 320–327. [CrossRef]
46. Asano, T.; Tanaka, T.; Suzuki, H.; Li, G.; Ohishi, T.; Kawada, M.; Yoshikawa, T.; Kaneko, M.K.; Kato, Y. A Defucosylated Anti-EpCAM Monoclonal Antibody (EpMab-37-mG(2a)-f) Exerts Antitumor Activity in Xenograft Model. *Antibodies* **2022**, *11*, 74. [CrossRef] [PubMed]
47. Tateyama, N.; Nanamiya, R.; Ohishi, T.; Takei, J.; Nakamura, T.; Yanaka, M.; Hosono, H.; Saito, M.; Asano, T.; Tanaka, T.; et al. Defucosylated Anti-Epidermal Growth Factor Receptor Monoclonal Antibody 134-mG(2a)-f Exerts Antitumor Activities in Mouse Xenograft Models of Dog Epidermal Growth Factor Receptor-Overexpressed Cells. *Monoclon. Antib. Immunodiagn. Immunother.* **2021**, *40*, 177–183. [CrossRef] [PubMed]
48. Takei, J.; Ohishi, T.; Kaneko, M.K.; Harada, H.; Kawada, M.; Kato, Y. A defucosylated anti-PD-L1 monoclonal antibody 13-mG(2a)-f exerts antitumor effects in mouse xenograft models of oral squamous cell carcinoma. *Biochem. Biophys. Rep.* **2020**, *24*, 100801. [CrossRef] [PubMed]
49. Kato, Y.; Yamada, S.; Furusawa, Y.; Itai, S.; Nakamura, T.; Yanaka, M.; Sano, M.; Harada, H.; Fukui, M.; Kaneko, M.K. PMab-213: A Monoclonal Antibody for Immunohistochemical Analysis Against Pig Podoplanin. *Monoclon. Antib. Immunodiagn. Immunother.* **2019**, *38*, 18–24. [CrossRef]
50. Furusawa, Y.; Yamada, S.; Itai, S.; Sano, M.; Nakamura, T.; Yanaka, M.; Fukui, M.; Harada, H.; Mizuno, T.; Sakai, Y.; et al. PMab-210: A Monoclonal Antibody Against Pig Podoplanin. *Monoclon. Antib. Immunodiagn. Immunother.* **2019**, *38*, 30–36. [CrossRef]
51. Furusawa, Y.; Yamada, S.; Itai, S.; Nakamura, T.; Yanaka, M.; Sano, M.; Harada, H.; Fukui, M.; Kaneko, M.K.; Kato, Y. PMab-219: A monoclonal antibody for the immunohistochemical analysis of horse podoplanin. *Biochem. Biophys. Rep.* **2019**, *18*, 100616. [CrossRef] [PubMed]
52. Furusawa, Y.; Yamada, S.; Itai, S.; Nakamura, T.; Takei, J.; Sano, M.; Harada, H.; Fukui, M.; Kaneko, M.K.; Kato, Y. Establishment of a monoclonal antibody PMab-233 for immunohistochemical analysis against Tasmanian devil podoplanin. *Biochem. Biophys. Rep.* **2019**, *18*, 100631. [CrossRef] [PubMed]
53. Kato, Y.; Kaneko, M.K.; Kuno, A.; Uchiyama, N.; Amano, K.; Chiba, Y.; Hasegawa, Y.; Hirabayashi, J.; Narimatsu, H.; Mishima, K.; et al. Inhibition of tumor cell-induced platelet aggregation using a novel anti-podoplanin antibody reacting with its platelet-aggregation-stimulating domain. *Biochem. Biophys. Res. Commun.* **2006**, *349*, 1301–1307. [CrossRef] [PubMed]
54. Chalise, L.; Kato, A.; Ohno, M.; Maeda, S.; Yamamichi, A.; Kuramitsu, S.; Shiina, S.; Takahashi, H.; Ozone, S.; Yamaguchi, J.; et al. Efficacy of cancer-specific anti-podoplanin CAR-T cells and oncolytic herpes virus G47Delta combination therapy against glioblastoma. *Mol. Ther. Oncol.* **2022**, *26*, 265–274. [CrossRef]
55. Ishikawa, A.; Waseda, M.; Ishii, T.; Kaneko, M.K.; Kato, Y.; Kaneko, S. Improved anti-solid tumor response by humanized anti-podoplanin chimeric antigen receptor transduced human cytotoxic T cells in an animal model. *Genes Cells* **2022**, *27*, 549–558. [CrossRef]
56. Tamura-Sakaguchi, R.; Aruga, R.; Hirose, M.; Ekimoto, T.; Miyake, T.; Hizukuri, Y.; Oi, R.; Kaneko, M.K.; Kato, Y.; Akiyama, Y.; et al. Moving toward generalizable NZ-1 labeling for 3D structure determination with optimized epitope-tag insertion. *Acta Crystallogr. D Struct. Biol.* **2021**, *77*, 645–662. [CrossRef]
57. Kaneko, M.K.; Ohishi, T.; Nakamura, T.; Inoue, H.; Takei, J.; Sano, M.; Asano, T.; Sayama, Y.; Hosono, H.; Suzuki, H.; et al. Development of Core-Fucose-Deficient Humanized and Chimeric Anti-Human Podoplanin Antibodies. *Monoclon. Antib. Immunodiagn. Immunother.* **2020**, *39*, 167–174. [CrossRef]
58. Fujii, Y.; Matsunaga, Y.; Arimori, T.; Kitago, Y.; Ogasawara, S.; Kaneko, M.K.; Kato, Y.; Takagi, J. Tailored placement of a turn-forming PA tag into the structured domain of a protein to probe its conformational state. *J. Cell. Sci.* **2016**, *129*, 1512–1522. [CrossRef]

59. Abe, S.; Kaneko, M.K.; Tsuchihashi, Y.; Izumi, T.; Ogasawara, S.; Okada, N.; Sato, C.; Tobiume, M.; Otsuka, K.; Miyamoto, L.; et al. Antitumor effect of novel anti-podoplanin antibody NZ-12 against malignant pleural mesothelioma in an orthotopic xenograft model. *Cancer Sci.* **2016**, *107*, 1198–1205. [CrossRef]
60. Kaneko, M.K.; Abe, S.; Ogasawara, S.; Fujii, Y.; Yamada, S.; Murata, T.; Uchida, H.; Tahara, H.; Nishioka, Y.; Kato, Y. Chimeric Anti-Human Podoplanin Antibody NZ-12 of Lambda Light Chain Exerts Higher Antibody-Dependent Cellular Cytotoxicity and Complement-Dependent Cytotoxicity Compared with NZ-8 of Kappa Light Chain. *Monoclon. Antib. Immunodiagn. Immunother.* **2017**, *36*, 25–29. [CrossRef]
61. Ito, A.; Ohta, M.; Kato, Y.; Inada, S.; Kato, T.; Nakata, S.; Yatabe, Y.; Goto, M.; Kaneda, N.; Kurita, K.; et al. A Real-Time Near-Infrared Fluorescence Imaging Method for the Detection of Oral Cancers in Mice Using an Indocyanine Green-Labeled Podoplanin Antibody. *Technol. Cancer Res. Treat.* **2018**, *17*, 1533033818767936. [CrossRef]
62. Tamura, R.; Oi, R.; Akashi, S.; Kaneko, M.K.; Kato, Y.; Nogi, T. Application of the NZ-1 Fab as a crystallization chaperone for PA tag-inserted target proteins. *Protein Sci.* **2019**, *28*, 823–836. [CrossRef]
63. Shiina, S.; Ohno, M.; Ohka, F.; Kuramitsu, S.; Yamamichi, A.; Kato, A.; Motomura, K.; Tanahashi, K.; Yamamoto, T.; Watanabe, R.; et al. CAR T Cells Targeting Podoplanin Reduce Orthotopic Glioblastomas in Mouse Brains. *Cancer Immunol. Res.* **2016**, *4*, 259–268. [CrossRef] [PubMed]
64. Kuwata, T.; Yoneda, K.; Mori, M.; Kanayama, M.; Kuroda, K.; Kaneko, M.K.; Kato, Y.; Tanaka, F. Detection of Circulating Tumor Cells (CTCs) in Malignant Pleural Mesothelioma (MPM) with the "Universal" CTC-Chip and An Anti-Podoplanin Antibody NZ-1.2. *Cells* **2020**, *9*, 888. [CrossRef] [PubMed]
65. Nishinaga, Y.; Sato, K.; Yasui, H.; Taki, S.; Takahashi, K.; Shimizu, M.; Endo, R.; Koike, C.; Kuramoto, N.; Nakamura, S.; et al. Targeted Phototherapy for Malignant Pleural Mesothelioma: Near-Infrared Photoimmunotherapy Targeting Podoplanin. *Cells* **2020**, *9*, 1019. [CrossRef]
66. Fujii, Y.; Kaneko, M.; Neyazaki, M.; Nogi, T.; Kato, Y.; Takagi, J. PA tag: A versatile protein tagging system using a super high affinity antibody against a dodecapeptide derived from human podoplanin. *Protein Expr. Purif.* **2014**, *95*, 240–247. [CrossRef] [PubMed]
67. Kato, Y.; Kaneko, M.K.; Kunita, A.; Ito, H.; Kameyama, A.; Ogasawara, S.; Matsuura, N.; Hasegawa, Y.; Suzuki-Inoue, K.; Inoue, O.; et al. Molecular analysis of the pathophysiological binding of the platelet aggregation-inducing factor podoplanin to the C-type lectin-like receptor CLEC-2. *Cancer Sci.* **2008**, *99*, 54–61. [CrossRef]
68. Kato, Y.; Vaidyanathan, G.; Kaneko, M.K.; Mishima, K.; Srivastava, N.; Chandramohan, V.; Pegram, C.; Keir, S.T.; Kuan, C.T.; Bigner, D.D.; et al. Evaluation of anti-podoplanin rat monoclonal antibody NZ-1 for targeting malignant gliomas. *Nucl. Med. Biol.* **2010**, *37*, 785–794. [CrossRef]
69. Itai, S.; Ohishi, T.; Kaneko, M.K.; Yamada, S.; Abe, S.; Nakamura, T.; Yanaka, M.; Chang, Y.W.; Ohba, S.I.; Nishioka, Y.; et al. Anti-podocalyxin antibody exerts antitumor effects via antibody-dependent cellular cytotoxicity in mouse xenograft models of oral squamous cell carcinoma. *Oncotarget* **2018**, *9*, 22480–22497. [CrossRef]

Disclaimer/Publisher's Note: The statements, opinions and data contained in all publications are solely those of the individual author(s) and contributor(s) and not of MDPI and/or the editor(s). MDPI and/or the editor(s) disclaim responsibility for any injury to people or property resulting from any ideas, methods, instructions or products referred to in the content.

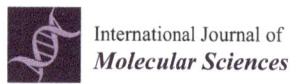

Review

Targeting *KRAS* G12C Mutation in Colorectal Cancer, A Review: New Arrows in the Quiver

Javier Ros [1,2,†], Caterina Vaghi [1,3,4,†], Iosune Baraibar [1,2], Nadia Saoudi González [1,2], Marta Rodríguez-Castells [1,2], Ariadna García [1,2], Adriana Alcaraz [1,2], Francesc Salva [1,2], Josep Tabernero [1,2] and Elena Elez [1,2,*]

1. Medical Oncology, Vall d'Hebron Institute of Oncology (VHIO), 08035 Barcelona, Spain; caterina.vaghi@unimi.it (C.V.)
2. Medical Oncology, Vall d'Hebron Universite Hospital, 08035 Barcelona, Spain
3. Department of Oncology and Hemato-Oncology, University of Milan, 20122 Milan, Italy
4. Department of Hematology, Oncology, and Molecular Medicine, Grande Ospedale Metropolitano Niguarda, 20162 Milan, Italy
* Correspondence: meelez@vhio.net
† These authors contributed equally to this work.

Citation: Ros, J.; Vaghi, C.; Baraibar, I.; Saoudi González, N.; Rodríguez-Castells, M.; García, A.; Alcaraz, A.; Salva, F.; Tabernero, J.; Elez, E. Targeting *KRAS* G12C Mutation in Colorectal Cancer, A Review: New Arrows in the Quiver. *Int. J. Mol. Sci.* **2024**, *25*, 3304. https://doi.org/10.3390/ijms25063304

Academic Editor: Donatella Delle Cave

Received: 22 February 2024
Revised: 13 March 2024
Accepted: 13 March 2024
Published: 14 March 2024

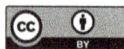

Copyright: © 2024 by the authors. Licensee MDPI, Basel, Switzerland. This article is an open access article distributed under the terms and conditions of the Creative Commons Attribution (CC BY) license (https://creativecommons.org/licenses/by/4.0/).

Abstract: Kirsten rat sarcoma virus oncogene homolog (*KRAS*) is the most frequently mutated oncogene in human cancer. In colorectal cancer (CRC), *KRAS* mutations are present in more than 50% of cases, and the *KRAS* glycine-to-cysteine mutation at codon 12 (*KRAS* G12C) occurs in up to 4% of patients. This mutation is associated with short responses to standard chemotherapy and worse overall survival compared to non-G12C mutations. In recent years, several *KRAS* G12C inhibitors have demonstrated clinical activity, although all patients eventually progressed. The identification of negative feedback through the EGFR receptor has led to the development of KRAS inhibitors plus an anti-EGFR combination, thus boosting antitumor activity. Currently, several KRAS G12C inhibitors are under development, and results from phase I and phase II clinical trials are promising. Moreover, the phase III CodeBreaK 300 trial demonstrates the superiority of sotorasib-panitumumab over trifluridine/tipiracil, establishing a new standard of care for patients with colorectal cancer harboring *KRAS* G12C mutations. Other combinations such as adagrasib-cetuximab, divarasib-cetuximab, or FOLFIRI-panitumumab-sotorasib have also shown a meaningful response rate and are currently under evaluation. Nonetheless, most of these patients will eventually relapse. In this setting, liquid biopsy emerges as a critical tool to characterize the mechanisms of resistance, consisting mainly of acquired genomic alterations in the MAPK and PI3K pathways and tyrosine kinase receptor alterations, but gene fusions, histological changes, or conformational changes in the kinase have also been described. In this paper, we review the development of KRAS G12C inhibitors in colorectal cancer as well as the main mechanisms of resistance.

Keywords: KRAS G12C colorectal cancer; liquid biopsy; mechanism of resistance; KRAS inhibitor; pocket

1. Introduction

Kirsten rat sarcoma virus oncogene homolog (*KRAS*) is the most frequently mutated oncogene in human cancer. In colorectal cancer (CRC), *KRAS* mutations are present in more than 50% of cases [1,2]. The recommended backbone treatment for *KRAS*-mutant colorectal cancer included a fluoropyrimidine-based regimen in combination with oxaliplatin and/or irinotecan and the addition of an anti-VEGF in the first and second line [2]. EGFR inhibitors are not recommended in *RAS*-mutant CRC due to their limited clinical activity. Beyond the second line, trifluridine/tipiracil (-TAS-102-, a combination of trifluridine, a cytotoxic nucleic acid analogue, and tipiracil, a thymidine phosphorylase inhibitor), regorafenib (an oral multikinase inhibitor that blocks VEGFR1-3, KIT, RET, RAF1, BRAF, PDGFR, and FGFR), and recently the combination TAS-102-bevacizumab have demonstrated clinical benefit and are considered the standard of care [3–5]. However, not all patients respond to such treatments in the refractory setting and overall survival remains poor. The prognostic impact of a *RAS* mutation is already well-established, demonstrating worse overall survival compared with those tumors with a *RAS/BRAF* wild-type profile [6–10]. In colorectal cancer, the *KRAS* glycine-to-cysteine mutation at codon 12 (*KRAS* G12C) occurs in up to 4% of patients and is associated with poorer overall survival (OS) in the first and second line when treated with chemotherapy. In addition, in the refractory setting among patients treated with TAS-102, *KRAS* G12C mutations were biomarkers for reduced OS benefit from TAS-102 [11–13]. Indeed, median overall survival (mOS) among patients with *KRAS* G12C tumors was 16.1 and 9.7 months in the first and second line, whereas mOS for those patients with non-G12C *KRAS*-mutated tumors was 18.3 and 11.4 months in the first and second line, respectively [12,13].

The most frequent *KRAS* mutation in colorectal cancer is the G12D mutation that can be found in up to 42% of colorectal tumors. The G12D mutation has been shown to have an intermediate intrinsic and GAP-mediated GTP hydrolysis rate compared to other G12 and G13 mutants, with mutations such as G12A significantly reducing intrinsic hydrolysis, and G12C exhibiting wild-type levels [14]. *KRAS* G12D mutations have been shown to elicit distinct gene and protein expression profiles compared with other *KRAS* mutations in a tissue-specific manner [15,16].

Importantly, the KRAS G12C protein cycles between an "on" state, in which a guanosine triphosphate (GTP) is attached, and an "off" state in which the GTP loses one phosphate, turning into guanosine diphosphate (GDP). In its active state, KRAS increases downstream oncogenic signaling and cell growth. The G12C mutation impairs GTP hydrolysis, which shifts KRAS to the active GTP-binding state, promoting tumorigenesis and metastases [17,18]. This dynamic conformational change exposes a pocket that can be targeted with specific inhibitors. Indeed, in the last few years, several KRAS G12C inhibitors, including adagrasib, sotorasib, and divarasib among others, have been developed as monotherapy or in combination with anti-EGFR agents, demonstrating meaningful clinical activity. New combinations that boost antitumor efficacy and overcome acquired resistance are currently being developed. In this paper, we review the development of KRAS inhibitors in metastatic colorectal cancer, the already described mechanism of resistance, and novel combinations to overcome such resistances and boost the antitumoral effect.

2. The *RAS* Pathway and Downstream Signaling

RAS proteins are small, membrane-bound guanine nucleotide-binding proteins involved in several signaling pathways that ultimately regulate cell growth, motility, angiogenesis, and survival in various cancer types. They are associated with tumor progression and resistance to targeted therapies. In physiological conditions, RAS shifts between two conformational states: an active state, where an active guanosine-5′-triphosphate (GTP) is attached to the RAS protein, and an inactive state, where GTP is processed to become guanosine diphosphate (GDP). The initial step in RAS activation involves the activation of several receptor tyrosine kinases (RTKs), induced by ligand binding in the extracellular domain of RTKs. This leads to RTK dimerization and autophosphorylation. The activated receptors then interact with the growth factor receptor protein 2 (GRB2), recruiting guanine nucleotide exchange factors (GEFs), including the Son of Sevenless homolog (SOS). SOS promotes GDP/GTP exchange, inducing a conformational change that activates the kinase. This activation triggers different pathways, including RAF/MEK/ERK, PI3K/AKT/mTOR, and nuclear transcription factors involved in cell survival and metastases. The RAS cycle is ultimately switched off by GTPase-activating proteins (GAPs), which induce GTP hydrolysis, forming inactive RAS-GDP. The G12C mutation occurs at the 12th position of the *KRAS* gene, where glycine (G) is replaced by a cysteine (C) amino acid [17,18]. This mutation leads to the production of a mutated KRAS protein with altered function, which remains constitutively active. In this case, an allosteric pocket below the switch II region of the mutant cysteine was identified by Ostrem et al. [19]. G12C inhibitors preferentially bind RAS in the GDP-bound conformation, blocking the exchange with GTP and thus preventing the activation of the signaling cascade. Figure 1 pictures Ras signaling pathways and drugs associated with KRAS G12C inhibition.

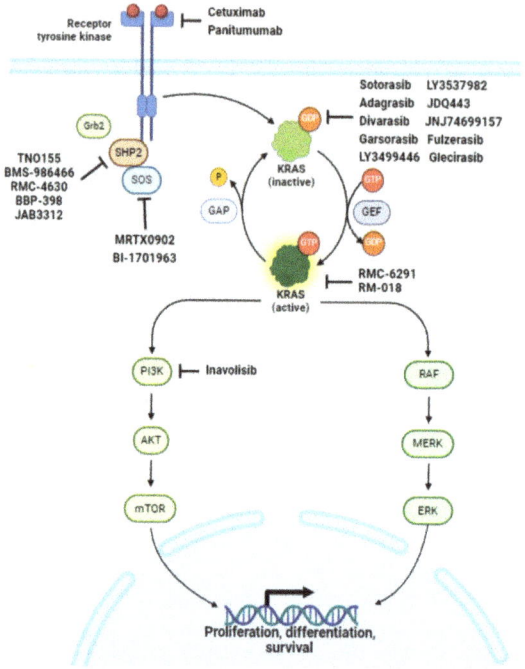

Figure 1. RAS signaling pathways and drugs associated with KRAS G12C inhibition.

3. Development of KRAS G12C Inhibitors

The emergence of KRAS G12C inhibitors represents a new therapeutic strategy in this population. In addition to the development of several inhibitors, upfront and acquired mechanisms of resistance have been identified and some strategies have been developed to overcome such resistance.

3.1. KRAS Inhibitors in Monotherapy

3.1.1. Sotorasib

After the discovery of compounds that covalently bind to the switch II pocket of KRAS G12C in its inactive GDP-bound state (off) and the understanding of the mechanism of KRAS G12C inhibition, sotorasib (AMG510) was developed and entered the clinical setting in 2018 as the first-in-class anti-KRAS G12C [19–23]. In the phase I/II CodeBreaK 100 trial, 129 patients with previously treated advanced solid tumors harboring the *KRAS* G12C mutation were enrolled in the phase I cohort [24]. Among them, 42 were heavily pretreated. In total, twenty-five patients received the expansion dose of 960 mg qd (from the Latin "quaque die", once a day), which was subsequently established as the recommended phase II trial dose (RP2D). No dose-limiting toxic effects occurred, nor did any treatment-related adverse event resulting in death. The most common treatment-related adverse events (TRAEs) were diarrhea, fatigue, nausea, and an increase in aspartate or alanine aminotransferase, occurring in 30%, 23%, 21%, 13%, and 12% of the total population, respectively. Regarding anti-tumor activity, three out of 42 mCRC patients (7.1%) responded, with all responses occurring in the cohort treated with the 960 mg qd dose. The disease control rate (DCR) was 73.8% in the total mCRC patients and 80% in the 960 mg qd cohort. The subsequent phase II cohort of the CodeBreaK 100 trial included 62 patients with a mean of three previous lines [25]. These patients received sotorasib 960 mg qd. After almost 2 years, with five patients still on the treatment, the objective response rate (ORR) was 9.7%, with tumor shrinkage in 66% of patients and a DCR of 82% of patients. The median progression free survival (mPFS) was 4 months. Grade 3 TRAEs occurred in six patients (10%); diarrhea, fatigue, nausea, and elevation of transaminases were confirmed as the most common. The only grade 4 event observed was an increase in blood creatinine phosphokinase. Apart from being safe and tolerable, sotorasib monotherapy demonstrated only modest anti-tumor activity in mCRC, especially if compared with other histologies such as NSCLC, in which sotorasib monotherapy achieved an ORR of 41% and a mPFS of 6.3 months [26]. Table 1 summarizes clinical trials evaluating KRAS G12C inhibition in patients with *KRAS* G12C-mutated colorectal cancer.

Table 1. Key clinical trials targeting KRAS G12C in mCRC, completed or with already published data.

Study Name/ID Phase	Population (n. of Patients)	Treatment Regimen (n. of Patients Treated)	Results	Grade 3 or Higher TRAEs
Clinical Trials Targeting KRAS G12C in mCRC, Completed or with Already Published Data				
CodeBreaK 100/NCT03600883 Phase I	advanced *KRAS* G12C mutant solid tumors (124, including 42 mCRC)	Sotorasib (AMG510)	limited to mCRC treated with any dose ORR 7.1% (3/42) DCR 73.8% (31/42) mPFS 4 mo	52.7%, in the overall population
CodeBreaK 100 (CRC expansion cohort)/NCT03600883 Phase II	advanced *KRAS* G12C mutant mCRC (62)	Sotorasib (AMG510) 960 mg qd	ORR 9.7% (6/62) DCR 82.3% (51/62) mPFS 4 mo	10% (6/62)
KRYSTAL-1/NCT03785249 Phase I/Ib	advanced *KRAS* G12C mutant solid tumors (25, including 4 mCRC)	Adagrasib (MRTX849)	limited to evaluable mCRC treated with 600 mg bid ORR 50% (1/2) DOR 4.2 mo	36% (9/25)
KRYSTAL-1 (monotherapy arm)/NCT03785249 Phase I/II	advanced *KRAS* G12C mutant mCRC (44)	Adagrasib (MRTX849) 600 mg bid	ORR 19% (8/43) DCR 86% (37/43) mPFS 5.6 mo	34% (15/43)
NCT04449874 Phase Ib	advanced *KRAS* G12C mutant solid tumors (137, including 55 mCRC)	Divarasib (GDC-6036)	limited to mCRC population ORR 29.1% (20/55) mPFS 5.6 mo limited to mCRC treated with 400 mg qd ORR 35.9% (14/39) mPFS 6.9 mo	7% (4/55)
pooled analysis of NCT05005234 and NCT05497336 Phase I	advanced *KRAS* G12C mutant solid tumors, including 45 mCRC	Fulzerasib (IBI531)	limited to mCRC patients treated with 600 mg bid ORR 43.8% (14/32) DCR 87.5% (28/32)	20% (9/32)
Clinical trials targeting EGFR-KRAS G12C in mCRC, completed or with already published data				
CodeBreaK 101/NCT04185883 Phase Ib	advanced *KRAS* G12C mutant mCRC (48)	Sotorasib (AMG510) + panitumumab	limited to patients treated with 960 mg qd ORR 30% (12/40) DCR 92.5% (37/40) mPFS 5.7 mo	27% (13/48)
CodeBreaK 101 (subprotocol H)/NCT04185883 Phase Ib	advanced *KRAS* G12C mCRC previously treated ≥1 prior treatment (33)	Sotorasib (AMG510) 960 mg qd + panitumumab + FOLFIRI (54)	ORR 58.1% DCR 93.5% mPFS 5.7 mo	45.5% (15/33)

Table 1. Cont.

Study Name/ID Phase	Population (n. of Patients)	Treatment Regimen (n. of Patients Treated)	Results	Grade 3 or Higher TRAEs
CodeBreaK 300/NCT05198934 Phase III	advanced KRAS G12C mutant mCRC (160)	Sotorasib (AMG510) 960 qd mg + panitumumab (53)	ORR 26.4% DCR 71.7% mPFS 5.6 mo	35.8% (19/53)
		Sotorasib (AMG510) 240 qd mg + panitumumab (53)	ORR 5.7% DCR 67.9% mPFS 3.9	30.2% (16/53)
		SOC (54)	ORR 0% DCR 46.3% mPFS 2.2 mo	43.1% (23/54)
KRYSTAL-1 (combination arm)/NCT03785249 Phase I/II	advanced KRAS G12C mutant mCRC (32)	Adagrasib (MRTX849) 600 mg bid + cetuximab	ORR 46% (13/28) DCR 100% (28/28) mPFS 6.9 mo mOS 13.4 mo	16% (5/32)
NCT04449874 (arm C) Phase Ib	advanced KRAS G12C mutant mCRC (29)	Divarasib (GDC-6036) at 400 mg qd (26) + cetuximab	limited to KRAS G12C inhibitor naive population ORR 62.5% (14/24) mPFS 8 mo	37.9% (11/29)
NCT04585035 Phase I/II	advanced KRAS G12C mutant solid tumors, including 29 mCRC	Garsorasib (D-1553) 600 mg bid (29) + cetuximab	ORR 51.7% (15/29) DCR 93.1% (27/29) mPFS 7.56 mo	10.3% (3/29)

ID: identification number; TRAEs: treatment-related adverse events; Mo: months; DOR: duration of response; ORR: overall response rate; mPFS: progression-free survival; qd: quaque die (once a day); bid: bis in die (2 times a day).

3.1.2. Adagrasib

The KRAS G12C inhibitor adagrasib (MRTX849) binds irreversibly and selectively to KRAS G12C in its inactive state [27]. In the phase I/Ib KRYSTAL-1 trial, where 25 patients with advanced, previously treated, solid tumors harboring KRAS G12C mutations were enrolled and treated with various expansion doses, four of them were affected with mCRC, with two receiving the RP2D of 600 mg bid (from the Latin "bis in die", two times a day). A toxicity profile consistent with sotorasib was observed, with nausea (80.0%), diarrhea (70.0%), vomiting (50.0%), and fatigue (45.0%) being the most prevalent TRAEs in the cohort treated with the RP2D. The most common grade 3/4 TRAE was fatigue (15.0%). In terms of pharmacokinetics, adagrasib displayed a longer half-life compared to sotorasib (23 h versus 5.5 h), along with a higher exposure dose dependency and ability to penetrate the central nervous system. Notably, one out of the two mCRC patients treated with the RP2D exhibited a partial response (PR), with a DOR lasting 4.2 months. Additional efficacy data came from the phase I/II trial KRYSTAL-1, in which 44 patients affected with mCRC were treated with adagrasib 600 mg bid, with 19% achieving PR, an mDOR of 4.3 months, and an mPFS of 5.6 months [28].

3.1.3. Divarasib

The clinical development of divarasib (GDC-6036) started in 2020. Compared to its predecessors, divarasib boasts a potency of five to twenty times greater and a selectivity of up to 50 times higher [29]. Notably, at equivalent nanomolar concentrations, divarasib achieves a higher relative alkylation of KRAS G12C compared to sotorasib and adagrasib. Furthermore, non-KRAS G12C proteins are alkylated at higher concentrations with divarasib compared to the other two drugs. In a phase I trial assessing the safety of divarasib, out of the 137 patients enrolled, 55 were diagnosed with mCRC [30]. Grade 3 or higher TRAEs were observed in 12% of the total population, including diarrhea, increased aspartate aminotransferase, nausea, vomiting, and fatigue. A long half-life of 17 h was observed.

Regarding efficacy in the mCRC population, a complete response (CR) or PR was observed in 29% of patients, including one CR. Importantly, higher ORR and mPFS of 36% and 6.9 months, respectively, emerged when analyzing only the subset of 39 patients treated with the RP2D of 400 mg qd. All partial responses were accompanied by a reduction in circulating tumor DNA (ctDNA) *KRAS* G12C allele frequency to less than 1% after 2 cycles. Co-occurring mutations in *APC* and *TP53* did not significantly impact the response. Analysis of pre- and post-treatment ctDNA from 16 responders revealed that at least one genomic alteration mechanistically linked to KRAS inhibitor resistance developed in nine patients. These alterations included *RAS* copy number gain or amplification, non-*KRAS* G12C mutations, alterations in receptor tyrosine kinases (RTKs) and mitogen-activated protein kinase (MAPK) pathway components, including *ERBB2* and *MET* amplifications, and *BRAF* mutations, respectively. Conversely, at least one pre-existing mutation in all *RAS* genes was found in six out of 25 patients in the total population with progressive disease (PD) as the best response, including one mCRC patient, with an adaptive increase and decrease in the allele variant frequency of the non-*KRAS* G12C and *KRAS* G12C mutations, respectively, in three out of these six. Again, a striking difference in efficacy endpoints between NSCLC and CRC was observed with divarasib, as higher ORR of 53.4% and mPFS of 13.1 months were achieved in NSCLC patients.

3.1.4. Other Inhibitors

The aggregate data of two phase I trials (NCT05005234, NCT05497336) in which Fulzerasib (IBI351) has been tested in 45 mCRC patients with *KRAS* G12C mutations have been reported. Among the 32 evaluable patients, an ORR of 43.8% (14/32) was observed. Grade 3 TRAEs occurred in nine patients (20.0%), with no drug-related adverse events leading to treatment discontinuation or death [31]. Finally, Garsorasib (D-1553) monotherapy demonstrated deep clinical activity and safety in heavily pretreated patients with *KRAS* G12C-mutated CRC. Based on this initial activity, the combination of Garsorasib and cetuximab was evaluated in a phase II trial [32]. This trial included 40 patients, 80% of them having received at least two previous lines. ORR was 45% with a DCR of 95%. mPFS was 7.6 months whereas OS data is still immature. No grade 4/5 TRAEs were reported [29].

3.2. A Step Forward in Boosting Antitumor Activity: Combining KRAS G12C Inhibitors with Anti-EGFR

From the outset, a notable discrepancy in efficacy emerged between patients with NSCLC and CRC in the early phases of trials involving sotorasib. Impressively, the best ORR reported was 41% in NSCLC compared to 9.7% in mCRC (CodeBreaK 100) [25,26]. Amodio et al. uncovered several variances at the cellular level, notably observing that colorectal cancer lines exhibited a higher basal level of phosphorylated-functional-receptor tyrosine kinases (RTKs) and maintained responsiveness to further activation of EGFR by growth factors [33]. In this milieu of concurrent mechanisms, inhibiting *KRAS* G12C can not result in quelling cell growth and proliferation. Moreover, a more pronounced rebound of the MAPK pathway following *KRAS* G12C inhibition was demonstrated in CRC compared to NSCLC cell lines. Consequently, the synergistic combination of *KRAS* G12C inhibitors and anti-EGFR therapies was investigated both in vitro and in colorectal patient-derived models, yielding significant tumor regression or even complete remission. Rayan et al. further explored adaptive resistance to *KRAS* G12C inhibitors, identifying the rebound of the MAPK pathway as a principal mechanism [34]. This rebound, characterized by marked induction of GTP-bound forms of wild-type HRAS and KRAS, which was otherwise abrogated by the knockdown of HRAS and NRAS, leads to MAPK pathway activation in a *KRAS* G12C-independent way, suggesting that it can not be overcome by escalating the dosage of *KRAS* G12C inhibitors. Instead, a strategy involving upstream and downstream inhibition, specifically with SHP2 or MEK inhibitors, resulted in a robust and sustained inhibition of MAPK signaling in vitro. This study suggested an alternative approach, consisting of a combination of *KRAS* G12C inhibitors with compounds targeting RTK signaling. These findings paved the way for the combination of KRAS G12C inhibitors with either panitumumab and cetuximab, and with other inhibitors along the MAPK pathway, which are currently under investigation in combination with KRAS G12C inhibitors in ongoing clinical trials [18,35].

3.2.1. Adagrasib Cetuximab

In the phase I/II trial KRYSTAL-1, adagrasib was also tested in combination with cetuximab in 32 patients [28]. Grade 3 or higher TRAEs were reported in 34% of the monotherapy group and 16% of the combination therapy group, with no grade 5 adverse events observed. However, 16% of patients receiving cetuximab discontinued the drug due to toxicity. The toxicity profile of the combination only differed in cetuximab-related adverse events, without any synergistic toxic effects observed. Notably, in patients receiving adagrasib with cetuximab, the ORR increased from 19% to 46%, along with a mPFS of 6.9 months, compared to adagrasib monotherapy. An exploratory analysis of ctDNA revealed a higher clearance of the KRAS G12C mutant allele after two cycles in the combination therapy group compared to the monotherapy group (88% vs. 55%), correlating with the different ORR. No association between response and PI3KCA and TP53 mutations were identified. The phase III KRYSTAL-10 trial comparing adagrasib plus cetuximab vs. second-line chemotherapy has completed recruitment.

3.2.2. Sotorasib Panitumumab

The combination of sotorasib and panitumumab has also been investigated [36,37]. The phase Ib trial, CodeBreaK 101, included cohorts specifically focused on mCRC patients, comprising a dose exploration cohort of eight patients to determine the RP2D of sotorasib in combination with panitumumab and a dose expansion cohort that included 40 patients [36]. In total, 27% of patients experienced TRAEs of grade $\geq$3, mostly attributed to panitumumab, including rash (6%), acneiform dermatitis (4%), and hypomagnesemia (4%). Panitumumab led to interruption or reduction more often than sotorasib (29% versus 15%), but no discontinuation of any drug due to a treatment-related adverse event was reported. In the exploratory cohort, which included 63% of patients previously treated with sotorasib monotherapy, ORR was 12% and the DCR was 80%. Conversely, in the expansion cohort (anti-KRAS naive), ORR and DCR were higher at 30% and 92%, respectively, with a mPFS of 5.7 months. Importantly, the study also evaluated the impact of sidedness but no difference in terms of response based on primary tumor location was observed.

The phase III trial CodeBreaK 300 tested sotorasib in the refractory setting at two different doses (960 mg and 240 mg qd), both in combination with panitumumab, and compared the results with the standard of care, consisting of either regorafenib or trifluridine/tiparacil [37]. Despite the RP2D having already been set at 960 mg qd, the alternative dose of 240 mg qd of sotorasib was tested due to its non-linear pharmacokinetic properties. The trial reached its primary endpoint by demonstrating the superiority of the combination of panitumumab and sotorasib at the two doses tested compared to the SOC in terms of PFS [5.7 versus 2.2 months, HR 0.49 (95% CI, 0.30 to 0.80; p = 0.006) and 3.9 versus 2.2, HR 0.58 (95% CI, 0.36 to 0.93; p = 0.03), respectively]. A significant difference in terms of ORR also emerged among the arms, in which CR/PR was achieved in 26%, 5.7%, and 0% of patients treated with sotorasib 960 mg qd and panitumumab, sotorasib 240 mg qd and panitumumab, and regorafenib or trifluridine/tiparacil, respectively. Data on overall survival is still immature. Regarding treatment-related events, a grade 3 or higher TRAE occurred in 35.8%, 30.2%, and 43% of patients treated with the combination of sotorasib and panitumumab at a dose of either 960 mg qd or 240 mg qd, respectively, and with the SOC. The most common grade 3 or higher TRAEs of regorafenib-trifluridine/tiparacil were neutropenia (23.5%), anemia (5.9%), and hypertension (5.9%), whereas for the combinations, the grade 3 or higher TRAEs were panitumumab-related dermatitis acneiform (11.3%), hypomagnesemia (5.7%), and rash (5.7%). Finally, sotorasib and panitumumab were also investigated in combination with FOLFIRI in 33 pretreated mCRC with at least one prior line of systemic therapy. ORR was 58%. More grade 3 or higher TRAEs were observed, up to 45%, mostly dermatologic [38].

3.2.3. Divarasib Cetuximab

Divarasib was also tested in combination with cetuximab in a cohort of 29 patients with *KRAS* G12C mutation mCRC, predominantly administrated at the dose of 400 mg qd [39]. Patients had been previously treated with at least two prior lines of systemic therapy, including KRAS G12C inhibitors in five patients. A similar frequency of grade 3 or higher TRAEs was observed with the combination and monotherapy (11%). However, a more complex toxicity profile emerged, as in addition to diarrhea, lipase elevation, hypomagnesemia, rash, and other anti-EGFR-related toxicities also occurred. Two grade 4 TRAEs were reported: one case of hypomagnesemia and one neutropenia. Among patients who have not previously received KRAS G12C inhibitors, the ORR was 62.5% and the mPFS was 8.1 months. Interestingly, three out of five patients pre-treated with KRAS G12C inhibitors achieved PR. CtDNA analysis revealed a significant and widespread decline in *KRAS* G12C variant allele frequency (VAF), with a KRAS G12C VAF below 0.5% after two cycles in 77% of patients, including one patient achieving stable disease (SD). At the time of disease progression, an acquired genomic alteration potentially related to adaptive resistance was identified in 13 out of 14 profiled patients; genomic alterations were consistent with those reported in patients receiving divarasib monotherapy.

3.3. Ongoing Clinical Trials and New KRAS G12C Inhibitors in Colorectal Cancer

Several clinical trials investigating the safety and efficacy of both well-established and new KRAS G12C inhibitors, alone, in combination with anti-EGFR, or combined with inhibitors of other upstream/downstream modulators of the MAPK pathway, are ongoing.

A combination of adagrasib and cetuximab is under further investigation in a phase III trial that compares the combination to chemotherapy in a second-line setting (KRYSTAL-10). The addition of irinotecan to adagrasib and cetuximab is under evaluation in a phase I trial, to explore the safety and activity of the combination (NCT05722327). Boosting KRAS G12C inhibition through targeting upstream/downstream effectors of the MAPK pathway is also under evaluation. The main MAPK pathway effectors targeted by combination compounds under evaluation include SHP2 (Src homology region 2-containing protein tyrosine phosphatase 2), a non-receptor-type protein tyrosine phosphatase encoded by the gene *PTPN11* that acts downstream of most receptor tyrosine kinases, and SOS1 (Son of Sevenless homolog 1), a GEF that switches RAS-GDP to its active conformational status. Simultaneous inhibition of SOS1 and KRAS, which was synergistic in preclinical models of *KRAS* G12C-mutated cancer cells [40], is now under clinical investigation in KRYSTAL-14 and other trials (such as NCT05578092). Similarly, the KRYSTAL-2, KontRASt-1, NCT05288205, and NCT06024174 are currently evaluating concurrent inhibition of KRAS and SHP2, as it boosted KRAS inhibition in preclinical models [34,41–43]. In addition, adagrasib is also under investigation in combination with the CDK4/6 (cycline-dependent kinase 4/6) inhibitor palbociclib in KRYSTAL-16, as it boosts KRAS inhibition due to the fact that KRAS is known to mediate cell proliferation partly through the Cyclin D family [44]. The concurrent inhibition of KRAS and CDK4/6 demonstrated increased antitumor activity in preclinical models [45]. Another putative target of combinational inhibition under clinical investigation in combination with garsorasib is the downstream effector of the MAPK pathway FAK (focal adhesive kinase), a non-receptor tyrosine kinase that promotes tumorigenesis. In fact, its concurrent blockade was found superior to anti-KRAS monotherapy in preclinical models [46].

The combination of divarasib and cetuximab, plus or minus chemotherapy, is under investigation in the INTRINSIC trial (NCT04929223), an umbrella trial evaluating the safety and efficacy of diverse targeted therapies in specific subpopulations of patients with mCRC, including those harboring *KRAS* G12C.

Several other anti-KRAS G12C compounds have been developed and are now being tested in phase I trials, mainly in combination with anti-EGFR therapy, anti-SHP2, anti-SOS1, or a pan RAS inhibitor. Pharmacodynamic and pharmacokinetic differences between these compounds might translate into differential efficacy. For example, JDQ443 and JNJ-74699157 interact with a different cysteine residue than other KRAS G12C inhibitors [47]. Thus, this suggests that they may be able to overcome mechanisms of resistance consisting of target mutations that have already been reported [47–49]. Conversely, RMC 6291 has a unique and innovative mechanism of action compared to other KRAS G12C inhibitors: it binds to cylophilin A and forms a binary complex which then blocks KRAS G12C in its GTP-bound state (on) in a tertiary complex, leading to the disruption of RAS effector binding and direct extinction of KRAS G12C (on) signaling [50]. Although it outperformed other anti-KRAS G12C (off) inhibitors in ex vivo models, clinical data are still awaited. Table 2 summarizes ongoing clinical trials evaluating KRAS G12C inhibition in patients with *KRAS* G12C-mutated colorectal cancer, and Table 3 summarizes the most relevant differences between adagrasib, sotorsaib, and divarsib.

Table 2. Key ongoing clinical trials evaluating KRAS G12C inhibitors, alone or in combination with other compounds.

Study ID/Name Phase	Treatment Regimen	Population
Ongoing clinical trials evaluating well established anti-KRAS G12C in combination with other compounds		
NCT04975256/KRYSTAL 14 Phase I/Ib	Adagrasib (MRTX849) + BI 1701963 (inhibitor of KRAS and SOS1 interaction)	advanced *KRAS* G12C mutant solid tumors
NCT05578092 Phase I/II	Adagrasib (MRTX849) + MRTX0902 (SOS1 inhibitor)	advanced solid tumors *KRAS* G12C mutant or harboring any mutations in MAPK pathway effectors
NCT05178888/KRYSTAL-16 Phase I/Ib	Adagrasib (MRTX849) + palbociclib	advanced *KRAS* G12C mutant solid tumors
NCT04330664/KRYSTAL-2 Phase I/II	Adagrasib (MRTX849) + TNO155 (SHP2 inhibitor)	advanced *KRAS* G12C mutant solid tumors
NCT04793958/KRYSTAL-10 Phase III	Adagrasib (MRTX849) + cetuximab vs chemotherapy	advanced *KRAS* G12C mutant mCRC
NCT05722327 Phase I	Adagrasib (MRTX849) + cetuximab and irinotecan	advanced *KRAS* G12C mutant mCRC
NCT06024174 Phase 1/2	Adagrasib (MRTX849) + BMS-986466 (SHP2 Inhibitor) +/− cetuximab	advanced *KRAS* G12C mutant NSCLC, PDCA, BTC and CRC
NCT04418661 Phase I	Adagrasib (MRTX849) + RMC-4630 (SHP2 inhibitor)	advanced *KRAS* G12C mutant solid tumors
NCT04892017 Phase I/II	DCC-3116 (ULK inhibitor) +/− trametinib, binimetinib, or sotorasib (AMG510)	advanced solid tumors harboring any mutation in RAS/MAPK pathway
NCT05480865/Argonaut Phase I	Sotorasib (AMG510) + BBP-398 (SHP2 inhibitor)	advanced *KRAS* G12C mutant solid tumors
NCT04929223/INTRINSIC Phase I/Ib	Divarasib (GDC-6036) + Cetuximab +/− FOLFOX or FOLFIRI (in *KRAS* G12C)	advanced mutant mCRC
NCT05497336 Phase Ib/III	Fulzerasib (IBI351) + cetuximab (phase Ib) and versus SOC (phase III in mCRC)	advanced *KRAS* G12C mutant solid tumors (phase Ib) pretreated *KRAS* G12C mutant mCRC (phase III)
NCT06166836 Phase Ib/II	Garsorasib (D-1553) + ifebemtinib (IN10018) (FAK inhibitor)	advanced *KRAS* G12C mutant solid tumors

Table 2. Cont.

Study ID/Name Phase	Treatment Regimen	Population
	Ongoing clinical trials evaluating other anti-KRAS G12C inhibitors	
NCT04165031 Phase I/II	LY3499446 +/− several compounds, based on histology (cetuximab in mCRC)	advanced KRAS G12C mutant solid tumors
NCT 04956640/LOXO-RAS-2000 Phase I/II	LY3537982 +/− several compounds, based on histology (cetuximab in mCRC)	advanced KRAS G12C mutant solid tumors
NCT04699188/KontRASt-01 Phase Ib/II	Opnurasib (JDQ443) +/− TNO155 (SHP2 inhibitor) + tislelizumab	advanced KRAS G12C mutant solid tumors
NCT05358249/KontRASt-03 Phase Ib/II	Opnurasib (JDQ443) + cetuximab (in mCRC)	advanced KRAS G12C mutant solid tumors
NCT05002270 Phase I/II	Glecirasib (JAB-21822)	advanced KRAS G12C mutant solid tumors
NCT05194995 Phase Ib/II	Glecirasib (JAB-21822) + cetuximab	advanced KRAS G12C CRC, small intestine cancer and appendiceal cancer
NCT05288205 Phase I/IIa	Glecirasib (JAB-21822) + JAB-3312 (SHP2 inhibitor)	advanced KRAS G12C mutant solid tumors
NCT04006301 Phase I	JNJ-74699157	advanced KRAS G12C mutant solid tumors
NCT05462717 Phase I	RMC-6291	advanced KRAS G12C mutant solid tumors
NCT06128551 Phase Ib	RMC-6291 + RMC-6236 (pan-RAS inhibitor)	advanced KRAS G12C mutant solid tumors
NCT06117371 Phase I/Ib	BEBT-607	advanced KRAS G12C mutant solid tumors
NCT06006793 Phase I	SY-5933	advanced KRAS G12C mutant solid tumors
NCT06006793 Phase I	BPI-421286	advanced KRAS G12C mutant solid tumors
NCT04973163 Phase Ia/Ib	BI 1823911	advanced KRAS G12C mutant solid tumors
NCT05410145 Phase I	D3S-001	advanced KRAS G12C mutant solid tumors
NCT05768321 Phase I	GEC255	advanced KRAS G12C mutant solid tumors
NCT05485974 Phase I	HBI-2438	advanced KRAS G12C mutant solid tumors

FAK: focal adhesion kinase; SHP: Src homology region 2-containing protein tyrosine phosphatase 2; SOS1: Son of Sevenless homolog 1.

Table 3. Summary of the most relevant differences between adagrasib, sotorsaib, and divarsib.

Name	Main Pharmacokinetics Characteristic of KRAS G12C Inhibitors		
	Sotorasib (AMG510)	Adagrasib (MRTX849)	Divarasib (GDC-6036)
Mechanism of action	covalent inhibitor of KRAS G12C	covalent inhibitor of KRAS G12C	covalent inhibitor of KRAS G12C
Half-life (hours)	5.5 ± 1.8	24	17.6 ± 2.7
Dose	960 mg qd	600 mg bid	400 mg qd
Median time to maximum concentration (hours)	1	6	2
Other features		CNS penetration	

qd: quaque die (once a day); bid: bis in die (2 times a day): CNS: central nervous system.

4. Mechanisms of Resistance

4.1. EGFR-Mediated Adaptive Feedback Reactivation of the RAS-MAPK Pathway

The first clinical results with KRAS G12C inhibitors in monotherapy suggested that the KRAS G12C inhibition was lineage-specific. Colorectal cancer cell lines have high basal RTK activation compared to NSCLC cell lines, and in colorectal cancer, G12C inhibition promotes higher phospho-ERK rebound than in NSCLC. Amodio et al. identified EGFR signaling as the main mechanism of resistance to KRAS G12C inhibitors, paving the way to a new strategy of combinatorial targeting of both EGFR and KRAS G12C. This was proven to be highly effective in patient-derived organoids and xenografts [33]. Figure 2 summarizes the mechanisms of resistance and proposed therapeutic strategies to overcome it.

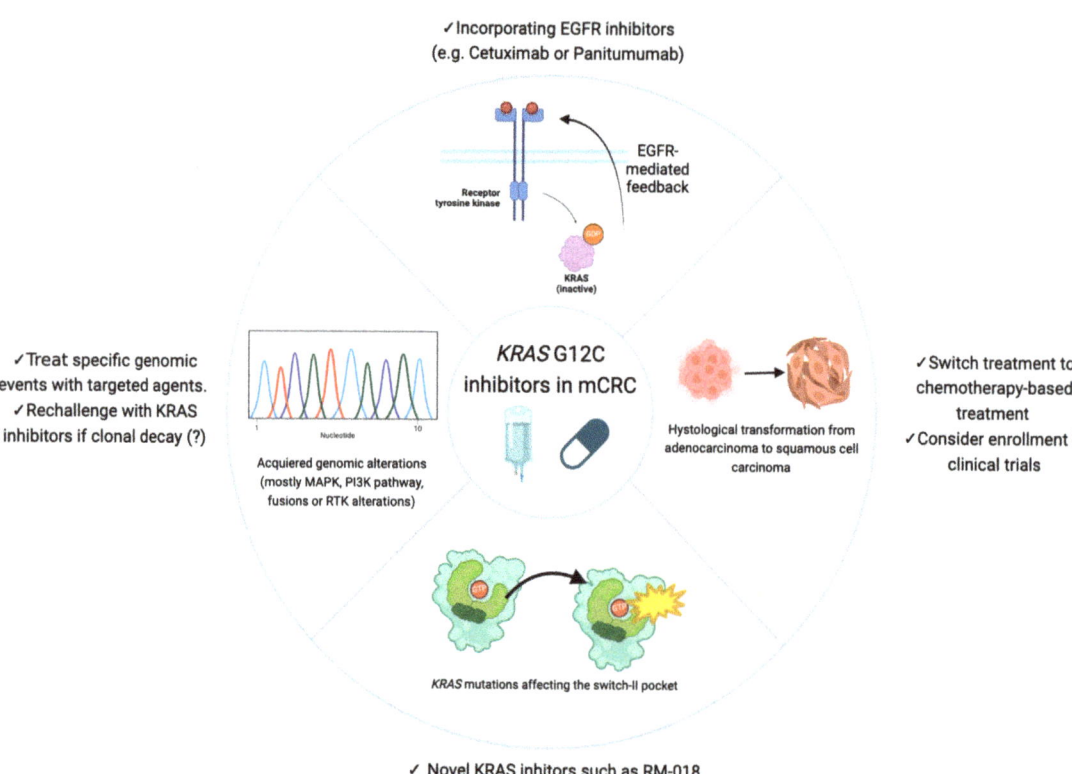

Figure 2. Summary of mechanisms of resistance and proposed therapeutic strategies to overcome it.

4.2. Acquired Genomic Events

From the results of paired plasma sample analyses from patients treated with divarasib +/− cetuximab, up to 90% had at least one acquired genomic alteration associated with treatment resistance [30,39]. Most common genomic mechanisms of resistance included genomic *KRAS* alterations (including mutations in non-G12C KRAS, BRAF-V600E, HRAS, MAP2K1, and KRAS, NRAS, and BRAF amplifications) that led to KRAS oncogenic activation, but also alterations in the PI3K and RTK pathways components, including *EGFR*, *MYC*, and *MET* amplifications and *ALK* and *RET* fusions [30,39]. Similar data has been reported with adagrasib +/− cetuximab, where genomic acquired mechanisms of resistance were detectable in more than 70% of the patients, mostly affecting genes coding for MAPK and PI3K pathway effectors and RTKs [51]. Importantly, responses were observed regardless of EGFR expression. Among patients treated with sotorasib monotherapy, genomic acquired mechanisms were also common (71%), and mostly involved RTK genes (27%), above all *EGFR*, *ERBB2*, and *KIT* [52]. In fact, more than 30% of the patients had more than three genomic mechanisms of resistance. New RTK alterations frequently emerged at progression in CRC, highlighting the potential role of combining KRAS G12C inhibitors with upstream inhibitors such as SHP2 or EGFR inhibitors. Finally, deep mutational scanning (in silico) demonstrates drug-specific patterns of resistance, with some mutations conferring resistance to adagrasib but not to sotorasib, and vice versa [49]. These pieces of evidence demonstrate the distinctiveness and complexity of the secondary resistance to KRAS G12C inhibition and pave the way to overcoming it through the development of both novel KRAS inhibitors with alternative modes of binding and different allele specificities, and effective combination therapy regimens with inhibitors of other effectors in the MAPK pathway. Both these strategies are already under investigation [41,47,48,50]. On the contrary, besides promising pre-clinical evidence of effective concurrent blockading of PI3K/AKT/mTOR signaling, no clinical trial is currently ongoing to our knowledge [43,53].

4.3. KRAS Switch-II Pocket Mutations

Most of the patients treated with KRAS G12C inhibitors will develop polyclonal genomic alterations as a central acquired mechanism of resistance. Notably, several *KRAS* mutations including R68S, H95R, and Y96D mutations affect the switch-II pocket, to which KRAS G12C inhibitors bind, conferring resistance to these drugs [49,54]. In patient-derived *KRAS* G12C models, a novel functionally distinct tricomplex KRAS G12C active-state inhibitor (RM-018) has been tested preclinically and successfully inhibited KRAS G12C/Y96D, thus overcoming this mechanism of resistance. Collectively, mutations that disrupt covalent drug binding can lead to clinical resistance to KRAS G12C inhibitors.

4.4. Histological Switch

In two out of ten patients (one patient with CRC and the other with non-small cell lung carcinoma) treated with adagrasib monotherapy, from whom paired tumor tissue was available, the histologic transformation from adenocarcinoma to squamous cell carcinoma was observed without any identifiable genomic mechanism of resistance [49]. Studies in G12C and G12D *KRAS*-mutant lung cancer mouse models and organoids treated with KRAS inhibitors reveal that tumors invoke a lineage plasticity program to switch from adenocarcinoma to squamous via transcriptomic and epigenomic changes, modulating the response to KRAS inhibition [55].

5. Discussion

KRAS G12C mutations are present in a small percentage of metastatic colorectal cancer patients [9]. However, it is associated with a poor response to standard treatments and shorter overall survival compared with non-G12C mutations [12,13]. Thus, the development of targeted agents that can improve these outcomes is paramount. In the last decade, several KRAS G12C inhibitors have emerged. Nonetheless, the understanding of the underlying biology of these tumors has also been crucial in identifying and overcoming mechanisms of resistance. Early on, after the first patients were treated with KRAS G12C inhibitors, it was observed that, like *BRAF*-mutated tumors [56,57], when blocking the *KRAS* mutation, negative adaptive feedback through the EGFR receptor emerges, leading to resistance [33]. Thus, subsequent studies included either cetuximab or panitumumab to overcome this mechanism of resistance. Indeed, with this combination, clinical outcomes improved as the drugs boost the antitumor effect. In this scenario, adagrasib and sotorasib are the first inhibitors being developed and the ones that are in a more advanced stage. The CodeBreaK 300 trial, combining sotorasib and panitumumab, has been the first phase III randomized trial to demonstrate the benefit of a KRAS inhibitor over standard treatment in colorectal cancer [38]. Currently, the KRYSTAL-10 trial, a randomized phase III trial comparing adagrasib plus cetuximab vs. chemotherapy, has finished recruitment, and results are awaited in the upcoming months. In addition, new KRAS inhibitors such as divarasib or garsorasib have also demonstrated deep clinical activity not only in monotherapy, with disease control rates of 84% and 95%, respectively, but also in combination with anti-EGFR agents. When divarasib was combined with cetuximab, the DCR increased to 95.8% [30,39]. However, data from these trials, despite being promising, need to be carefully interpreted as they come from small, non-randomized phase I and phase II clinical trials. However, it could be expected that the combination of these new KRAS inhibitors plus anti-EGFR may improve the patients' clinical outcomes significantly. Regarding treatment-related adverse events, the toxicity profile is similar and manageable among different KRAS G12C inhibitors, mostly low-grade gastrointestinal adverse events and rash.

On the other hand, despite the addition of anti-EGFR to overcome the EGFR-mediated adaptive feedback reactivation of the RAS-MAPK pathway following KRAS G12C inhibition, eventually all patients will progress. In this regard, liquid biopsy has been demonstrated to be a reliable tool in colorectal cancer to monitor response, to forecast prognosis, and to identify genomic mechanisms of resistance [58–63]. Circulating tumor DNA from the KRYSTAL-1 and CodeBreaK 100 trials has been demonstrated to be able to identify multiple acquired pathological genomic alterations among patients treated with KRAS G12C inhibitors, with or without anti-EGFR, in up to 70% of the patients, but particularly among patients treated with the combination [51,52]. In addition, through ctDNA, it has been identified that patients receiving the double combination have larger decreases in ctDNA, and this was associated with deeper responses. Indeed, those patients with a mutant allele fraction clearance (MAFC) higher than 90% achieve an ORR of 47% and 67% with adagrasib and adagrasib-cetuximab, respectively, whereas patients with a MAFC lower than 90% have an ORR of 8% and 33% with adagrasib and adagrasib-cetuximab, respectively [51]. Similar results were also observed in phase 1b, where divarasib and cetuximab were combined, in which patients with higher MAFC achieve higher ORR compared with patients with lower MAFC [39]. Based on these results, it is clear that ctDNA can be used to track tumor dynamics and identify mechanisms of resistance. In this regard, it could be hypothesized that, similar to the *RAS* wild-type and *BRAF* story in which rechallenge (anti-EGFR and BRAF inhibitor plus anti-EGFR, respectively) guided with liquid biopsy has been demonstrated to improve clinical outcomes [64–67]. If there is a resistance to clonal decay, perhaps the reintroduction of KRAS G12C inhibitors may be effective in a well-selected population. However, liquid biopsy has also highlighted that RTK alterations are commonly found in this scenario, which opens a window of opportunity to test new drugs such as SHP2 inhibitors or combinations with immune checkpoint inhibitors. Lastly, less common but also important mechanisms of resistance need to be discussed, such as the histological switch after a KRAS inhibitor-based combination or the conformational changes of the switch-II pocket produced by specific acquired *KRAS* mutations. The first scenario highlights the importance of obtaining, when possible, tumor tissue upon progression, as this tissue can be informative in helping make decisions such as changes to a specific chemotherapy regimen based on histological differentiation. The second scenario is also a window of opportunity to test new tricomplex inhibitors that can block KRAS activation even when conventional inhibitors are not able to because of three-dimensional structural changes. Finally, the combination of chemotherapy with KRAS G12C inhibitors has also demonstrated deep clinical responses. The phase 1b CodeBreaK 101 subprotocol H is currently evaluating the combination of FOLFIRI plus sotorasib plus panitumumab in the refractory setting with an ORR of 58% and a DCR of 93%, including patients previously treated with KRAS G12C inhibitors, thus suggesting that rechallenge with KRAS G12C inhibitors in combination with chemotherapy may lead to responses even among patients who have previously progressed to a KRAS G12C inhibitor [38].

Finally, many studies have pointed out the role of the gut microbiome as a prognostic and predictive biomarker in colorectal cancer [68,69]. In colorectal cancer, *Fusobacterium nucleatum* has been related to genetic and epigenetic lesions, such as microsatellite instability, the CpG island methylator phenotype, and genome mutations in colorectal cancer tissues [70]. Indeed, *F. nucleatum* could promote proliferation and metabolism, remodel the immune microenvironment, and facilitate metastasis and chemoresistance in the tumorigenesis and development of CRC [68]. In addition, *F. nucleatum* is enriched in *KRAS* G12-mutant CRC tumor tissues and contributes to colorectal tumorigenesis. Thus, personalized modulation of the gut microbiota may provide a more targeted strategy for CRC treatment.

All in all, the landscape of KRAS G12C inhibitors in colorectal cancer is changing faster, and the identification of mechanisms of resistance has been paramount in boosting the antitumor activity of these combinations. Despite data from randomized phase III trials still being scarce, data from phase II trials evaluating new molecules are promising.

6. Conclusions

Even though *KRAS* G12C mutations represent a small percentage of all mCRC (around 4%), the development of KRAS G12C inhibitors has demonstrated meaningful clinical activity. Currently, there is only one randomized phase III trial demonstrating benefit over trifluridine/tipiracil, but ongoing trials, combining KRAS inhibitors with anti-EGFR, show promising results and may increase therapeutic options in different settings in the upcoming years. In addition, the identification of mechanisms of resistance has led to new treatment strategies to overcome acquired mechanisms of resistance such as conformational changes of the switch-II pocket, acquired genomic events, or histological changes. In this scenario, liquid biopsy may help to track tumor responses, identify mechanisms of resistance, and track clonal decay to develop new treatment strategies. There are new arrows in the quiver for *KRAS*-mutated colorectal cancer.

Author Contributions: Conceptualization J.R. and C.V.; resources, J.R., C.V., I.B., N.S.G., M.R.-C., A.G., A.A., F.S., J.T. and E.E.; writing—original draft preparation, J.R. and C.V.; writing—review and editing, J.R., C.V., I.B., N.S.G., M.R.-C., A.G., A.A., F.S., J.T. and E.E.; supervision, E.E. All authors have read and agreed to the published version of the manuscript.

Funding: This research received no external funding.

Conflicts of Interest: J.R. declares personal financial interests in the form of speaking/travel grants or accommodation from Amgen, Merck, Pierre-Fabre, Servier, and Sanofi. C.V. declares no conflicts of interest. N.S.G. declares accommodation and travel expenses from AMGEN and MERCK and personal speaker honoraria from AMGEN. F.S. reports personal financial interests, honoraria for advisory roles, travel grants, and research grants (over the past 5 years) from Hoffman–La Roche, Sanofi Aventis, Amgen, Merck Serono, Servier, and Bristol-Myers Squibb. I.B. has received accommodation and travel expenses from Amgen, Merck, Sanofi, and Servier; and personal speaker honoraria from Astra Zeneca. M.R.-C. declares personal speaker honoraria from ROVI and accommodation expenses from BMS, Amgen, and Merck. A.G. declares no conflicts of interest. A.A. declares no conflicts of interest. J.T. reports personal financial interest in the form of scientific consultancy roles at Array Biopharma, AstraZeneca, Bayer, Boehringer Ingelheim, Chugai, Daiichi Sankyo, and F. Hoffmann-La. E.E. reports roles as a consultant/advisor and/or honoraria, travel grants, and research grants from Amgen, Bayer, Hoffman-La Roche, Merck Serono, Sanofi, Pierre Fabre, MSD, Organon, Novartis, and Servier, and reports institutional research funding from Amgen Inc., Array Biopharma Inc., AstraZeneca Pharmaceuticals LP, BeiGene, Boehringer Ingelheim, Bristol Myers Squibb, Celgene, Debiopharm International SA, F. Hoffmann-La Roche Ltd., Genentech Inc., HalioDX SAS, Hutchison Medi Pharma International, Janssen-Cilag SA, MedImmune, Menarini, Merck Health KGAA, Merck Sharp & Dohme, Merus NV, Mirati, Novartis Farmacéutica SA, Pfizer, Pharma Mar, Sanofi Aventis Recherche & Développement, Servier, and Taiho Pharma USA Inc. Roche Ltd., Genentech Inc, Halio DXSAS, Hutchison Medi Pharma International, Ikena Oncology, Inspirna Inc, IQVIA, Lilly, Menarini, Merck Serono, Merus, MSD, Mirati, Neophore, Novartis, Ona Therapeutics, Orion Biotechnology, Peptomyc, Pfizer, Pierre Fabre, Samsung Bioepis, Sanofi, Scandion Oncology, Scorpion Therapeutics, Seattle Genetics, Servier, Sotio Biotech, Taiho, Tessa Therapeutics, and Thera Myc. Stocks: Oniria Therapeutics and also educational collaboration with medex/HMP, Medscape Education, MJH Life Sciences, Peer View Institute for Medical Education and Physicians Education Resource (PER).

References

1. Muzny, D.M.; Bainbridge, M.N.; Chang, K.; Dinh, H.H.; Drummond, J.A.; Fowler, G.; Kovar, C.L.; Lewis, L.R.; Morgan, M.B.; Newsham, I.F.; et al. Comprehensive Molecular Characterization of Human Colon and Rectal Cancer. *Nature* **2012**, *487*, 330. [CrossRef]
2. Cervantes, A.; Adam, R.; Roselló, S.; Arnold, D.; Normanno, N.; Taïeb, J.; Seligmann, J.; De Baere, T.; Osterlund, P.; Yoshino, T. et al. Metastatic Colorectal Cancer: ESMO Clinical Practice Guideline for Diagnosis, Treatment and Follow-up ☆. *Ann. Oncol* **2023**, *34*, 10–32. [CrossRef] [PubMed]
3. Mayer, R.J.; Van Cutsem, E.; Falcone, A.; Yoshino, T.; Garcia-Carbonero, R.; Mizunuma, N.; Yamazaki, K.; Shimada, Y.; Tabernero, J.; Komatsu, Y.; et al. Randomized Trial of TAS-102 for Refractory Metastatic Colorectal Cancer. *N. Engl. J. Med.* **2015**, *372*, 1909–1919. [CrossRef] [PubMed]
4. Prager, G.W.; Taieb, J.; Fakih, M.; Ciardiello, F.; Van Cutsem, E.; Elez, E.; Cruz, F.M.; Wyrwicz, L.; Stroyakovskiy, D.; Pápai, Z. et al. Trifluridine–Tipiracil and Bevacizumab in Refractory Metastatic Colorectal Cancer. *N. Engl. J. Med.* **2023**, *388*, 1657–1667 [CrossRef] [PubMed]
5. Grothey, A.; Van Cutsem, E.; Sobrero, A.; Siena, S.; Falcone, A.; Ychou, M.; Humblet, Y.; Bouché, O.; Mineur, L.; Barone, C. et al. Regorafenib Monotherapy for Previously Treated Metastatic Colorectal Cancer (CORRECT): An International, Multicentre, Randomised, Placebo-Controlled, Phase 3 Trial. *Lancet* **2013**, *381*, 303–312. [CrossRef] [PubMed]
6. Henry, J.T.; Coker, O.; Chowdhury, S.; Shen, J.P.; Morris, V.K.; Dasari, A.; Raghav, K.; Nusrat, M.; Kee, B.; Parseghian, C.; et al Comprehensive Clinical and Molecular Characterization of KRAS G12C -Mutant Colorectal Cancer. *JCO Precis. Oncol.* **2021**, *6*, 613–621. [CrossRef] [PubMed]
7. Jones, R.P.; Sutton, P.A.; Evans, J.P.; Clifford, R.; McAvoy, A.; Lewis, J.; Rousseau, A.; Mountford, R.; McWhirter, D.; Malik, H.Z. Specific Mutations in KRAS Codon 12 Are Associated with Worse Overall Survival in Patients with Advanced and Recurrent Colorectal Cancer. *Br. J. Cancer* **2017**, *116*, 923–929. [CrossRef]
8. Lee, J.K.; Sivakumar, S.; Schrock, A.B.; Madison, R.; Fabrizio, D.; Gjoerup, O.; Ross, J.S.; Frampton, G.M.; Napalkov, P.; Montesion, M.; et al. Comprehensive Pan-Cancer Genomic Landscape of KRAS Altered Cancers and Real-World Outcomes in Solid Tumors. *NPJ Precis. Oncol.* **2022**, *6*, 91. [CrossRef]
9. Nassar, A.H.; Adib, E.; Kwiatkowski, D.J. Distribution of KRAS G12C Somatic Mutations across Race, Sex, and Cancer Type. *N. Engl. J. Med.* **2021**, *384*, 185–187. [CrossRef]
10. Schirripa, M.; Nappo, F.; Cremolini, C.; Salvatore, L.; Rossini, D.; Bensi, M.; Businello, G.; Pietrantonio, F.; Randon, G.; Fucà, G.; et al. KRAS G12C Metastatic Colorectal Cancer: Specific Features of a New Emerging Target Population. *Clin. Color. Cancer* **2020**, *19*, 219–225. [CrossRef]
11. Ciardiello, D.; Chiarazzo, C.; Famiglietti, V.; Damato, A.; Pinto, C.; Zampino, M.G.; Castellano, G.; Gervaso, L.; Zaniboni, A.; Oneda, E.; et al. Clinical Efficacy of Sequential Treatments in KRASG12C-Mutant Metastatic Colorectal Cancer: Findings from a Real-Life Multicenter Italian Study (CRC-KR GOIM). *ESMO Open* **2022**, *7*, 100567. [CrossRef] [PubMed]
12. Fakih, M.; Tu, H.; Hsu, H.; Aggarwal, S.; Chan, E.; Rehn, M.; Chia, V.; Kopetz, S. Real-World Study of Characteristics and Treatment Outcomes Among Patients with KRAS p.G12C-Mutated or Other KRAS Mutated Metastatic Colorectal Cancer. *Oncologist* **2022**, *27*, 663–674. [CrossRef] [PubMed]
13. Van de Haar, J.; Ma, X.; Ooft, S.N.; van der Helm, P.W.; Hoes, L.R.; Mainardi, S.; Pinato, D.J.; Sun, K.; Salvatore, L.; Tortora, G.; et al. Codon-Specific KRAS Mutations Predict Survival Benefit of Trifluridine/Tipiracil in Metastatic Colorectal Cancer. *Nat. Med.* **2023**, *29*, 605–614. [CrossRef] [PubMed]
14. Zeissig, M.N.; Ashwood, L.M.; Kondrashova, O.; Sutherland, K.D. Next Batter up! Targeting Cancers with KRAS-G12D Mutations. *Trends Cancer* **2023**, *9*, 955–967. [CrossRef] [PubMed]
15. Hammond, D.E.; Mageean, C.J.; Rusilowicz, E.V.; Wickenden, J.A.; Clague, M.J.; Prior, I.A. Differential Reprogramming of Isogenic Colorectal Cancer Cells by Distinct Activating KRAS Mutations. *J. Proteome Res.* **2015**, *14*, 1535–1546. [CrossRef] [PubMed]
16. Brubaker, D.K.; Paulo, J.A.; Sheth, S.; Gygi, S.P.; Lauffenburger, D.A.; Haigis, K.M. Proteogenomic Network Analysis of Context-Specific KRAS Signaling in Mouse-to-Human Cross-Species Translation. *Cell Syst.* **2019**, *9*, 258–270. [CrossRef]
17. Kwan, A.K.; Piazza, G.A.; Keeton, A.B.; Leite, C.A. The Path to the Clinic: A Comprehensive Review on Direct KRASG12C Inhibitors. *J. Exp. Clin. Cancer Res.* **2022**, *41*, 27. [CrossRef]
18. Ciardiello, D.; Maiorano, B.A.; Martinelli, E. Targeting KRASG12C in Colorectal Cancer: The Beginning of a New Era. *ESMO Open* **2023**, *8*, 100745. [CrossRef]
19. Ostrem, J.M.; Peters, U.; Sos, M.L.; Wells, J.A.; Shokat, K.M. K-Ras(G12C) Inhibitors Allosterically Control GTP Affinity and Effector Interactions. *Nature* **2013**, *503*, 548–551. [CrossRef]
20. Kargbo, R.B. Inhibitors of G12C Mutant Ras Proteins for the Treatment of Cancers. *ACS Med. Chem. Lett.* **2019**, *10*, 10. [CrossRef]
21. Lito, P.; Solomon, M.; Li, L.S.; Hansen, R.; Rosen, N. Cancer Therapeutics: Allele-Specific Inhibitors Inactivate Mutant KRAS G12C by a Trapping Mechanism. *Science* **2016**, *351*, 604–608. [CrossRef] [PubMed]
22. Patricelli, M.P.; Janes, M.R.; Li, L.S.; Hansen, R.; Peters, U.; Kessler, L.V.; Chen, Y.; Kucharski, J.M.; Feng, J.; Ely, T.; et al. Selective Inhibition of Oncogenic KRAS Output with Small Molecules Targeting the Inactive State. *Cancer Discov.* **2016**, *6*, 316–329. [CrossRef] [PubMed]

23. Canon, J.; Rex, K.; Saiki, A.Y.; Mohr, C.; Cooke, K.; Bagal, D.; Gaida, K.; Holt, T.; Knutson, C.G.; Koppada, N.; et al. The Clinical KRAS(G12C) Inhibitor AMG 510 Drives Anti-Tumour Immunity. *Nature* **2019**, *575*, 217–223. [CrossRef] [PubMed]
24. Hong, D.S.; Fakih, M.G.; Strickler, J.H.; Desai, J.; Durm, G.A.; Shapiro, G.I.; Falchook, G.S.; Price, T.J.; Sacher, A.; Denlinger, C.S.; et al. KRASG12C Inhibition with Sotorasib in Advanced Solid Tumors. *N. Engl. J. Med.* **2020**, *383*, 1207. [CrossRef] [PubMed]
25. Fakih, M.G.; Kopetz, S.; Kuboki, Y.; Kim, T.W.; Munster, P.N.; Krauss, J.C.; Falchook, G.S.; Han, S.W.; Heinemann, V.; Muro, K.; et al. Sotorasib for Previously Treated Colorectal Cancers with KRASG12C Mutation (CodeBreaK100): A Prespecified Analysis of a Single-Arm, Phase 2 Trial. *Lancet Oncol.* **2022**, *23*, 115–124. [CrossRef]
26. Dy, G.K.; Govindan, R.; Velcheti, V.; Falchook, G.S.; Italiano, A.; Wolf, J.; Sacher, A.G.; Takahashi, T.; Ramalingam, S.S.; Dooms, C.; et al. Long-Term Outcomes and Molecular Correlates of Sotorasib Efficacy in Patients With Pretreated KRAS G12C-Mutated Non–Small-Cell Lung Cancer: 2-Year Analysis of CodeBreaK 100. *J. Clin. Oncol.* **2023**, *41*, 3311. [CrossRef] [PubMed]
27. Ou, S.H.I.; Jänne, P.A.; Leal, T.A.; Rybkin, I.I.; Sabari, J.K.; Barve, M.A.; Bazhenova, L.; Johnson, M.L.; Velastegui, K.L.; Cilliers, C.; et al. First-in-Human Phase I/IB Dose-Finding Study of Adagrasib (MRTX849) in Patients with Advanced KRAS G12CSolid Tumors (KRYSTAL-1). *J. Clin. Oncol.* **2022**, *40*, 2530–2538. [CrossRef] [PubMed]
28. Yaeger, R.; Weiss, J.; Pelster, M.S.; Spira, A.I.; Barve, M.; Ou, S.-H.I.; Leal, T.A.; Bekaii-Saab, T.S.; Paweletz, C.P.; Heavey, G.A.; et al. Adagrasib with or without Cetuximab in Colorectal Cancer with Mutated KRAS G12C. *N. Engl. J. Med.* **2023**, *388*, 44–54. [CrossRef]
29. Purkey, H. Discovery of GDC-6036, a Clinical Stage Treatment for KRAS G12C-Positive Cancers. *Cancer Res.* **2022**, *82* (Suppl. S12), ND11. [CrossRef]
30. Sacher, A.; LoRusso, P.; Patel, M.R.; Miller, W.H.; Garralda, E.; Forster, M.D.; Santoro, A.; Falcon, A.; Kim, T.W.; Paz-Ares, L.; et al. Single-Agent Divarasib (GDC-6036) in Solid Tumors with a KRAS G12C Mutation. *N. Engl. J. Med.* **2023**, *389*, 710–721. [CrossRef]
31. Yuan, Y.; Deng, Y.; Jin, Y.; Pan, Y.; Wang, C.; Wang, Z.; Zhang, Z.; Meng, X.; Hu, Y.; Zhao, M.; et al. Efficacy and Safety of IBI351 (GFH925) Monotherapy in Metastatic Colorectal Cancer Harboring KRASG12C Mutation: Preliminary Results from a Pooled Analysis of Two Phase I Studies. *J. Clin. Oncol.* **2023**, *41*, 3586. [CrossRef]
32. Xu, R.-H.; Xu, Y.; Yan, D.; Munster, P.; Ruan, D.; Deng, Y.; Pan, H.; Underhill, C.R.; Richardson, G.; Nordman, I.; et al. 55O Safety and Efficacy of D-1553 in Combination with Cetuximab in KRAS G12C Mutated Colorectal Cancer (CRC): A Phase II Study. *Ann. Oncol.* **2023**, *34*, S410–S411. [CrossRef]
33. Amodio, V.; Yaeger, R.; Arcella, P.; Cancelliere, C.; Lamba, S.; Lorenzato, A.; Arena, S.; Montone, M.; Mussolin, B.; Bian, Y.; et al. EGFR Blockade Reverts Resistance to KRASG12C Inhibition in Colorectal Cancer. *Cancer Discov.* **2020**, *10*, 1129–1139. [CrossRef] [PubMed]
34. Ryan, M.B.; Coker, O.; Sorokin, A.; Fella, K.; Barnes, H.; Wong, E.; Kanikarla, P.; Gao, F.; Zhang, Y.; Zhou, L.; et al. KRASG12C-Independent Feedback Activation of Wild-Type RAS Constrains KRASG12C Inhibitor Efficacy. *Cell Rep.* **2022**, *39*, 110993. [CrossRef]
35. Nusrat, M.; Yaeger, R. KRAS Inhibition in Metastatic Colorectal Cancer: An Update. *Curr. Opin. Pharmacol.* **2023**, *68*, 102343. [CrossRef]
36. Kuboki, Y.; Fakih, M.; Strickler, J.; Yaeger, R.; Masuishi, T.; Kim, E.J.; Bestvina, C.M.; Kopetz, S.; Falchook, G.S.; Langer, C.; et al. Sotorasib with Panitumumab in Chemotherapy-Refractory KRASG12C-Mutated Colorectal Cancer: A Phase 1b Trial. *Nat. Med.* **2024**, *30*, 265–270. [CrossRef] [PubMed]
37. Fakih, M.G.; Salvatore, L.; Esaki, T.; Modest, D.P.; Lopez-Bravo, D.P.; Taieb, J.; Karamouzis, M.V.; Ruiz-Garcia, E.; Kim, T.-W.; Kuboki, Y.; et al. Sotorasib plus Panitumumab in Refractory Colorectal Cancer with Mutated KRAS G12C. *N. Engl. J. Med.* **2023**, *389*, 2125–2139. [CrossRef]
38. Hong, D.S.; Kuboki, Y.; Strickler, J.H.; Fakih, M.; Houssiau, H.; Price, T.J.; Elez, E.; Siena, S.; Chan, E.; Nolte-Hippenmeyer, J.; et al. Sotorasib (Soto) plus Panitumumab (Pmab) and FOLFIRI for Previously Treated KRAS G12C-Mutated Metastatic Colorectal Cancer (MCRC): CodeBreaK 101 Phase 1b Safety and Efficacy. *J. Clin. Oncol.* **2023**, *41*, 3513. [CrossRef]
39. Desai, J.; Alonso, G.; Kim, S.H.; Cervantes, A.; Karasic, T.; Medina, L.; Shacham-Shmueli, E.; Cosman, R.; Falcon, A.; Gort, E.; et al. Divarasib plus Cetuximab in KRAS G12C-Positive Colorectal Cancer: A Phase 1b Trial. *Nat. Med.* **2024**, *30*, 271. [CrossRef]
40. Hillig, R.C.; Sautier, B.; Schroeder, J.; Moosmayer, D.; Hilpmann, A.; Stegmann, C.M.; Werbeck, N.D.; Briem, H.; Boemer, U.; Weiske, J.; et al. Discovery of Potent SOS1 Inhibitors That Block RAS Activation via Disruption of the RAS–SOS1 Interaction. *Proc. Natl. Acad. Sci. USA* **2019**, *116*, 2551–2560. [CrossRef]
41. Negrao, M.V.; Cassier, P.A.; Solomon, B.; Schuler, M.; Rohrberg, K.; Cresta, S.; Dooms, C.; Tan, D.S.W.; Loong, H.H.; Amatu, A.; et al. MA06.03 KontRASt-01: Preliminary Safety and Efficacy of JDQ443 + TNO155 in Patients with Advanced, KRAS G12C-Mutated Solid Tumors. *J. Thorac. Oncol.* **2023**, *18*, S117–S118. [CrossRef]
42. Ryan, M.B.; de la Cruz, F.F.; Phat, S.; Myers, D.T.; Wong, E.; Shahzade, H.A.; Hong, C.B.; Corcoran, R.B. Vertical Pathway Inhibition Overcomes Adaptive Feedback Resistance to KrasG12C Inhibition. *Clin. Cancer Res.* **2020**, *26*, 1617–1643. [CrossRef] [PubMed]
43. Matsubara, H.; Miyoshi, H.; Kakizaki, F.; Morimoto, T.; Kawada, K.; Yamamoto, T.; Obama, K.; Sakai, Y.; Taketo, M.M. Efficacious Combination Drug Treatment for Colorectal Cancer That Overcomes Resistance to KRAS G12C Inhibitors. *Mol. Cancer Ther.* **2019**, *22*, 529–538. [CrossRef] [PubMed]

44. Sommerhalder, D.; Thevathasan, J.; Ianopulos, X.; Volinn, W.; Hong, D. Abstract CT242: KRYSTAL-16: A Phase I/Ib Trial of Adagrasib (MRTX849) in Combination with Palbociclib in Patients with Advanced Solid Tumors with KRASG12C Mutation. *Cancer Res.* **2022**, *82*, CT242. [CrossRef]
45. Hallin, J.; Engstrom, L.D.; Hargi, L.; Calinisan, A.; Aranda, R.; Briere, D.M.; Sudhakar, N.; Bowcut, V.; Baer, B.R.; Ballard, J.A.; et al. The KRASG12C Inhibitor MRTX849 Provides Insight toward Therapeutic Susceptibility of KRAS-Mutant Cancers in Mouse Models and Patients. *Cancer Discov.* **2020**, *10*, 54–71. [CrossRef] [PubMed]
46. Zhang, B.; Zhang, Y.; Zhang, J.; Liu, P.; Jiao, B.; Wang, Z.; Ren, R. Focal Adhesion Kinase (FAK) Inhibition Synergizes with KRAS G12C Inhibitors in Treating Cancer through the Regulation of the FAK–YAP Signaling. *Adv. Sci.* **2021**, *8*, 2100250. [CrossRef] [PubMed]
47. Wang, J.; Martin-Romano, P.; Cassier, P.; Johnson, M.; Haura, E.; Lenox, L.; Guo, Y.; Bandyopadhyay, N.; Russell, M.; Shearin, E.; et al. Phase I Study of JNJ-74699157 in Patients with Advanced Solid Tumors Harboring the KRAS G12C Mutation. *Oncologist* **2022**, *27*, 536–553. [CrossRef]
48. Weiss, A.; Lorthiois, E.; Barys, L.; Beyer, K.S.; Bomio-Confaglia, C.; Burks, H.; Chen, X.; Cui, X.; De Kanter, R.; Dharmarajan, L.; et al. Discovery, Preclinical Characterization, and Early Clinical Activity of JDQ443, a Structurally Novel, Potent, and Selective Covalent Oral Inhibitor of KRAS G12C. *Cancer Discov.* **2022**, *12*, 1500–1517. [CrossRef]
49. Awad, M.M.; Liu, S.; Rybkin, I.I.; Arbour, K.C.; Dilly, J.; Zhu, V.W.; Johnson, M.L.; Heist, R.S.; Patil, T.; Riely, G.J.; et al. Acquired Resistance to KRAS G12C Inhibition in Cancer. *N. Engl. J. Med.* **2021**, *384*, 2382–2393. [CrossRef]
50. Cregg, J.; Nichols, R.J.; Yang, Y.C.; Schulze, C.J.; Wang, Z.; Dua, R.; Jiang, J.; Nasholm, N.; Knox, J.E.; Seamon, K.; et al. Abstract ND07: Discovery of RMC-6291, a Tri-Complex KRASG12C(ON) Inhibitor. *Cancer Res.* **2023**, *83*, ND07. [CrossRef]
51. Pelster, M.S.; Yaeger, R.; Klempner, S.J.; Ou, S.-H.I.; Spira, A.I.; Jänne, P.A.; Uboha, N.V.; Gaffar, Y.A.; Newman, G.; Paweletz, C.P.; et al. 549O Adagrasib with or without Cetuximab in Patients with KRASG12C-Mutated Colorectal Cancer (CRC): Analysis of Tumor Biomarkers and Genomic Alterations. *Ann. Oncol.* **2023**, *34*, S410. [CrossRef]
52. Prenen, H.; Fakih, M.; Falchook, G.; Strickler, J.; Hindoyan, A.; Anderson, A.; Ang, A.; Kurata, T.; Price, T. SO-39 Evaluation of Acquired Resistance to Sotorasib in KRAS p.G12C-Mutated Colorectal Cancer: Exploratory Plasma Biomarker Analysis of CodeBreaK 100. *Ann. Oncol.* **2022**, *33*, S373. [CrossRef]
53. Yaeger, R.; Mezzadra, R.; Sinopoli, J.; Bian, Y.; Marasco, M.; Kaplun, E.; Gao, Y.; Zhao, H.; Paula, A.D.C.; Zhu, Y.; et al. Molecular Characterization of Acquired Resistance to KRASG12C–EGFR Inhibition in Colorectal Cancer. *Cancer Discov.* **2023**, *13*, 41–55. [CrossRef] [PubMed]
54. Tanaka, N.; Lin, J.J.; Li, C.; Ryan, M.B.; Zhang, J.; Kiedrowski, L.A.; Michel, A.G.; Syed, M.U.; Fella, K.A.; Sakhi, M.; et al. Clinical Acquired Resistance to KRASG12C Inhibition through a Novel KRAS Switch-II Pocket Mutation and Polyclonal Alterations Converging on RAS–MAPK Reactivation. *Cancer Discov.* **2021**, *11*, 1913–1922. [CrossRef] [PubMed]
55. Tong, X.; Patel, A.S.; Kim, E.; Li, H.; Chen, Y.; Li, S.; Liu, S.; Dilly, J.; Kapner, K.S.; Zhang, N.; et al. Adeno-to-Squamous Transition Drives Resistance to KRAS Inhibition in LKB1 Mutant Lung Cancer. *Cancer Cell* **2024**, *42*, 413–428.e7. [CrossRef] [PubMed]
56. Corcoran, R.B.; Ebi, H.; Turke, A.B.; Coffee, E.M.; Nishino, M.; Cogdill, A.P.; Brown, R.D.; Pelle, P.D.; Dias-Santagata, D.; Hung, K.E.; et al. EGFR-Mediated Reactivation of MAPK Signaling Contributes to Insensitivity of BRAF-Mutant Colorectal Cancers to RAF Inhibition with Vemurafenib. *Cancer Discov.* **2012**, *2*, 227–235. [CrossRef] [PubMed]
57. Prahallad, A.; Sun, C.; Huang, S.; Di Nicolantonio, F.; Salazar, R.; Zecchin, D.; Beijersbergen, R.L.; Bardelli, A.; Bernards, R. Unresponsiveness of Colon Cancer to BRAF(V600E) Inhibition through Feedback Activation of EGFR. *Nature* **2012**, *483*, 100–103. [CrossRef]
58. Tie, J.; Wang, Y.; Tomasetti, C.; Li, L.; Springer, S.; Kinde, I.; Silliman, N.; Tacey, M.; Wong, H.L.; Christie, M.; et al. Circulating Tumor DNA Analysis Detects Minimal Residual Disease and Predicts Recurrence in Patients with Stage II Colon Cancer. *Sci. Transl. Med.* **2016**, *8*, 346ra92. [CrossRef]
59. Montagut, C.; Dalmases, A.; Bellosillo, B.; Crespo, M.; Pairet, S.; Iglesias, M.; Salido, M.; Gallen, M.; Marsters, S.; Tsai, S.P.; et al. Identification of a Mutation in the Extracellular Domain of the Epidermal Growth Factor Receptor Conferring Cetuximab Resistance in Colorectal Cancer. *Nat. Med.* **2012**, *18*, 221–223. [CrossRef]
60. Montagut, C.; Argilés, G.; Ciardiello, F.; Poulsen, T.T.; Dienstmann, R.; Kragh, M.; Kopetz, S.; Lindsted, T.; Ding, C.; Vidal, J.; et al. Efficacy of Sym004 in Patients With Metastatic Colorectal Cancer With Acquired Resistance to Anti-EGFR Therapy and Molecularly Selected by Circulating Tumor DNA Analyses: A Phase 2 Randomized Clinical Trial. *JAMA Oncol.* **2018**, *4*, e175245. [CrossRef]
61. Ros, J.; Matito, J.; Villacampa, G.; Comas, R.; Garcia, A.; Martini, G.; Baraibar, I.; Saoudi, N.; Salvà, F.; Martin, A.; et al. Plasmatic BRAF-V600E Allele Fraction as a Prognostic Factor in Metastatic Colorectal Cancer Treated with BRAF Combinatorial Treatments. *Ann. Oncol.* **2023**, *34*, 543–552. [CrossRef] [PubMed]
62. Parseghian, C.M.; Loree, J.M.; Morris, V.K.; Liu, X.; Clifton, K.K.; Napolitano, S.; Henry, J.T.; Pereira, A.A.; Vilar, E.; Johnson, B.; et al. Anti-EGFR-Resistant Clones Decay Exponentially after Progression: Implications for Anti-EGFR Re-Challenge. *Ann. Oncol.* **2019**, *30*, 243–249. [CrossRef] [PubMed]
63. Reinert, T.; Henriksen, T.V.; Christensen, E.; Sharma, S.; Salari, R.; Sethi, H.; Knudsen, M.; Nordentoft, I.; Wu, H.T.; Tin, A.S.; et al. Analysis of Plasma Cell-Free DNA by Ultradeep Sequencing in Patients With Stages I to III Colorectal Cancer. *JAMA Oncol.* **2019**, *5*, 1124–1131. [CrossRef] [PubMed]

4. Sartore-Bianchi, A.; Pietrantonio, F.; Lonardi, S.; Mussolin, B.; Rua, F.; Crisafulli, G.; Bartolini, A.; Fenocchio, E.; Amatu, A.; Manca, P.; et al. Circulating Tumor DNA to Guide Rechallenge with Panitumumab in Metastatic Colorectal Cancer: The Phase 2 CHRONOS Trial. *Nat. Med.* **2022**, *28*, 1612–1618. [CrossRef] [PubMed]
5. Ji, J.; Wang, C.; Fakih, M. Rechallenge With BRAF and Anti-EGFR Inhibitors in Patients With Metastatic Colorectal Cancer Harboring BRAFV600E Mutation Who Progressed on Cetuximab and Encorafenib With or Without Binimetinib: A Case Series. *Clin. Color. Cancer* **2022**, *21*, 267–271. [CrossRef] [PubMed]
6. Ros, J.; Vivancos, A.; Tabernero, J.; Élez, E. Circulating Tumor DNA, and Clinical Features to Guide Rechallenge with BRAF Inhibitors in BRAF-V600E Mutated Metastatic Colorectal Cancer. *Ann. Oncol.* **2023**, *35*, 240–241. [CrossRef] [PubMed]
7. Akhoundova, D.; Pietge, H.; Hussung, S.; Kiessling, M.; Britschgi, C.; Zoche, M.; Rechsteiner, M.; Weber, A.; Fritsch, R.M. Targeting Secondary and Tertiary Resistance to BRAF Inhibition in BRAF V600E–Mutated Metastatic Colorectal Cancer. *JCO Precis. Oncol.* **2021**, *5*, 1082–1087. [CrossRef]
8. Wang, N.; Fang, J.Y. Fusobacterium Nucleatum, a Key Pathogenic Factor and Microbial Biomarker for Colorectal Cancer. *Trends Microbiol.* **2023**, *31*, 159–172. [CrossRef]
9. Marmorino, F.; Piccinno, G.; Rossini, D.; Ghelardi, F.; Murgioni, S.; Salvatore, L.; Nasca, V.; Antoniotti, C.; Daniel, F.; Schietroma, F.; et al. Gut Microbiome Composition as Predictor of the Efficacy of Adding Atezolizumab to First-Line FOLFOXIRI plus Bevacizumab in Metastatic Colorectal Cancer: A Translational Analysis of the AtezoTRIBE Study. *J. Clin. Oncol.* **2023**, *41*, 3534. [CrossRef]
10. Zhu, H.; Li, M.; Bi, D.; Yang, H.; Gao, Y.; Song, F.; Zheng, J.; Xie, R.; Zhang, Y.; Liu, H.; et al. Fusobacterium Nucleatum Promotes Tumor Progression in KRAS p.G12D-Mutant Colorectal Cancer by Binding to DHX15. *Nat. Commun.* **2024**, *15*, 1688. [CrossRef]

Disclaimer/Publisher's Note: The statements, opinions and data contained in all publications are solely those of the individual author(s) and contributor(s) and not of MDPI and/or the editor(s). MDPI and/or the editor(s) disclaim responsibility for any injury to people or property resulting from any ideas, methods, instructions or products referred to in the content.

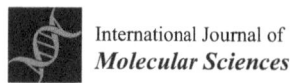

Review

Exosomes in Colorectal Cancer: From Physiology to Clinical Applications

Stefan Titu [1,2], Vlad Alexandru Gata [2,3], Roxana Maria Decea [4], Teodora Mocan [1,5,*], Constantin Dina [6], Alexandru Irimie [1,2] and Cosmin Ioan Lisencu [2,3]

1. Faculty of Medicine, "Iuliu Hatieganu" University of Medicine and Pharmacy, 400126 Cluj-Napoca, Romania
2. Department of Surgical Oncology, The Oncology Institute "Prof. Dr. Ion Chiricuta" Cluj-Napoca, 400015 Cluj-Napoca, Romania
3. Department of Oncological Surgery and Gynecological Oncology, "Iuliu Hațieganu" University of Medicine and Pharmacy, 400012 Cluj-Napoca, Romania
4. Department of Physiology, Faculty of Medicine, "Iuliu Hațieganu" University of Medicine and Pharmacy, 400012 Cluj-Napoca, Romania
5. Nanomedicine Department, Regional Institute of Gastroenterology and Hepatology, 400126 Cluj-Napoca, Romania
6. Faculty of Medicine, Ovidius University, 900527 Constanta, Romania
* Correspondence: teodora.mocan@umfcluj.ro

Abstract: Exosomes are nanosized vesicles that have been found to be involved in many diseases. Exosomes can mediate communication between cells in a variety of ways. Certain types of mediators derived from cancer cells can play a crucial role in the development of this pathology, promoting tumor growth, invasion, metastasis, angiogenesis, and immunomodulation. Exosomes in the bloodstream show promise as a future tool for detecting cancer at an early stage. The sensitivity and specificity of clinical exosome biomarkers need to be enhanced. Knowledge of exosomes is not only important for understanding the significance of cancer progression but also for providing clinicians with useful information for the diagnosis, treatment, and discovery of methods to prevent cancer from recurring. The widespread adoption of diagnostic tools based on exosomes may revolutionize cancer diagnosis and treatment. Tumor metastasis, chemoresistance, and immunity are all aided by exosomes. A potential new approach to cancer therapy involves preventing metastasis by inhibiting miRNA intracellular signaling and blocking the formation of pre-metastatic niches. For colorectal patients, exosomes represent a promising area of investigation for improving the diagnosis, treatment, and management. Reported data demonstrate that the serum expression level of certain exosomal miRNA is significantly higher in primary colorectal cancer patients. The present review discusses mechanisms and clinical implications of exosomes in colorectal cancer.

Keywords: exosome; cancer; colorectal cancer; exosomal miRNA; lncRNA

1. Exosomes

Exosomes are nanosized vesicles that have been found to be involved in many diseases. They are secreted by various cell types upon the fusion of multivesicular bodies and the plasma membrane [1]. Exosomes are typically 40–150 nm in diameter and carry nucleic acids, proteins, lipids, and metabolites [2]. Exosomes eventually generate multivesicular endosomes (MVEs) that are secreted into the extracellular space to travel to other cells [3]. Originally, when released from cells, exosomes were considered cellular garbage collectors following cell degradation or loss of cellular homeostasis without playing an important role in the surrounding body cells. However, more recent findings have showed that they mediate cell–cell communication, being loaded with proteins, lipids and nucleic acids that are delivered to target cells, and they are able to alter the biological behavior of the recipient cells [4]. Various surface molecules are shown to be responsible for the interaction between

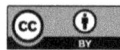

extracellular vesicles and recipient cells for their uptake. After they bind to the target cell, several processes may occur, receptor–ligand interaction, endocytosis and/or phagocytosis or membrane fusion and further load delivery into the cytosol and the subsequent change in the physiological state of the recipient cell [4]. There have been several studies where all membrane-bound vesicles are largely cited as extracellular vesicles and not particularly referred to as exosomes, microvesicles or other subtypes. Nevertheless, it is necessary to clearly distinguish exosomes from other extracellular vesicles in order to comprehend their action and compare various study results [5]. The biogenesis of exosomes involves their origin in endosomes, and they exhibit membrane protein expression profiles involved in membrane transport and fusion such as Rab GTPases, annexins and flotillin, components of the ESCRT complex, integrins and tetraspanins, including CD9, CD63, and CD81 [6].

One of the basic functions of exosomes is the elimination of excessive proteins or undesirable molecules from the cell, but they are important mediators of intercellular communication and are involved in various pathways being biologically active vesicles released into the extracellular environment [1].

Exosome engineering through genetic and chemical methods for targeted drug delivery may help increase their therapeutic applicability as clinical biomarkers [7]. There are still a lot of aspects to be considered for the design of new cancer treatment strategies, but exosomes exhibit great potential in precision cancer medicine. Figure 1 is broadly depicting all clinical applications that exosomes may have.

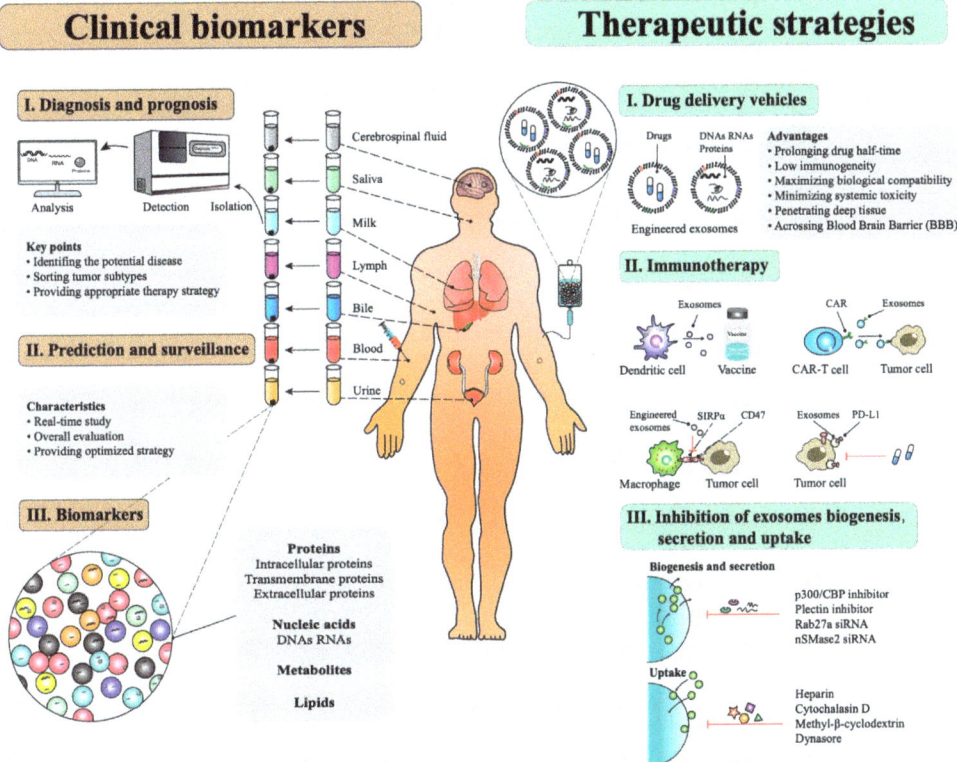

Figure 1. Key applications of exosomes. Reprinted with permission from Zhu, L. et al., 2000 [7].

As exosomes have proved their key role in cancer processes, there are three main research areas with clear participation in cancer progression: exosomes can modulate host immune response and induce immune tolerance; exosome crosstalk with the tumor microenvironment promotes tumor growth and progression; and their significant role in metastasis [2].

More exosomes are produced and released by cancer cells than by healthy ones, and the molecules found in exosomes released by tumor cells are very different from those found in healthy ones. Recent studies have shown that there are substantial differences between colorectal cancer (CRC) patients and healthy controls in the levels of certain microRNAs (miRNAs), long non-coding RNA (lncRNAs), and proteins found in exosomes isolated from blood (NCs). Some research suggests that these exosomal molecules can serve as markers for colorectal cancer.

2. The Role of Exosomes in Human Disease in General and Cancer in Particular

2.1. Exosome Modulation of the Immune System

There have been various studies on the role exosomes play in immune regulation, with a more recent one focusing on how exosomes regulate the immune response [8].

It has been demonstrated that human Epstein–Barr virus-infected B cells secrete exosomes carrying Major Histocompatibility Complex (MHC) classes I and II, thus indicating their potential implication in the modulation of immune responses [9]. This finding has triggered numerous other studies that have confirmed that exosomes secreted by antigen-presenting cells, for example, DCs, express class I, class II MHC, adhesion, and co-stimulatory molecules. Such features allow exosomes to directly activate CD8+ and CD4+ T-cells and induce a strong immune response [1]. Peptide-pulsed dendritic cells release immunogenic exosomes and stimulate a strong CD8+ T-cell-dependent anti-tumor immune response [10].

Exosomes derived from cancer cells express tumor antigens able to activate dendritic cells, therefore determining immune priming and triggering a specific cytotoxic response superior to the immunogenicity of tumor cell lysates or soluble antigens in vaccines [11]. It has been shown that one intraperitoneal injection of tumor peptide-loaded dendritic cell-derived exosomes can trigger a very powerful immune response that could lead to tumor growth delay or tumor rejection [12]. While this could be attributed to high antigen density, it is also due to the presence of heat shock proteins as seen in the case of exosomes produced by melanoma cells [13,14].

Exosomes trigger immune response suppression, leading to the low immunogenicity observed in several studies. Exosomes derived from cancer cells can suppress natural killer cells by downregulating NKG2D expression [15].

Dendritic cell maturation is impaired in vivo by tumor cell-derived exosomes, therefore leading to immunosuppression. Breast cancer cell-derived exosomes are internalized by bone marrow myeloid precursors, impairing dendritic cell differentiation by promoting IL6 overexpression and Stat3 phosphorylation [16]. Subsequent research showed that bone marrow precursor cells isolated from an IL6 knockout (KO) model can differentiate into dendritic cells following treatment with exosomes derived from cancer cells. Altogether, these study results indicate the immunosuppressive potential of tumor cell-derived exosomes via NK and DC modulation. Still, not all findings can identify the effector molecules initiating the modulation of the immune response [2].

2.2. Exosomes and Cancer

Cancer progression is determined by the crosstalk between cancer cells and the neighboring cells. This type of cell-to-cell communication is based on dynamic information exchange, inducing a pro-tumor microenvironment where carcinogenesis occurs and the immune response is modulated in order to promote tumor progression and survival [1].

Exosomes are essential components of the intercellular microenvironment, acting as regulators of cell-to-cell communication. It has been widely demonstrated that exosomes can induce phenotypic changes in neighboring cells through the activation of specific cell-signaling pathways leading to cancer progression [17].

Extensive studies have been carried out on intracellular communication, mainly during tumor development. Exosome-associated RNAs, miRNAs, proteins, DNAs, and even metabolites are able to determine changes in the outcome of recipient cells via autocrine and paracrine signaling mechanisms. Exosomal proteins are able to modulate the outcome of exosome-secreting cells through autocrine signaling. More specifically, chronic myeloid leukemia-derived exosomes contain TGFβ1, a cytokine that binds to the TGFβ1 receptor in leukemia cells and further promotes tumor growth by the activation of ERK, AKT and anti-apoptotic pathways in producer cells [5].

Some of their characteristics make exosomes superior to other extracellular vesicles for use as therapeutic agents, such as their stability in vivo and in vitro, bioavailability, good distribution into the surrounding body fluids, their ability to successfully cross the blood–brain barrier, good tolerance and regulation of gene expression by transferring miRNA and siRNA into target cells. All these features indicate their potential role in anti-cancer vaccines as well as natural liposomes for targeted delivery with various options for novel cancer therapies [1].

Mitochondrial DNA components were detected in exosomes, resulting from the culture supernatant of myoblasts and chromosomal DNA (vide infra). Chromosomal DNA was identified in cell culture supernatant in both human and mouse biological fluids, such as blood, seminal fluid, and urine. DNA-loaded exosomes could enhance DNA stability after it leaves the cell [18]. Such findings promote the use of exosomes as novel biomarkers in liquid biopsies, assisting the diagnosis and monitoring of cancer patients [19]. Blood plasma exosomes containing circulating DNA are complex agents in cancer therapies, isolating cancer-specific DNA for circulating cancer cell-derived exosomes [20].

Fibroblast-derived exosomes were shown to stimulate the protrusion of breast cancer cells (BCC) as well as their motility and metastasis dependent on tetraspanins, namely Cd81, which are common EV-associated markers. A study on a mouse model showed that tumor exosomes influence cancer metastasis based on the core PCP pathway in breast cancer cells, indicating that PCP components are almost mutually distributed in the protrusions of single, motile and malignant cells. Exosome activity is associated with the Wnt11 produced in breast cancer cells, and exosomes secreted from fibroblast are internalized by BCCs and further loaded with Wnt11. Therefore, exosomes secreted from fibroblasts play an important role in mediating the mobilization of autocrine Wnt-PCP signaling in BCCs, stimulating invasive behavior and metastasis in murine models [21].

In a recent study, cancer-associated fibroblasts demonstrated enhanced exosome production following gemcitabine injection, which also influenced exosome content by an increase in the presence of SNAIL1 and miR-146a. After treating pancreatic cancer cells with gemcitabine-derived CAF exosomes, cancer cells showed resistance to therapy and increased proliferation. Such results emphasize the ability of stromal cell-derived exosomes to enhance pro-cancer properties, including migration and resistance to therapy [22].

3. Exosomes and Colon Cancer—Reported Associations

Exosomes are often employed as a novel reservoir for disease biomarker discovery, especially in cancers. There have been reports showing the usefulness of exosomal miRNA-103, tripartite motif-containing 3 protein, glypican-1 proteoglycan protein and hepatocyte growth factor-regulated tyrosine kinase substrate protein in colon cancers. As a result, exosomes proved their potential as tumor markers for various types of cancers, including colorectal cancer [23–25].

As cancer cells secrete more exosomes than normal cells, there is a significant difference between molecules found in tumor cell-derived exosomes and those in normal cells. It has been demonstrated that there is a significant difference in certain miRNAs, lncRNAs and proteins in blood-derived exosomes between patients with colorectal patients and healthy subjects. Such exosomal molecules could be used as predictors for colorectal cancer [24].

The serum expression level of exosomal miRNA (let-7a, miR-1229, miR-1246, miR-150, miR-21, miR-223, and miR-23a) was significantly higher in primary colorectal cancer patients, including those with early-stage disease than in healthy subjects, being substantially downregulated following tumor excision. Those seven miRNAs also showed significantly higher secretion by colon cancer cell lines when compared to the healthy colon-derived cell line.

Their high sensitivity was validated by receiver operating characteristic (ROC) analysis [26].

Exosome and CRC Metastasis

It has been stated that 90% of cancer deaths are caused by metastasis. Commonly, colorectal cancer spreads to distant organs (liver, lung, lymph nodes). In the case of patients with distant metastasis, the five-year survival rate is a grim 10%. It is thus very important to detect metastasis early in order to increase the survival of these patients [24].

MiR-203 demonstrated the existence of a link between tumor and host cells, with exosomal miR-203 presented as a novel biomarker to predict metastasis mainly as a promotor of monocyte differentiation to M2-TAMs and the subsequent formation of pre-metastatic niches. There have been significant clinical findings showing the dual functions of miR-203 in the progression of colorectal cancer [27].

Enhanced IRF-2 serum levels in CRC patients with lymph node metastasis present themselves as a novel biomarker for metastasis. Exosomal IRF-2 is able to activate lymph node metastases by remodeling the lymphatic network [28].

Shao et al. demonstrated that serum extracellular vesicles containing miR-21 in colon cancer cells are new macrophage regulators leading to the creation of an inflammatory pre-metastatic niche in colon cancer liver metastasis. While cancer develops, primary CRC cells secrete serum extracellular vesicles containing miR-21 that are transported by the blood flow to the liver where they are engulfed by macrophages. The serum extracellular vesicles deliver the miR-21 load, and by targeting the TLR7 pathway, they polarize macrophages enhancing the synthesis and release of pro-inflammatory cytokines such as IL-6, thus paving the way for a permissive inflammatory pre-metastatic niche in the liver where circulating CRC cells can survive, colonize and subsequently develop macrometastasis [29].

Recent research has shown that miR-375 controls the expression of MMP2 and other genes involved in the epithelial–mesenchymal transition (EMT), such as SNAIL. Colorectal cancer cells proliferate, invade, and migrate when miR-375 is suppressed. Loss of function of the tumor suppressor miR-374 in colorectal cancer (CRC) promotes proliferation, invasion, migration, and intrahepatic metastasis through activation of the PIK3/AKT pathway. To a large extent, miR-374 inhibition upregulates the expression of its targets, which include the transcription factors SNAIL, SLUG, and ZEB1 as well as NCAD and VIM [30].

The regulation of ZEB transcription factors in CRC cells is primarily mediated by two members of the miR-200 family: miR-200c and miR-429. MiR-200c inhibition of ZEB1 expression leads to EMT inactivation and decreased CRC cell invasion and migration. Because of its ability to target ONECUT2, MiR-429 could suppress cell migration and invasion, reversing TGFb's EMT-inducing effects. MiR-429 is, however, substantially downregulated in colorectal cancer [31].

Because of its ability to target ONECUT2, MiR-429 could suppress cell migration and invasion, reversing TGFb's EMT-inducing effects. In contrast, miR-429 is considerably downregulated in colorectal cancer [32].

In addition, the loss of ASCL2 function, a target of WNT signaling, can activate the miR-200 cluster, which in turn inhibits the ZEB and SNAIL families of transcription factors and controls the plasticity from EMT to mesenchymal–epithelial transition (MET) [33].

It has been found that the upregulation of the ZEB2 target gene is associated with CRC invasion and metastasis when other tumor suppressors, particularly miR-335, miR-132, and miR-192, are downregulated [34–36].

Takano et al. stated that CRC cell-derived exosomal miR-203 promotes the differentiation of monocytes into M2-tumor-associated macrophages (TAMs) involved in colorectal cancer metastasis to the liver [27].

Table 1 summarizes the roles of exosomes in colorectal metastatic disease. One can distinguish the important clinical aspects in which exosomes are involved as well as opposite effects (anticancer/cancer promoter) reported for different exosomes.

Table 1. Exosomes in colorectal metastatic disease.

Name	Role	Clinical Implication
miR-203	promotor of monocyte differentiation to M2-TAMs	carcinogenesis and progression by promoting tumor growth, proliferation, antiapoptotic mechanisms, and migration [27]
IRF-2	vascular endothelial growth factor C	activate lymph node metastases by remodeling the lymphatic network [28]
miR-21	TLR7 pathway	polarize macrophages enhancing synthesis and release of pro-inflammatory cytokines such as IL-6 [29]
miR-375	controls expression of MMP2 (and other genes involved in the epithelial-mesenchymal transition (EMT)), SNAIL gene	promotes proliferation, invasion, migration, and intrahepatic metastasis through activation of the PIK3/AKT pathway [30]
miR-200c	inhibition of ZEB1 expression	EMT inactivation and decreased CRC cell invasion and migration [31]
miR-429	target ONECUT2	suppress cell migration and invasion [32]
miR-335 miR-132 miR-192	upregulation of the ZEB2	CRC invasion and metastasis [27]

4. Exosomal Elements as Predictive Markers for Colon Cancer

Efforts have been made to employ miRNAs in serum or plasma as diagnostic biomarkers for more cancers. There are still decisions to be made regarding the type of miRNAs to be selected as markers. The particular properties of exosomes, such as their ability to embed specific miRNAs, their stability in the blood flow, their reproducible detection, and especially their ability to reflect the properties of cancer cells, promote them as important tools in the design of highly sensitive diagnostic strategies for the rapid and non-invasive monitoring of cancer evolution [26].

Exosomal miRNAs could be a biomarker of colorectal cancer. A recent RNA sequencing study on exosomes in colorectal cancer patients indicated high miRNA-139-3p, let-7b-3p and miRNA-145-3p expression in plasma exosomes [37].

Elevated exosomal miRNA-19a levels in the serum of colorectal patients were indicative of cancer recurrence [38].

Moreover, exosomal miRNA-17-92a expression in the blood was associated with cancer recurrence. Certain exosomal miRNAs such as miRNA-1229, miRNA-1246, miRNA-21, miRNA-23a, let-7a, miRNA-223 and miRNA-150 demonstrated great transfer by serum exosomes in colorectal cancer patients, but they were significantly lower following surgical excision [26].

MiRNA-1246, miRNA-21 and miRNA-23a stand out as powerful diagnostic biomarkers of colorectal cancer [39].

Figure 2 illustrates one method to be implemented in the future to analyze cargoes of exosomes in order to highlight different types of miRNA embedded as biomarkers for colorectal cancer.

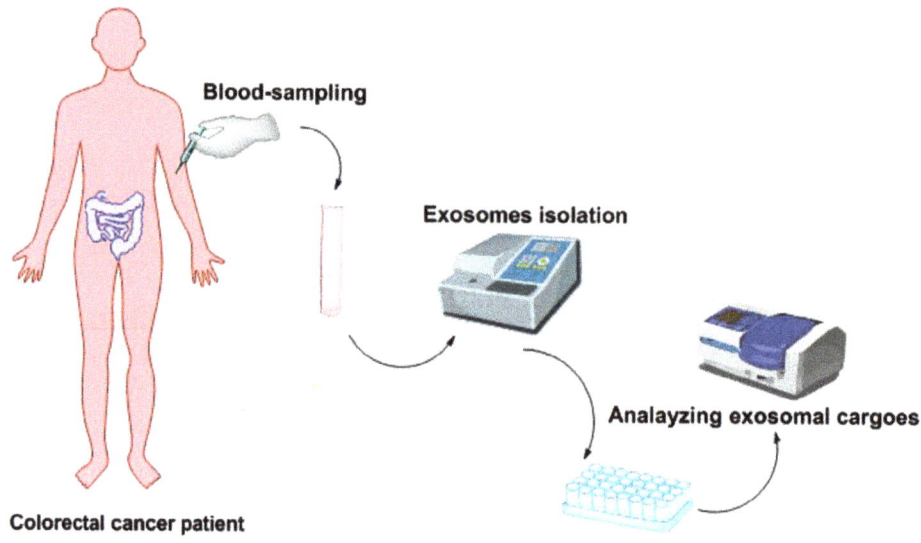

Figure 2. Method for highlighting types of biomarkers of colorectal cancer patient. Reprinted with permission from Ahmadi, M et al., 2021 [40].

Table 2 shows the types of exosomal miRNAs that are potential cancer diagnostic biomarkers in colorectal cancer. The studies discussed the use of lncRNA-loaded CRC-derived exosomes as diagnostic biomarkers.

Table 2. Potential cancer diagnostic biomarkers miRNA in colorectal cancer. Adapted with permission from Ahmadi, M et al., 2021 [40].

miRNA Type	Isolated from	Level of miRNA in CRC
mrRNA-23a; miRNA-301a	Serum	High
miRNA-486-5p	Plasma	High
miRNA-6803-5p	Serum	High
miRNA-125a-3p	Plasma	High
miRNA-150-5p	Serum	Low

In another study, Zou et al. observed significantly lower serum exosomal miR-150-5p levels in colorectal cancer patients, therefore being appropriate diagnosis indicators. Diagnostic accuracy was boosted by the combined use of miR-150-5p and the carcinoembryonic antigen. Altogether, these findings emphasize the potential of exosomal miRNAs in diagnosing colorectal cancer [41].

LncRNA is a non-coding RNA that has a size of more than 200 nt in length, and it was found in the blood exosomes of patients diagnosed with colorectal cancer. The results in one study showed an overexpression of lncRNA differentially expressed. This could lead in using lncRNA as a tumor marker due to its non-invasive character, high sensitivity and specificity, as well as stability. It is also highly correlated with aggressive tumor behavior and poor prognosis. Such results provide the grounds for the design of an early diagnostic and prognostic biomarker for colorectal cancer and the corresponding novel therapeutic strategies [42].

In their study, Hu et al. study demonstrated that exosomal lncRNAs, namely LNCV6_98602, LNCV6_98390, LNCV_108266, LNCV6_116109, LNCV6_38772, and LNCV6_84003 plasma expression, was significantly higher in patients with colorectal cancer, promoting them as potential diagnostic biomarkers for this type of cancer [43].

Barbagallo et al. showed in two types of CRC cell lines (HCT-116, Caco-2) that urothelial cancer associated 1 (UCA1), also a lncRNA, can act as a RNA regulator for colorectal cancer progression by modulating the ceRNA network, thus upregulating ANLN, BIRC5, IPO7, KIF2A and KIF23 in two ways: (1) miRNAs sponge effects determining negative expression, and (2) the direct binding of mRNAs to 3′-UTRs to protect them from degradation. Such elaborate RNA-based regulatory signaling for cancer control suggests the design of novel anticancer therapies targeting UCA1 [44].

Granulocytic myeloid-derived suppressor cells were shown to enhance the capability of colorectal cancer cells for self-renewal and differentiation as a result of exosomes and exosomal S100A9 influence in the tumor microenvironment, mainly under hypoxic conditions. Hyperoxia reduces the stemness of colon cancer cells via the inhibition of the production of GM-Exo. Elevated plasma concentration of exosomal S100A9 was linked to the occurrence and recurrence of colorectal cancer. The production of block MDSC exosomes could be used as a new approach for colorectal therapy [45].

The results demonstrate the potential use of exosomal proteins as biomarkers of colorectal cancer.

5. Detection and Screening Based on Exosomal Components

The carcinoembryonic antigen (CEA) was also observed in the serum exosomes of colorectal patients [46]. The value of the area under the curve (AUC) of serum exosomal CEA (0.9354) was greater than that of serum CEA (0.8557). It is thus more significant to detect serum exosomal CEA in order to predict distant metastasis in colorectal cancer. The overexpression of interferon regulatory factor 2 (IRF-2) was observed in the serum exosomes of colorectal cancer patients with lymph node metastasis [28].

From a mechanistic view, exosomal IRF-2 triggers lymph node metastasis by remodeling the lymphatic network. Certain miRNAs were differentially expressed in the plasma exosomes of patients with locally advanced rectal cancer, therefore promoting themselves as potential biomarkers for the poor prognosis of colorectal cancer [47].

Among them, there was a correlation between low miR-181a-5p levels and high miR-30d-5p levels in plasma exosomes and lymph node metastases and liver metastases. There is still no clear definition of the roles these RNAs play in colorectal cancer [24].

In their study, Jun et al. were able to identify several candidate targets with a miRNA–mRNA network (mRNA: CBFB, CDH3, ETV4, FOXQ1, FUT1, GCNT2, GRIN2D, KIAA1549, KRT80, LZTS1, SLC39A10, SPTBN2, ZSWIM4; and exosomal miRNA: hsa-miR-126, hsa-miR-139, hsa-miR-141, hsa-miR-29c, and hsa-miR-423), which could be used as potential biomarkers in the diagnosis of colorectal cancer with the presence of an exosomal miRNA–mRNA network in cancer progression. Their results pave the way for new diagnostic and treatment strategies of colorectal cancer [48].

6. Targeting Exosomal Components—Drugs, Nanostructures, Polymers

There have been great attempts to enhance the innate properties of exosomes and to enhance the manufacturing process of exosomes or exosome mimetics. Exosome-based drug delivery tools were divided into three subgroups based on the extent of human manipulation and their natural feel compared with cell-derived exosomes. Frequent protein components that exosomes contain include cytoskeletal (such as actin), cytosolic (for example GAPDH), heat shock (HSP90), antigen presentation (MHC-I, -II), and membrane proteins (CD9, CD63) together with proteins involved in vesicle trafficking (Tsg101) [49].

In the tumor microenvironment (TME), fibroblasts are a major component. MicroRNAs regulate multiple signaling pathways, causing fibroblasts at the primary tumor site to take on a new phenotype and transform into CAFs. Cancer-associated fibroblasts (CAFs) are distinct from normal fibroblasts (NFs) due to their pro-tumorigenic properties and high expression of smooth muscle actin (28). To promote tumor growth, CAFs secrete a variety of pro-inflammatory molecules, such as interleukins, chemokines, and extracellular matrix (ECM) components.

Oxaliplatin (Oxa) is a common chemotherapeutic agent for colorectal cancer treatment. The exosome-mediated crosstalk between CRC-associated fibroblasts (CAFs) and CRC cells have demonstrated important roles in chemoresistance to Oxa. It was also confirmed that oncogene miR-21, one of the most oncogenic miRNAs, was enriched in the exosomes from CAFs [50].

After overexpression in exosomes, miR-21 is transported to colorectal cancer cells and enhances AKT phosphorylation strongly related to chemoresistance to Oxa. In another study, lncRNA H19 was expressed to a great extent in the CAFs of colorectal cancer patients which also increased with cancer progression. LncRNA H19, as a oncofetal transcript, has been shown to promote SIRT1-mediated autophagy in colorectal cancer (CRC) cells, which in turn confers resistance to 5-fluorouracil [51].

One of the most common causes of therapeutic failure is resistance to therapy. The various mechanisms of exomes were shown to determine drug resistance in several recent studies. Exosomes can guide miRNAs, lncRNAs and proteins to the target cells and trigger signal transmission between drug-resistant cells and sensitive cells, stromal cells and tumor cells, which can lead to the drug resistance of tumor cells [52,53].

Other examples of resistance were observed in the microenvironment of ovarian cancer, where exosomes derived from tumor-associated adipocytes and tumor-associated fibroblasts are able to transport miR-21 to ovarian cells, downregulating APAF1 expression and inhibiting tumor apoptosis, thus leading to resistance to paclitaxel [54].

In colorectal cancer, CAF-derived exosomes loaded with miR-92a-3p are aimed at FBXW7 and MOAP1 in the tumor microenvironment and further activate the WNT/β-catenin pathway, inhibit mitochondrial apoptosis, leading to cell stemness, epithelial–mesenchymal transition, tumor metastasis and resistance to 5-FU/L-OHP [55].

Tumors are able to stray from attacks from the immune system by various mechanisms that allow them to avoid being detected. The immunomodulatory potential makes exosomes useful in novel immunological strategies to improve antitumor immunity.

Cancer immunotherapy using chimeric antigen receptor (CAR) is a promising therapeutic approach. The clinical use of CAR-modified T cell (CAR-T) therapy in solid tumors was not as successful as in hematological malignancies, such as acute lymphoid leukemia, mainly due to side effects such as cytokine release syndrome (CRS), cytokine storm and on-target/off-tumor responses [56].

7. Future Directions

Because of their notable accuracy across a wide range of biological datasets, microRNAs have emerged as promising leads in the search for additional CRC cancer biomarkers. The value of serum miRNAs throughout CRC diagnosis, prognosis, and treatment response has been the subject of a plethora of recent papers. Compared to traditional markers such as carcinoembryonic antigen (CEA) and CA19-9, a panel of six miRNAs (miR-21, let-7g, miR-31, miR-92a, miR-181b, and miR-203) has been shown to be a potential marker for CRC diagnosis with over 40% specificity and sensitivity [57].

The absence of trustworthy methods for cancer detection has led to a drawback in the development of colorectal cancer. There is a need for highly efficient detection techniques in order to lower the risk of cancer-associated mortality. More and more findings have demonstrated the strong correlation between the initiation and progression of colorectal cancer and the differentially expressed exosomal RNAs and proteins. These molecules are able to influence the oncogenesis, metastasis, chemoresistance and recurrence of colorectal cancer, thus being potential candidates for this type of cancer. There are several advantages offered by exosomes as novel tumor markers: (i) they could be superior to conventional techniques in terms of sensitivity and specificity; (ii) their bioactive molecular content, without much serum involvement; (iii) they are characterized by high stability and their contents do not degrade in the extracellular environment; and (iv) they are secreted by a variety of body liquids, and thus, they can be extracted in a non-invasive manner. The

Food and Drug Administration has already approved the use of certain exosome-based diagnostic kits in clinical trials [24].

Nevertheless, there are certain drawbacks to the use of exosomes as tumor markers. For example, it is essential to rapidly and meticulously isolate exosomes from a sample prior to using them as biomarkers. The present isolation techniques have their own limitations, being bulky, lengthy, including contaminations, and they are expensive. The purity of exosomes is of great importance and the presence of impurities, such as proteins and RNAs in exosomal compounds has been reported, which may have a negative impact on the accuracy of exosome-based diagnosis. It is thus crucial to design highly accurate separation methods to enable the transition of exosome detection to clinical applications. Another aspect is the term "exosomes" itself, which is not recommended nomenclature anymore due to the wide vesicle heterogeneity depending on the purification method, which has dictated the quality and accuracy of the final product. The different results have led to standardization issues, and thus, studies cannot be compared. It is necessary to eliminate all deviations in order to successfully employ exosomes as biomarkers [24].

There are multiple mechanisms by which exosomes act as mediators of intercellular communication. Those derived from colorectal cancer cells are essential mediators in this type of cancer influencing tumor formation by enhancing growth, invasion, metastasis, angiogenesis and immunomodulation. Regardless the stage of the condition, exosomes can transport certain biomolecules into the blood, therefore promoting themselves as promising biomarkers for cancer stage. As exosomes are released into various biofluids, they could be used as a novel diagnostic biomarker in colorectal cancer. There are still a few aspects that need to be thoroughly explained, such as the processes of separation, characterization and validation [40].

8. Conclusions

Several studies have investigated the potential of exosomes as diagnostic and prognostic biomarkers in cancer in general and colorectal cancer in specific and as targets for novel therapeutic interventions. However, further research is needed to fully understand the complex roles of exosomes in colorectal cancer and to translate this knowledge into clinical practice. Overall, exosomes represent a promising area of investigation for improving the diagnosis, treatment, and management of colorectal cancer.

It has become increasingly evident that there are several key aspects regarding the underlying mechanisms of exosome-mediated crosstalk in the tumor microenvironment, distant cell interactions, exosome heterogeneity, and molecular mechanisms that are responsible for resistance and metastasis. Our understanding of exosome-mediated therapy-resistance in different cancers will be directed by the tumor context, which will be directed by the design of different research approaches in this new vast area of study based on the tumor context. The translation of these findings into the clinical realm will provide a novel and effective treatment modality for future cancer patients.

Due to their quantity and heterogeneity, exosome biomarkers can produce false positives and negatives in diagnosis and prognosis. Clinical exosome biomarker sensitivity and specificity must be improved.

Blocking the formation of pre-metastatic niches and inhibiting miRNAs intracellular signaling to prevent metastasis may be used as a novel cancer therapy strategy.

Author Contributions: Conceptualization: S.T., V.A.G. and T.M.; Writing—original draft preparation: S.T., R.M.D. and C.I.L.; Writing—review and editing: S.T., V.A.G. and R.M.D.; Supervision: T.M., C.D. and A.I.; Final approval: T.M., C.D., A.I. and C.I.L. All authors have read and agreed to the published version of the manuscript.

Funding: The authors would like to acknowledge support from the National Authority for Scientific Research and Innovation Romania, CNCS-UEFISCDI, cod PN-III-P2-2.1-PED-2021-0073.

Institutional Review Board Statement: Not applicable.

Informed Consent Statement: Not applicable.

Data Availability Statement: Not applicable.

Conflicts of Interest: The authors declare no conflict of interest.

References

1. De Toro, J.; Herschlik, L.; Waldner, C.; Mongini, C. Emerging roles of exosomes in normal and pathological conditions: New insights for diagnosis and therapeutic applications. *Front. Immunol.* **2015**, *6*, 203. [CrossRef]
2. Ruivo, C.F.; Adem, B.; Silva, M.; Melo, S.A. The Biology of Cancer Exosomes: Insights and New PerspectivesBiology of Cancer Exosomes. *Cancer Res.* **2017**, *77*, 6480–6488. [CrossRef]
3. Zhang, H.; Lu, J.; Liu, J.; Zhang, G.; Lu, A. Advances in the discovery of exosome inhibitors in cancer. *J. Enzym. Inhib. Med. Chem.* **2020**, *35*, 1322–1330. [CrossRef]
4. Tkach, M.; Théry, C. Communication by extracellular vesicles: Where we are and where we need to go. *Cell* **2016**, *164*, 1226–1232. [CrossRef]
5. Zhang, L.; Yu, D. Exosomes in cancer development, metastasis, and immunity. *Biochim. Biophys. Acta BBA Rev. Cancer* **2019**, *1871*, 455–468. [CrossRef]
6. Kowal, J.; Arras, G.; Colombo, M.; Jouve, M.; Morath, J.P.; Primdal-Bengtson, B.; Dingli, F.; Loew, D.; Tkach, M.; Théry, C. Proteomic comparison defines novel markers to characterize heterogeneous populations of extracellular vesicle subtypes. *Proc. Natl. Acad. Sci. USA* **2016**, *113*, E968–E977. [CrossRef]
7. Zhu, L.; Sun, H.; Wang, S.; Huang, S.; Zheng, Y.; Wang, C.; Hu, B.; Qin, W.; Zou, T.; Fu, Y. Isolation and characterization of exosomes for cancer research. *J. Hematol. Oncol.* **2020**, *13*, 152. [CrossRef]
8. Robbins, P.D.; Morelli, A.E. Regulation of immune responses by extracellular vesicles. *Nat. Rev. Immunol.* **2014**, *14*, 195–208. [CrossRef]
9. Raposo, G.; Nijman, H.W.; Stoorvogel, W.; Liejendekker, R.; Harding, C.V.; Melief, C.J.; Geuze, H.J. B lymphocytes secrete antigen-presenting vesicles. *J. Exp. Med.* **1996**, *183*, 1161–1172. [CrossRef]
10. Théry, C.; Duban, L.; Segura, E.; Véron, P.; Lantz, O.; Amigorena, S. Indirect activation of naïve CD4 T cells by dendritic cell–derived exosomes. *Nat. Immunol.* **2002**, *3*, 1156–1162. [CrossRef]
11. Wolfers, J.; Lozier, A.; Raposo, G.; Regnault, A.; Théry, C.; Masurier, C.; Flament, C.; Pouzieux, S.; Faure, F.; Tursz, T. Tumor-derived exosomes are a source of shared tumor rejection antigens for CTL cross-priming. *Nat. Med.* **2001**, *7*, 297–303. [CrossRef]
12. Vega, V.L.; Rodriguez-Silva, M.; Frey, T.; Gehrmann, M.; Diaz, J.C.; Steinem, C.; Multhoff, G.; Arispe, N.; De Maio, A. Hsp70 translocates into the plasma membrane after stress and is released into the extracellular environment in a membrane-associated form that activates macrophages. *J. Immunol.* **2008**, *180*, 4299–4307. [CrossRef]
13. Benson, M.J.; Dillon, S.R.; Castigli, E.; Geha, R.S.; Xu, S.; Lam, K.; Noelle, R.J. Cutting edge: The dependence of plasma cells and independence of memory B cells on BAFF and APRIL. *J. Immunol.* **2008**, *180*, 3655–3659. [CrossRef]
14. Lv, L.; Wan, Y.; Lin, Y.; Zhang, W.; Yang, M.; Li, G.; Lin, H.; Shang, C.; Chen, Y.; Min, J. Anticancer drugs cause release of exosomes with heat shock proteins from human hepatocellular carcinoma cells that elicit effective natural killer cell antitumor responses in vitro. *J. Biol. Chem.* **2012**, *287*, 15874–15885. [CrossRef]
15. Clayton, A.; Mitchell, J.P.; Court, J.; Mason, M.D.; Tabi, Z. Human tumor-derived exosomes selectively impair lymphocyte responses to interleukin-2. *Cancer Res.* **2007**, *67*, 7458–7466. [CrossRef]
16. Yu, S.; Liu, C.; Su, K.; Wang, J.; Liu, Y.; Zhang, L.; Li, C.; Cong, Y.; Kimberly, R.; Grizzle, W.E.; et al. Tumor exosomes inhibit differentiation of bone marrow dendritic cells. *J. Immunol.* **2007**, *178*, 6867–6875. [CrossRef]
17. Raimondo, S.; Saieva, L.; Corrado, C.; Fontana, S.; Flugy, A.; Rizzo, A.; De Leo, G.; Alessandro, R. Chronic myeloid leukemia-derived exosomes promote tumor growth through an autocrine mechanism. *Cell Commun. Signal.* **2015**, *13*, 8. [CrossRef]
18. Kalluri, R. The biology and function of exosomes in cancer. *J. Clin. Investig.* **2016**, *126*, 1208–1215. [CrossRef]
19. Choi, D.; Lee, T.H.; Spinelli, C.; Chennakrishnaiah, S.; D'Asti, E.; Rak, J. *Extracellular Vesicle Communication Pathways as Regulatory Targets of Oncogenic Transformation, Seminars in Cell & Developmental Biology*; Elsevier: Amsterdam, The Netherlands, 2017; pp. 11–22.
20. Thierry, A.; El Messaoudi, S.; Gahan, P.; Anker, P.; Stroun, M. Origins, structures, and functions of circulating DNA in oncology. *Cancer Metastasis Rev.* **2016**, *35*, 347–376. [CrossRef]
21. Luga, V.; Zhang, L.; Viloria-Petit, A.M.; Ogunjimi, A.A.; Inanlou, M.R.; Chiu, E.; Buchanan, M.; Hosein, A.N.; Basik, M.; Wrana, J.L. Exosomes mediate stromal mobilization of autocrine Wnt-PCP signaling in breast cancer cell migration. *Cell* **2012**, *151*, 1542–1556. [CrossRef]
22. Richards, K.E.; Zeleniak, A.E.; Fishel, M.L.; Wu, J.; Littlepage, L.E.; Hill, R. Cancer-associated fibroblast exosomes regulate survival and proliferation of pancreatic cancer cells. *Oncogene* **2017**, *36*, 1770–1778. [CrossRef]
23. Sun, Y.; Zheng, W.; Guo, Z.; Ju, Q.; Zhu, L.; Gao, J.; Zhou, L.; Liu, F.; Xu, Y.; Zhan, Q. A novel TP53 pathway influences the HGS-mediated exosome formation in colorectal cancer. *Sci. Rep.* **2016**, *6*, 28083. [CrossRef]
24. Xiao, Y.; Zhong, J.; Zhong, B.; Huang, J.; Jiang, L.; Jiang, Y.; Yuan, J.; Sun, J.; Dai, L.; Yang, C. Exosomes as potential sources of biomarkers in colorectal cancer. *Cancer Lett.* **2020**, *476*, 13–22. [CrossRef]

25. Lu, F.; Chen, S.; Shi, W.; Su, X.; Wu, H.; Liu, M. GPC1 promotes the growth and migration of colorectal cancer cells through regulating the TGF-β1/SMAD2 signaling pathway. *PLoS ONE* **2022**, *17*, e0269094. [CrossRef]
26. Ogata-Kawata, H.; Izumiya, M.; Kurioka, D.; Honma, Y.; Yamada, Y.; Furuta, K.; Gunji, T.; Ohta, H.; Okamoto, H.; Sonoda, H. Circulating exosomal microRNAs as biomarkers of colon cancer. *PLoS ONE* **2014**, *9*, e92921. [CrossRef]
27. Takano, Y.; Masuda, T.; Iinuma, H.; Yamaguchi, R.; Sato, K.; Tobo, T.; Hirata, H.; Kuroda, Y.; Nambara, S.; Hayashi, N.; et al. Circulating exosomal microRNA-203 is associated with metastasis possibly via inducing tumor-associated macrophages in colorectal cancer. *Oncotarget* **2017**, *8*, 78598–78613. [CrossRef]
28. Sun, B.; Zhou, Y.; Fang, Y.; Li, Z.; Gu, X.; Xiang, J. Colorectal cancer exosomes induce lymphatic network remodeling in lymph nodes. *Int. J. Cancer* **2019**, *145*, 1648–1659. [CrossRef]
29. Shao, Y.; Chen, T.; Zheng, X.; Yang, S.; Xu, K.; Chen, X.; Xu, F.; Wang, L.; Shen, Y.; Wang, T. Colorectal cancer-derived small extracellular vesicles establish an inflammatory premetastatic niche in liver metastasis. *Carcinogenesis* **2018**, *39*, 1368–1379. [CrossRef]
30. Chen, Y.; Jiang, J.; Zhao, M.; Luo, X.; Liang, Z.; Zhen, Y.; Fu, Q.; Deng, X.; Lin, X.; Li, L.; et al. microRNA-374a suppresses colon cancer progression by directly reducing CCND1 to inactivate the PI3K/AKT pathway. *Oncotarget* **2016**, *7*, 41306–41319. [CrossRef]
31. Hur, K.; Toiyama, Y.; Takahashi, M.; Balaguer, F.; Nagasaka, T.; Koike, J.; Hemmi, H.; Koi, M.; Boland, C.R.; Goel, A. MicroRNA-200c modulates epithelial-to-mesenchymal transition (EMT) in human colorectal cancer metastasis. *Gut* **2013**, *62*, 1315–1326. [CrossRef]
32. Sun, Y.; Shen, S.; Liu, X.; Tang, H.; Wang, Z.; Yu, Z.; Li, X.; Wu, M. MiR-429 inhibits cells growth and invasion and regulates EMT-related marker genes by targeting Onecut2 in colorectal carcinoma. *Mol. Cell. Biochem.* **2014**, *390*, 19–30. [CrossRef]
33. Tian, Y.; Pan, Q.; Shang, Y.; Zhu, R.; Ye, J.; Liu, Y.; Zhong, X.; Li, S.; He, Y.; Chen, L.; et al. MicroRNA-200 (miR-200) cluster regulation by achaete scute-like 2 (Ascl2): Impact on the epithelial-mesenchymal transition in colon cancer cells. *J. Biol. Chem.* **2014**, *289*, 36101–36115. [CrossRef]
34. Sun, Z.; Zhang, Z.; Liu, Z.; Qiu, B.; Liu, K.; Dong, G. MicroRNA-335 inhibits invasion and metastasis of colorectal cancer by targeting ZEB2. *Med. Oncol.* **2014**, *31*, 982. [CrossRef]
35. Zheng, Y.B.; Luo, H.P.; Shi, Q.; Hao, Z.N.; Ding, Y.; Wang, Q.S.; Li, S.B.; Xiao, G.C.; Tong, S.L. miR-132 inhibits colorectal cancer invasion and metastasis via directly targeting ZEB2. *World J. Gastroenterol.* **2014**, *20*, 6515–6522. [CrossRef]
36. Geng, L.; Chaudhuri, A.; Talmon, G.; Wisecarver, J.L.; Are, C.; Brattain, M.; Wang, J. MicroRNA-192 suppresses liver metastasis of colon cancer. *Oncogene* **2014**, *33*, 5332–5340. [CrossRef]
37. Min, L.; Zhu, S.; Chen, L.; Liu, X.; Wei, R.; Zhao, L.; Yang, Y.; Zhang, Z.; Kong, G.; Li, P. Evaluation of circulating small extracellular vesicles derived miRNAs as biomarkers of early colon cancer: A comparison with plasma total miRNAs. *J. Extracell. Vesicles* **2019**, *8*, 1643670. [CrossRef]
38. Matsumura, T.; Sugimachi, K.; Iinuma, H.; Takahashi, Y.; Kurashige, J.; Sawada, G.; Ueda, M.; Uchi, R.; Ueo, H.; Takano, Y. Exosomal microRNA in serum is a novel biomarker of recurrence in human colorectal cancer. *Br. J. Cancer* **2015**, *113*, 275–281. [CrossRef]
39. Lalkhen, A.G.; McCluskey, A. Clinical tests: Sensitivity and specificity. *Contin. Educ. Anaesth. Crit. Care Pain* **2008**, *8*, 221–223. [CrossRef]
40. Ahmadi, M.; Jafari, R.; Mahmoodi, M.; Rezaie, J. The tumorigenic and therapeutic functions of exosomes in colorectal cancer: Opportunity and challenges. *Cell Biochem. Funct.* **2021**, *39*, 468–477. [CrossRef]
41. Zou, S.; Chen, Y.; Ge, Z.; Qu, Y.; Cao, Y.; Kang, Z. Downregulation of serum exosomal miR-150-5p is associated with poor prognosis in patients with colorectal cancer. *Cancer Biomark.* **2019**, *26*, 69–77. [CrossRef]
42. Liu, T.; Zhang, X.; Gao, S.; Jing, F.; Yang, Y.; Du, L.; Zheng, G.; Li, P.; Li, C.; Wang, C. Exosomal long noncoding RNA CRNDE-h as a novel serum-based biomarker for diagnosis and prognosis of colorectal cancer. *Oncotarget* **2016**, *7*, 85551–85563. [CrossRef]
43. Hu, D.; Zhan, Y.; Zhu, K.; Bai, M.; Han, J.; Si, Y.; Zhang, H.; Kong, D. Plasma Exosomal Long Non-Coding RNAs Serve as Biomarkers for Early Detection of Colorectal Cancer. *Cell. Physiol. Biochem.* **2018**, *51*, 2704–2715. [CrossRef]
44. Barbagallo, C.; Brex, D.; Caponnetto, A.; Cirnigliaro, M.; Scalia, M.; Magnano, A.; Caltabiano, R.; Barbagallo, D.; Biondi, A.; Cappellani, A. LncRNA UCA1, upregulated in CRC biopsies and downregulated in serum exosomes, controls mRNA expression by RNA-RNA interactions. *Mol. Ther. Nucleic Acids* **2018**, *12*, 229–241. [CrossRef]
45. Wang, Y.; Yin, K.; Tian, J.; Xia, X.; Ma, J.; Tang, X.; Xu, H.; Wang, S. Granulocytic Myeloid-Derived suppressor cells promote the stemness of colorectal cancer cells through exosomal S100A9. *Adv. Sci.* **2019**, *6*, 1901278. [CrossRef]
46. Yokoyama, S.; Takeuchi, A.; Yamaguchi, S.; Mitani, Y.; Watanabe, T.; Matsuda, K.; Hotta, T.; Shively, J.E.; Yamaue, H. Clinical implications of carcinoembryonic antigen distribution in serum exosomal fraction—Measurement by ELISA. *PLoS ONE* **2017**, *12*, e0183337. [CrossRef]
47. Bjørnetrø, T.; Redalen, K.R.; Meltzer, S.; Thusyanthan, N.S.; Samiappan, R.; Jegerschöld, C.; Handeland, K.R.; Ree, A.H. An experimental strategy unveiling exosomal microRNAs 486-5p, 181a-5p and 30d-5p from hypoxic tumour cells as circulating indicators of high-risk rectal cancer. *J. Extracell. Vesicles* **2019**, *8*, 1567219. [CrossRef]
48. Ma, J.; Wang, P.; Huang, L.; Qiao, J.; Li, J. Bioinformatic analysis reveals an exosomal miRNA-mRNA network in colorectal cancer. *BMC Med. Genom.* **2021**, *14*, 60. [CrossRef]
49. Shao, J.; Zaro, J.; Shen, Y. Advances in Exosome-Based Drug Delivery and Tumor Targeting: From Tissue Distribution to Intracellular Fate. *Int. J. Nanomed.* **2020**, *15*, 9355–9371. [CrossRef]

50. Bhome, R.; Goh, R.W.; Bullock, M.D.; Pillar, N.; Thirdborough, S.M.; Mellone, M.; Mirnezami, R.; Galea, D.; Veselkov, K.; Gu, Q. et al. Exosomal microRNAs derived from colorectal cancer-associated fibroblasts: Role in driving cancer progression. *Aging* 2017, 9, 2666–2694. [CrossRef]
51. Ren, J.; Ding, L.; Zhang, D.; Shi, G.; Xu, Q.; Shen, S.; Wang, Y.; Wang, T.; Hou, Y. Carcinoma-associated fibroblasts promote the stemness and chemoresistance of colorectal cancer by transferring exosomal lncRNA H19. *Theranostics* 2018, 8, 3932–3948. [CrossRef]
52. Shedden, K.; Xie, X.T.; Chandaroy, P.; Chang, Y.T.; Rosania, G.R. Expulsion of small molecules in vesicles shed by cancer cells Association with gene expression and chemosensitivity profiles. *Cancer Res.* 2003, 63, 4331–4337.
53. Bach, D.; Hong, J.; Park, H.J.; Lee, S.K. The role of exosomes and miRNAs in drug-resistance of cancer cells. *Int. J. Cancer* 2017, 141, 220–230. [CrossRef]
54. Au Yeung, C.L.; Co, N.; Tsuruga, T.; Yeung, T.; Kwan, S.; Leung, C.S.; Li, Y.; Lu, E.S.; Kwan, K.; Wong, K. Exosomal transfer of stroma-derived miR21 confers paclitaxel resistance in ovarian cancer cells through targeting APAF1. *Nat. Commun.* 2016, 7, 11150 [CrossRef]
55. Hu, J.; Wang, W.; Lan, X.; Zeng, Z.; Liang, Y.; Yan, Y.; Song, F.; Wang, F.; Zhu, X.; Liao, W. CAFs secreted exosomes promote metastasis and chemotherapy resistance by enhancing cell stemness and epithelial-mesenchymal transition in colorectal cancer *Mol. Cancer* 2019, 18, 91. [CrossRef]
56. Wang, Z.; Wu, Z.; Liu, Y.; Han, W. New development in CAR-T cell therapy. *J. Hematol. Oncol.* 2017, 10, 53. [CrossRef]
57. Balacescu, O.; Sur, D.; Cainap, C.; Visan, S.; Cruceriu, D.; Manzat-Saplacan, R.; Muresan, M.-S.; Balacescu, L.; Lisencu, C.; Irimie, A. The Impact of miRNA in Colorectal Cancer Progression and Its Liver Metastases. *Int. J. Mol. Sci.* 2018, 19, 3711. [CrossRef]

Disclaimer/Publisher's Note: The statements, opinions and data contained in all publications are solely those of the individual author(s) and contributor(s) and not of MDPI and/or the editor(s). MDPI and/or the editor(s) disclaim responsibility for any injury to people or property resulting from any ideas, methods, instructions or products referred to in the content.

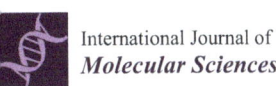

Case Report

Complete Metabolic Response to Combined Immune Checkpoint Inhibition after Progression of Metastatic Colorectal Cancer on Pembrolizumab: A Case Report

Carolin Krekeler [1,2,*], Klaus Wethmar [1,2], Jan-Henrik Mikesch [1,2], Andrea Kerkhoff [1,2], Kerstin Menck [1,2], Georg Lenz [1,2], Hans-Ulrich Schildhaus [3,4,5], Michael Wessolly [4,5], Matthias W. Hoffmann [6], Andreas Pascher [7], Inga Asmus [8], Eva Wardelmann [9] and Annalen Bleckmann [1,2]

1. Department for Medicine A, Hematology, Oncology, Hemostaseology and Pneumology, University Hospital Muenster, 48149 Muenster, Germany; annalen.bleckmann@ukmuenster.de (A.B.)
2. West German Cancer Center, University Hospital Muenster, 48149 Muenster, Germany
3. Institute of Pathology Nordhessen, 34119 Kassel, Germany
4. Institute of Pathology, University Hospital Essen, 45147 Essen, Germany
5. West German Cancer Center, University Hospital Essen, 45147 Essen, Germany
6. Department of General and Visceral Surgery, Raphaelsklinik Muenster, 48143 Muenster, Germany
7. Department of General, Visceral and Transplant Surgery, University Hospital Muenster, 48149 Muenster, Germany
8. Department of Nuclear Medicine, University Hospital Muenster, 48149 Muenster, Germany
9. Gerhard-Domagk-Institute of Pathology, University Hospital Muenster, 48149 Muenster, Germany
* Correspondence: carolin.krekeler@ukmuenster.de

Abstract: DNA mismatch repair deficient (dMMR) and microsatellite instable (MSI) metastatic colorectal cancer (mCRC) can be successfully treated with FDA- and EMA-approved immune checkpoint inhibitors (ICI) pembrolizumab and nivolumab (as single agents targeting the anti-programmed cell death protein-1 (PD-1)) or combinations of a PD-1 inhibitor with ipilimumab, a cytotoxic T-lymphocyte-associated protein 4 (CTLA-4)-targeting antibody. The best treatment strategy beyond progression on single-agent ICI therapy remains unclear. Here, we present the case of a 63-year-old male with Lynch-syndrome-associated, microsatellite instability-high (MSI-H) mCRC who achieved a rapid normalization of his tumor markers and a complete metabolic remission (CMR), currently lasting for ten months, on sequential ICI treatment with the combination of nivolumab and ipilimumab followed by nivolumab maintenance therapy after progression on single-agent anti-PD-1 ICI therapy. The therapy was well-tolerated, and no immune-related adverse events occurred. To the best of our knowledge, this is the first case of a sustained metabolic complete remission in an MSI-H mCRC patient initially progressing on single-agent anti-PD-1 therapy. Thus, dMMR mCRC patients might benefit from sequential immune checkpoint regimens even with long-term responses. However, further sophistication of clinical algorithms for treatment beyond progression on single-agent ICI therapy in MSI-mCRC is urgently needed.

Keywords: immune checkpoint inhibition; nivolumab; ipilimumab; microsatellite instability; metastatic colorectal cancer

1. Introduction

Mutations in the DNA repair genes *MLH1*, *MSH2*, *MSH6*, and *PMS2* may result in DNA-mismatch-repair-deficient cancer, characterized by a high mutational burden in repetitive DNA sequences, so-called microsatellites. Therefore, MMR deficiency is often associated with a high frequency of microsatellite instability, as found in various cancer entities [1].

While MMR deficiency is seen in about 10 to 15% of colorectal carcinomas, an underlying germline mutation in at least one DNA repair gene can be found in approximately

3% of all CRC patients [2,3]. Inherited MSI (hereditary non-polypous colorectal cancer; HNPCC, Lynch syndrome) is one of the most frequent tumor predisposition syndromes in CRC.

MSI-H mCRC responds poorly to cytotoxic treatment. Molecularly, genomic alterations in dMMR/MSI-H CRC lead to the creation of neoantigens and thus immunogenic epitopes on the cell surface. The microenvironment of dMMR/MSI-H CRC has been demonstrated to be enriched in tumor-infiltrating lymphocytes directed against these distinct tumor neoantigens, indicating ongoing immune surveillance in those cancers [4,5]. Nevertheless, an effective anti-tumor immune response is thwarted by an augmented expression of immune checkpoint molecules including PD-1, its ligand anti-programmed cell death protein-ligand 1 (PD-L1), and CTLA-4 and thus immunosuppressive features of the tumor immune ecosystem [6–9]. These immune escape mechanisms allow growth and progression of dMMR/MSI-H mCRC and are key barriers in anti-tumor immunity, as they inhibit T-cell anti-tumor responses [10].

Immune checkpoint inhibitors have revolutionized the treatment of solid tumors as they can overcome this blockade and strengthen anti-tumor immunity. For dMMR/MSI-H mCRC patients, ICI therapy has been shown to induce an effective anti-tumor immune response with long-term efficacy, while MSI stable tumors poorly respond to immunotherapy. Therefore, testing for MMR protein expression or MSI, preferably both, is mandatory.

More in detail, treatment of dMMR/MSI-H mCRC with a single anti-PD-1 agent, such as pembrolizumab (evaluated in KEYNOTE-164 [11,12] and KEYNOTE-177 trials [13]) or nivolumab (evaluated in the CHECKMATE-142 trial [14]), resulted in response rates of up to 32% and a median progression-free survival (PFS) and overall survival (OS) of 4.1/47.0 months for pembrolizumab and a 12-month overall survival rate of 73% for nivolumab, respectively [15,16]. Combined ICI therapy using the anti-PD-1 antibody nivolumab and the anti-CTLA-4 antibody ipilimumab has been demonstrated to increase the tumor infiltration with T-cells in melanomas [10]. In dMMR/MSI-H mCRC patients, the combined immune checkpoint blockade has shown increased objective response and disease control rates of 69% and 84%, respectively (median PFS/OS not reached at a minimum 24.2 months-follow-up; CHECKMATE-142 trial [17,18]). Hence, combined ICI treatment is already the current standard of care for MSI-H/dMMR mCRC patients in a first-line setting in the US and approved by the FDA.

However, the majority of patients with an initial response to single-agent ICI eventually develop progressive disease due to acquired ICI resistance [9,10,19–22]. The mechanisms of secondary resistance to ICI treatment are diverse and entity-specific [9]. Infiltration with tumor-suppressive cells, downregulation of major histocompatibility complexes (MHC) class I molecules, and thus, hampered antigen presentation, apotosis inhibition by hypoxia, alterations in gut microbiota, defective tp53 and INF-signal pathways, amplified WNT/ß-Catenin, and TGF-ß signaling, inducing an increased portion of cancer stem cells (CSCs) that impact the tumor environment, are factors that promote to the tumor-mediated ICI bypass [9,10,20].

With rising evidence to the underlying mechanisms of hampered ICI efficacy, therapeutic approaches to restore the immune system and boost ICI efficacy, such as CSC-directed therapy or fecal microbial transplantation, are increasing, but currently remain experimental.

At present, there is no general recommendation for further treatment options, and especially not for an adjustment of the immunotherapeutic regimen in dMRR/MSI-H mCRC patients progressing on single-agent anti-PD-1 ICI therapy.

Here, we report on the clinical course of a patient with KRAS-mutated dMMR/MSI-H mCRC successfully treated with dual checkpoint inhibition using nivolumab and ipilimumab after initial progression under single anti-PD-1 agent pembrolizumab.

2. Case Presentation

A 63-year-old male was diagnosed with a pT3, pN1c, pMx, L0, V0, Pn0, UICC (version 8) stage IIIB high-grade (G3), KRAS-mutated (Q61K) adenocarcinoma of the ascending colon in December 2019. Figure 1 illustrates the relevant timepoints of the diagnostic assessments and treatment strategies.

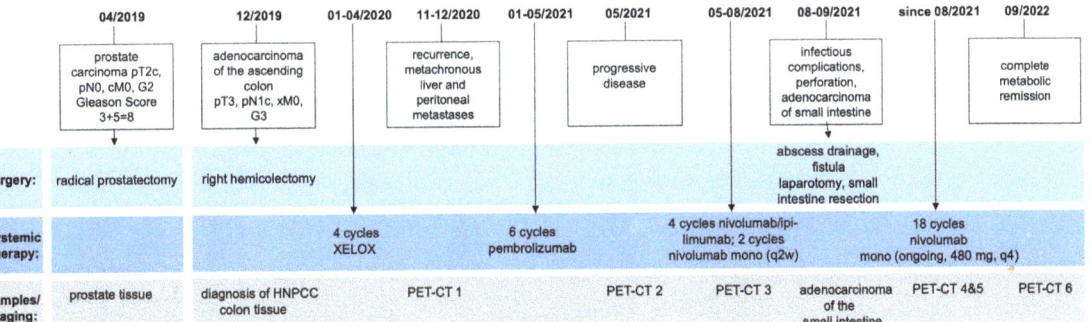

Figure 1. Timeline of the patient's treatment and course of the disease including obtained samples and imaging performed.

Histopathological work-up revealed the loss of MSH6 expression in the tumor tissue (Figure 2), and germline testing detected a frame-shift mutation in *MSH6 gene*, implicating Lynch syndrome. The patient was treated with four adjuvant courses of XELOX (capecitabine and oxaliplatin) after initial right hemicolectomy prior to initiating further care in our department. Post-treatment imaging showed no further evidence of disease.

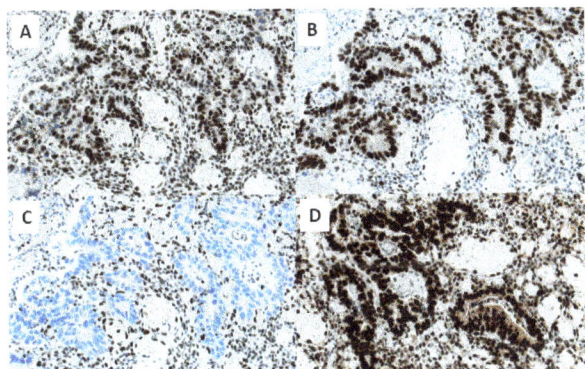

Figure 2. Immunohistochemistry reveals loss of MSH-6 mismatch repair protein in the tumor tissue immunohistochemical staining of mismatch repair proteins in tumor tissue of the small intestine shows an isolated nuclear loss of MSH6 (**C**), whereas MSH2 (**A**), MLH1 (**B**), and PMS2 (**D**) are strongly expressed (original magnification ×200, scale bar ≅ 50 µm). Nuclear staining was assessed in comparison to lymphocytes serving as internal positive control.

Eight months prior to the diagnosis of the dMMR/MSI-H colon carcinoma, the patient had already been diagnosed with prostate carcinoma (initial Gleason-Score 3 + 3 = 6) and high-grade prostate intraepithelial neoplasia (PIN). The lesions were regularly monitored via MRI and 3-monthly biopsies were performed while chemotherapy with capecitabine and oxaliplatin (XELOX) was applied. In July 2020, biopsies revealed a rising Gleason score (3 + 5 = 8), and the patient underwent robotic-assisted radical prostatectomy. As expected from the germline variants observed in the colon cancer samples, the immunohistochemical workup also revealed a loss of MSH6 expression in the prostate cancer tissue. Postoperative PSA-levels were always normal.

In November 2020, the first follow-up imaging by computed tomography (CT) showed multiple liver nodules, suspicious for diffuse liver metastases. At that time, the patient was admitted to our emergency department with melaena, infrapubic swelling, and severe periumbilical pain. Colonoscopy and balloon-assisted enteroscopy were inconclusive, while positron emission tomography and computed tomography (PET/CT, Figure 3a) showed local tumor recurrence at the site of the ileocolic anastomosis as well as massive disease progression with diffuse peritoneal carcinomatosis, subcutaneous lesions in the lower left abdomen at former laparoscopic port sites, one bone lesion in the tenth rib on the right, and multiple metastases to the liver and abdominal lymph nodes.

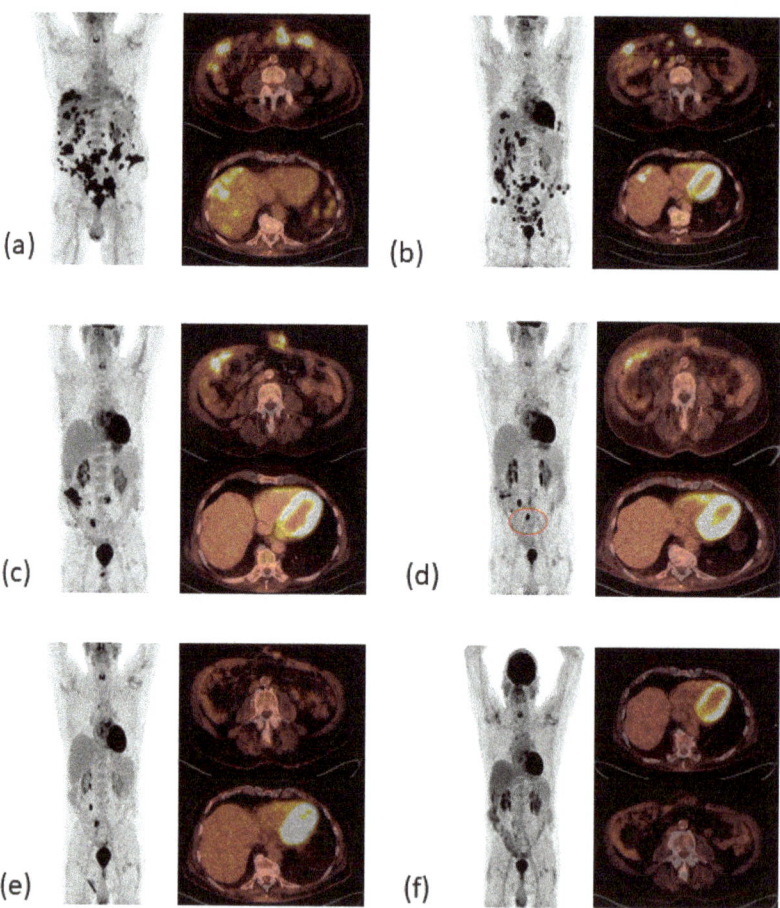

Figure 3. PET-CT images therapeutic response resulting in complete metabolic remission. (**a**) Local relapse and metachronous metastatic disease (December 2020). (**b**) Mixed response in April 2021 after six cycles pembrolizumab. (**c**) PR with decrease of metabolic activity and complete metabolic remission (CMR) of liver and bone metastases in June 2021. (**d**) Sustained CMR of liver metastases. Postoperative increased metabolic activity of one lymph node (red circle) in November 2021. (**e**) PR of the subcutaneous metastases, sustained CMR of liver metastases in March 2022. (**f**) CMR in September 2022.

Treatment with pembrolizumab was initiated at a fixed dose of 200 mg every three weeks (q3). Pembrolizumab was well tolerated, brought a rapid clinical improvement after the first dose with a decrease in abdominal swelling and pain, and reduced levels of the tumor markers carcinoembryonic antigen (CEA) and carbohydrate antigen 19-9 (CA 19-9, see Figure 4). A CT scan after three weeks of treatment confirmed the partial remission of the metastatic lesions (images not shown). However, after seven cycles of pembrolizumab monotherapy the CEA and CA 19-9 levels increased again to 19 ng/mL and 687 U/mL, respectively, and the patient developed indurated painful subcutaneous metastases of the abdominal wall. PET/CT imaging confirmed the suspected disease progression (Figure 3b).

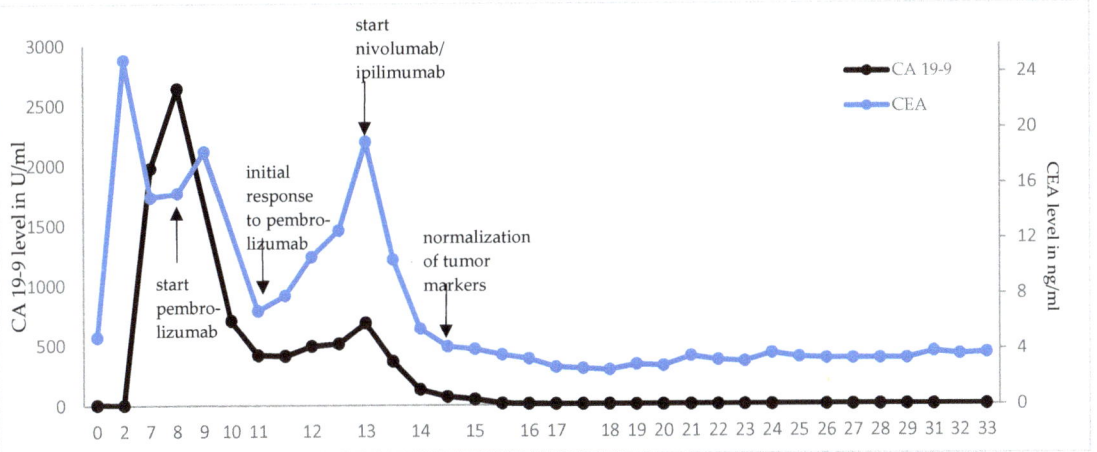

Figure 4. Dynamics of tumor markers after initiation of ICI therapy. CEA and CA 19-9 were monitored in regular blood draws. Rising tumor marker levels were seen after initial decrease under pembrolizumab monotherapy, matching with the image-confirmed disease progression. Treatment with ipilimumab and pembrolizumab led to a rapid decline and eventually normalization of CEA and CA 19-9 levels, respectively. Under ongoing nivolumab monotherapy, both markers are persistently in normal ranges.

In May 2021, the patient began a four-course treatment with the combination of the anti-PD-1 antibody nivolumab (3 mg/kg body weight) and the anti-CTLA-4 antibody ipilimumab (1 mg/kg body weight). This was chosen in view of the rapid initial clinical and serological response to pembrolizumab and the long-lasting clinical benefit seen with the combined blockade of PD-1 and CTLA-4 [14], which had just been approved for treatment of MSI-high CRC after failure of one line of chemotherapy [17]. The treatment was well tolerated, except for initial severe periumbilical pain that was controlled by oral opioids, and an inflammation of the abdominal wall after the third cycle of treatment that was thought to be immune-mediated. With this suspicion in mind, 10 mg oral prednisolone per day was applied together with the fourth cycle of combined ICI therapy. CA 19-9 and CEA levels declined rapidly, the latter returning to normal after three therapy cycles. A PET-CT scan revealed partial remission with a complete metabolic remission of the bone lesion and regression of all other metastases (Figure 3c).

After four cycles of nivolumab and ipilimumab, the patient was admitted to the emergency room with clinical signs of an acute abdomen showing elevated C-reactive protein (CRP) levels (20.5 mg/dL; normal range < 0.5 mg/dL) and an indurated abdominal swelling caused by abscesses in the abdominal wall at the sites of the former subcutaneous and peritoneal metastases. The abscesses were drained, intravenous antibiotic treatment was initiated, and the condition of the patient improved. The nivolumab maintenance therapy was continued at a constant dose of 240 mg every three weeks (q3w). However, a few days later, the patient was re-admitted to the hospital with progressive swelling of the right abdominal wall, rising CRP levels, and severe abdominal pain. An MRI with an oral contrast agent revealed a phlegmonous abdominal wall with multiple enteral fistulas and abscesses at sites of former metastases. That condition was most likely caused by rapid, treatment-induced tumor necrosis with subsequent superinfection. The abscesses were drained, dead and infected tissue was surgically debrided, and a combined antimycotic and antibiotic treatment was administered. Under the combined interventional and conservative treatment, the patient's condition improved, and the laboratory parameters returned to normal.

Although desired by the patient, the surgical excision of the fistulas and reconstruction of the abdominal wall was not recommended due to the marked local inflammation and the ongoing immunotherapy with nivolumab.

With the patient's consent and on his insistence, a laparotomy was performed, during which the perforated small bowel sections and the fistulas were removed and the abdominal wall was reconstructed (Figure 5).

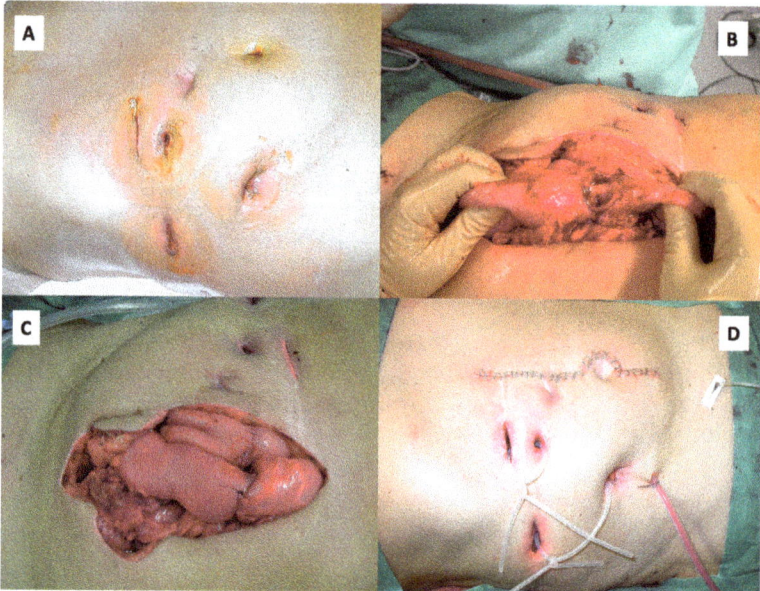

Figure 5. Laparotomy, fistula excision and abdominal wall reconstruction. Abdomen prior to surgery with multiple entero-cutaneous fistulas. (**A**) Necrotic former tumor tissue in the small intestine (**B**). After fistula excision, multiple end-to-end enterostomies were performed (**C**). Finally, the abdominal wall was reconstructed (**D**).

The histopathological work-up showed necrosis in former tumor lesions and one vital adenocarcinoma of the small intestine, again with an immunohistochemical-confirmed loss of MSH6 expression. The postoperative PET-CT scan (Figure 3d) indicated a persisting therapeutic response, although with a new metabolically active lymph node in the surgical site (SUV$_{max}$ 34.6) that was interpreted as a postoperative reactive lymphadenopathy.

After nine cycles of single-agent nivolumab 240 mg, q2w the condition of the patient was excellent, the tumor markers remained normal, and a PET-CT confirmed an ongoing PR in March 2022 (Figure 3e). The nivolumab maintenance therapy was, therefore, adjusted to a four-week interval with a flat dose of 480 mg. In September 2022, during an incisional hernia repair, no signs of a relapse were observed. In addition, after a total duration of 17 months of second-line dual ICI therapy, including 14 months of nivolumab maintenance therapy, PET-CT imaging (Figure 3f) first showed a complete metabolic remission (CMR) and no morphological evidence of residual disease in September 2022. Since then, the patient has remained in ongoing complete metabolic remission with tumor markers CEA and CA 19-9 within normal ranges during the 24-month follow-up after initiation of relapse-directed treatment.

To further investigate the underlying causes and mechanisms of this excellent response to combined anti-CTLA-4 and anti-PD-L1 blockade after progression under single agent PD-1 inhibiting therapy, we performed a molecular pathological analysis of the tumor tissue. We found no distinct *CD274*/PD-L1 mutation, which might possibly have reduced the efficacy of pembrolizumab, but not that of nivolumab due to the different binding sites. The tumor harbored a JAK2-mutation (R1063H, ClinVar: CN169374), which is described as a gain of function mutation (https://ckb.jax.org/geneVariant/show?geneVariantId=7650 (accessed on 29 June 2023)). In addition, 12 HLA class I somatic mutations were found in the tumor tissue (Table 1). Individually, none of the mutations have been described as pathogenic variant in molecular analysis databases. However, the frequency of mutations at the *HLA* gene loci was increased by a factor of 7.5 compared with the expected frequency of random gene mutations ($p < 0.01$). Nonetheless, the impact of the combination of several *HLA* mutations, and especially an eventual upregulation of *HLA* class I expression on antigen-presenting cells by the mutations, remains elusive.

Table 1. Multiple *HLA* mutations were observed during molecular pathological analysis of colon tumor tissue, which might contribute to the high efficacy of combined ICI therapy in this patient. All variants are, individually, of benign or indeterminate potential.

Locus (Transcript ID)	Start Position	End Position	Type of Variant	Affected DNA Section	Encoded Gene
			Substitution		
	29726903	29726904	AA > CT	ncRNA	
Chr.6 p22.1	29943483	29943484	AC > CG	Exon	HLA-A
(ENST00000396634.5)	29943494	29943495	GT > CG	Exon	HLA-A
	29944153	29944154	CA > TG	Exon	HLA-A
			SNV		
	29944118	29944118	T > A	Intron	HLA-A
	29944151	29944151	C > G	Exon	HLA-A
			Substitution		
	31271152	31271154	CAG > GTC	Exon	HLA-C
Chr. 6 p21.33	31356226	31356227	TC > GT	Promotor	
(ENST00000376228.9)	31356246	31356248	CCG > GTC	Promotor	
	31356748	31356749	CC > TG	Promotor	
			SNV		
	31271082	31271082	G > C	Exon	HLA-C
	31271089	31271089	C > G	Exon	HLA-C

3. Discussion

Here, we present a case of a complete metabolic and serologic remission in a patient with dMMR/MSI-H mCRC and Lynch syndrome-associated prostate cancer under treatment with combined anti-PD-1 and anti-CTLA-4 blockade with nivolumab and ipilimumab after progression under pembrolizumab monotherapy.

Treatment of mCRC with dMMR/MSI-H has traditionally been challenging due to the poor response to conventional chemotherapeutic therapy [23,24]. The development of FDA- and EMA-approved single agent immunotherapeutic drugs targeting PD-1, such as nivolumab and pembrolizumab, has revolutionized the therapeutic strategies in dMMR/MSI-H mCRC, refractory or relapsed after cytotoxic treatment, due to high objective response rates (ORR) and sustained responses [11,14]. Compared to the therapy with a single agent anti-PD-1 antibody, the combination of nivolumab (targeting PD-1) and ipilimumab (targeting CTLA-4) applied in the phase II CheckMate-142 trial yielded an increased ORR of 55% in patients previously treated with chemotherapy and showed a manageable safety profile [14,25]. Thus, dual checkpoint blockade was approved by the FDA in a first-line setting and by the EMA in dMMR/MSI-H mCRC after prior fluoropyrimidine-based treatment.

The use of pembrolizumab as a first line treatment in dMMR/MSI-H mCRC was shown to be superior to 5-fluoruracil-based therapy with regard to progression-free survival [19]. However, the combination of nivolumab and ipilimumab studied in the CHECKMATE-142 trial [17] showed a superior and durable responses, and thus, constitutes the new first line standard treatment in dMMR/MSI-H mCRC in the US, but is not yet authorized by the EMA.

Treating patients with progression after initial response to immune checkpoint inhibitors remains a major challenge. As every antibody directed against PD-1 binds to a distinct epitope, sequential therapy with another PD-1 blocker after progression on an anti-PD-1 antibody may be an option, although clear evidence for antibody-specific mechanisms of resistance is lacking [26,27]. Recent data for such sequential treatment with a single-agent anti-PD-1 drug or a combined use with a CTLA-4 inhibitor showed non-uniform responses ranging from durable response to massive disease progression [28–31].

Analysis of tumors with acquired resistance to anti-PD-1 antibodies demonstrated epigenetic changes, such as histone marks, DNA methylation, and miRNA signatures, eventually leading to an altered microenvironment and immune escape [32]. Furthermore, there is evidence that the tumor cells can escape immune surveillance by upregulating immune-suppressive molecules including lymphocyte-activation gene (LAG-3) and CTLA-4 as well as by the absence or decreased infiltration of (CD-8 positive) tumor-infiltrating leukocytes or the increased presence of immunosuppressive cells, such as regulatory T cells and myeloid-derived suppressor cells, in the tumor microenvironment [33,34]. Thus, the addition of a second immune checkpoint inhibitor like the anti-CTLA-4 antibody ipilimumab may help to overcome acquired resistance to the PD-1 blockade. There are emerging data showing long-term disease control after re-challenging immunotherapy with CTLA-4 and PD-1 antibodies in patients whose tumors had progressed on single agent PD-1 blockade in melanoma [35,36], hepatocellular carcinoma [37], non-small cell lung cancer [38], and urothelial cancer [39].

Moreover, loss of antigen expression, for example via defects in interferon-γ pathway due to mutations in JAK2-signaling [40], is an alternative mechanism of immune escape. We found one pathogenic somatic gain-of-function mutation in our patient. The mutation variant (JAK2 R1063H) lies within the protein kinase domain 2 of the JAK2-protein and results in, among other things, increased transcriptional activity. Gain of function mutations in JAK2-signaling are described as being associated with a significant increase in PD-L1 expression, which can affect response to immunotherapy [41,42].

Recently, downregulation of HLA class-I molecules was described as being associated with an inferior response to ICI therapy due to the impaired interaction with the antigen-presenting machinery at the protein level [43–45]. On the other hand, high HLA evolutionary divergence, and thus, the physiochemical sequence divergence between HLA-I alleles, has not only been shown to enable the presentation of more diverse immunopeptidomes, but to be associated with better survival [46,47]. The distinct HLA phenotype resulting from the various HLA mutations observed in our patient might have, thus, possibly led to (a) HLA protein defects resulting in alternative/increased epitope presentation, (b) an upregulation of the HLA-expression itself, or (c) a higher evolutionary divergence, and thus, increased diversity of neoepitopes. Hence, the patients' HLA variant might have conceivably contributed to higher immunogenicity and thus to an improved response to combined checkpoint inhibition compared with anti-PD-1 monotherapy. Moreover, it may have been crucial for the sustained CMR of this case of metastasized HNPCC-associated MSH6 deficient CRC under dual immune blockade. Future work on larger patient cohorts is required to resolve the predominant molecular mechanisms predicting response to dual checkpoint-inhibition after progress under PD-1 blockade.

In the literature, we found two other cases of dMMR/MSI-H CRC treated with sequential combined nivolumab and ipilimumab therapy after progression on single-agent pembrolizumab. In line with our findings, the re-challenge with immunotherapy led to partial responses of patients with dMMR/MSI-H mCRC in other case studies [48,49]. Winer et al. treated a 64-year-old patient with Lynch syndrome associated mCRC and urothelial carcinoma with the anti-PD-L1 antibody atezolizumab after progression on pembrolizumab and subsequently with ipilimumab and nivolumab after clinical progression marked by rising tumor markers. Even if the patient had similar clinical features (age, Lynch-syndrome, and multiple HNPCC-associated cancer entities) and a lower tumor burden (liver metastases only) compared to our patient, only a partial metabolic response and stabilized but strongly elevated CEA levels were reached [49]. Das et al. reported a 30% tumor mass reduction in an MSI-H mCRC female patient (Lynch-syndrome association not indicated) after four cycles of combined checkpoint inhibition and nivolumab maintenance therapy [48].

To our knowledge, this is the first published case describing a PET-CT-confirmed metabolic complete remission and serologic normalization of tumor markers CEA and CA 19-9. The causes for this excellent response, especially in comparison to the patient case reported by Winer et al., with a patient comparable in disease manifestation and demographics, remain uncertain. Possibly, the patient's good performance status at most points of the therapy, limited pre-existing illnesses (ischemic stroke without remains, hyperlipidemia), and the limited co-medication (ASS, rosuvastation, ezetimib) have contributed to an undelayed therapy administration and might have, thus, also contributed to this excellent therapeutic response. Moreover, the ethnicity of our patient might have influenced the response to ICI therapy, as non-Hispanic white patients are known to show higher response rates [50,51]. Hence, demographics and treatment characteristics might have impacted the therapy response. Finally, following a single case description, the results may not automatically be applied to a larger cohort.

Molecular pathologic analyses and examination for MSI are implemented in the clinical and diagnostic algorithms of mCRC. During the last decade, a variety of characteristic mutations resulting in signal pathway activation, and thus, driving tumor growth, became targetable. This case study underlines the high importance of molecular analyses and a patient-individual treatment regimen based on the underlying tumor biology. Precision medicine, and thus, the combination of drugs based on molecular tumor characteristics, will become increasingly important in the foreseeable future. As they can provide tumor control even in advanced therapy lines, clinicians should assess the molecular characteristics in mCRC for potential molecularly based therapy options as for the patient in our case study.

ICI treatment has superseded conventional cytotoxic treatment in MSI-H mCRC and has been implemented as a first-line standard in current guidelines. Despite the limitations of a single case report mentioned here, the rapid and ongoing therapy response in overcoming the acquired PD-1 resistance by adding an anti-CTLA-4 antibody may be a promising strategy for other patients with Lynch syndrome-associated CRC. However, for the inclusion of sequential ICI treatment beyond progression on single-agent anti-PD-1 therapy, future clinical trial evaluation is warranted, as patients with disease progression on single-agent anti-PD-1 therapies have been excluded in recent trials and especially in the CHECKMATE-142 trial.

The combination of drugs seems to reduce the immune escape phenomena associated with a single-target directed ICI therapy as multiple resistance mechanisms are required, achieves higher ORR and will, thus, become the first-line standard in the first-line setting in the foreseeable future [18].

4. Conclusions

Post-progression treatment of dMMR/MSI-H mCRC on anti-PD-1 therapy remains a major challenge. The addition of an anti-CTLA-4 drug might help to overcome initial or acquired resistance to ICI monotherapy and is able to provide a durable response this patient collective. Our patient with Lynch syndrome treated with four courses of nivolumab/ipilimumab combined and subsequent nivolumab maintenance therapy achieved an ongoing complete metabolic remission with normalized tumor markers.

Even if the predominant mechanisms and molecular features leading to the high effectiveness of sequential double-immune checkpoint blockade in individual patients are not yet fully understood, specific HLA mutations have emerged as biomarkers for the ICI response. The high frequency of HLA mutations observed in the tumor sample of our patient might have contributed to the excellent therapeutic response. Prospective HLA-genotyping may help to better understand the biological impact of distinct single mutations, and especially the combined effects of multiple HLA aberrations.

Prospective clinical trials are needed to confirm the effectiveness and safety of combined immunotherapy after progression on single agent ICI in dMMR/MSI-H mCRC, comparing sequential ICI therapy to a re-initiation of conventional chemotherapy, and to evaluate the significance of HLA gene mutations in predicting responses to checkpoint blockade.

Author Contributions: Conceptualization, C.K. and A.B.; methodology, C.K. and A.B.; software, C.K., E.W. and A.B.; writing—original draft preparation, C.K.; writing—review and editing, K.W., K.M., J.-H.M., A.K., K.M., G.L., H.-U.S., M.W., M.W.H., A.P., I.A., E.W. and A.B.; visualization, C.K., I.A., M.W.H., E.W. and A.B.; supervision, A.B. All authors have read and agreed to the published version of the manuscript.

Funding: This research received no external funding.

Institutional Review Board Statement: The study was conducted in accordance with the Declaration of Helsinki, and approved by the Joint Ethics Committee of the Physician's Chamber Westphalia-Lippe and the University of Münster, No. 2020-172-b-S for studies involving humans.

Informed Consent Statement: Informed consent was obtained from the patient involved in the case report. The study was approved by the Joint Ethics Committee of the Physician's Chamber Westphalia-Lippe and the University of Münster, No. 2020-172-b-S.

Data Availability Statement: The data presented in this study are available on request from the corresponding author. The data are not publicly available due to privacy reasons.

Acknowledgments: We thank the open access fund of the University of Muenster.

Conflicts of Interest: The authors declare no conflict of interest.

References

1. Zhao, P.; Li, L.; Jiang, X.; Li, Q. Mismatch Repair Deficiency/Microsatellite Instability-High as a Predictor for Anti-PD-1/PD-L1 Immunotherapy Efficacy. *J. Hematol. Oncol.* **2019**, *12*, 54. [CrossRef]
2. Pawlik, T.M.; Raut, C.P.; Rodriguez-Bigas, M.A. Colorectal Carcinogenesis: MSI-H Versus MSI-L. *Dis. Markers* **2004**, *20*, 199–206. [CrossRef]
3. Win, A.K.; Jenkins, M.A.; Dowty, J.G.; Antoniou, A.C.; Lee, A.; Giles, G.G.; Buchanan, D.D.; Clendenning, M.; Rosty, C.; Ahnen, D.J.; et al. Prevalence and Penetrance of Major Genes and Polygenes for Colorectal Cancer. *Cancer Epidemiol. Biomark. Prev.* **2017**, *26*, 404–412. [CrossRef]
4. Sahin, I.H.; Akce, M.; Alese, O.; Shaib, W.; Lesinski, G.B.; El-Rayes, B.; Wu, C. Immune Checkpoint Inhibitors for the Treatment of MSI-H/MMR-D Colorectal Cancer and a Perspective on Resistance Mechanisms. *Br. J. Cancer* **2019**, *121*, 809–818. [CrossRef] [PubMed]
5. Guidoboni, M.; Gafà, R.; Viel, A.; Doglioni, C.; Russo, A.; Santini, A.; Del Tin, L.; Macrì, E.; Lanza, G.; Boiocchi, M.; et al. Microsatellite Instability and High Content of Activated Cytotoxic Lymphocytes Identify Colon Cancer Patients with a Favorable Prognosis. *Am. J. Pathol.* **2001**, *159*, 297–304. [CrossRef]
6. Arai, Y.; Saito, H.; Ikeguchi, M. Upregulation of TIM-3 and PD-1 on CD4+ and CD8+ T Cells Associated with Dysfunction of Cell-Mediated Immunity after Colorectal Cancer Operation. *Yonago Acta Med.* **2012**, *55*, 1.
7. Jacobs, J.; Smits, E.; Lardon, F.; Pauwels, P.; Deschoolmeester, V. Immune Checkpoint Modulation in Colorectal Cancer: What's New and What to Expect. *J. Immunol. Res.* **2015**, *2015*, 158038. [CrossRef] [PubMed]
8. Amodio, V.; Mauri, G.; Reilly, N.M.; Sartore-Bianchi, A.; Siena, S.; Bardelli, A.; Germano, G. Mechanisms of Immune Escape and Resistance to Checkpoint Inhibitor Therapies in Mismatch Repair Deficient Metastatic Colorectal Cancers. *Cancers* **2021**, *13*, 2638. [CrossRef]
9. Mortezaee, K.; Majidpoor, J.; Najafi, S.; Tasa, D. Bypassing Anti-PD-(L)1 Therapy: Mechanisms and Management Strategies. *Biomed. Pharmacother. Biomed. Pharmacother.* **2023**, *158*, 114150. [CrossRef]
10. Rouzbahani, E.; Majidpoor, J.; Najafi, S.; Mortezaee, K. Cancer Stem Cells in Immunoregulation and Bypassing Anti-Checkpoint Therapy. *Biomed. Pharmacother. Biomed. Pharmacother.* **2022**, *156*, 113906. [CrossRef]
11. Le, D.T.; Kim, T.W.; Van Cutsem, E.; Geva, R.; Jäger, D.; Hara, H.; Burge, M.; O'Neil, B.; Kavan, P.; Yoshino, T.; et al. Phase II Open-Label Study of Pembrolizumab in Treatment-Refractory, Microsatellite Instability–High/Mismatch Repair–Deficient Metastatic Colorectal Cancer: KEYNOTE-164. *J. Clin. Oncol.* **2020**, *38*, 11–19. [CrossRef]

2. Le, D.T.; Diaz, L.; Kim, T.W.; Van Cutsem, E.; Geva, R.; Jäger, D.; Hara, H.; Burge, M.; O'Neil, B.; Kavan, P.; et al. 432P Pembrolizumab (Pembro) for Previously Treated, Microsatellite Instability–High (MSI-H)/Mismatch Repair–Deficient (DMMR) Metastatic Colorectal Cancer (MCRC): Final Analysis of KEYNOTE-164. *Ann. Oncol.* **2021**, *32*, S550. [CrossRef]
3. Diaz, L.A.; Shiu, K.-K.; Kim, T.-W.; Jensen, B.V.; Jensen, L.H.; Punt, C.; Smith, D.; Garcia-Carbonero, R.; Benavides, M.; Gibbs, P.; et al. Pembrolizumab versus Chemotherapy for Microsatellite Instability-High or Mismatch Repair-Deficient Metastatic Colorectal Cancer (KEYNOTE-177): Final Analysis of a Randomised, Open-Label, Phase 3 Study. *Lancet Oncol.* **2022**, *23*, 659–670. [CrossRef] [PubMed]
4. Overman, M.J.; McDermott, R.; Leach, J.L.; Lonardi, S.; Lenz, H.-J.; Morse, M.A.; Desai, J.; Hill, A.; Axelson, M.; Moss, R.A.; et al. Nivolumab in Patients with Metastatic DNA Mismatch Repair-Deficient or Microsatellite Instability-High Colorectal Cancer (CheckMate 142): An Open-Label, Multicentre, Phase 2 Study. *Lancet Oncol.* **2017**, *18*, 1182–1191. [CrossRef] [PubMed]
5. Overman, M.J.; Bergamo, F.; McDermott, R.S.; Aglietta, M.; Chen, F.; Gelsomino, F.; Wong, M.; Morse, M.; Van Cutsem, E.; Hendlisz, A.; et al. Nivolumab in Patients with DNA Mismatch Repair-Deficient/Microsatellite Instability-High (DMMR/MSI-H) Metastatic Colorectal Cancer (MCRC): Long-Term Survival According to Prior Line of Treatment from CheckMate-142. *J. Clin. Oncol.* **2018**, *36*, 554. [CrossRef]
6. Overman, M.J.; Lonardi, S.; Wong, K.Y.M.; Lenz, H.-J.; Gelsomino, F.; Aglietta, M.; Morse, M.A.; Van Cutsem, E.; McDermott, R.; Hill, A.; et al. Durable Clinical Benefit With Nivolumab Plus Ipilimumab in DNA Mismatch Repair–Deficient/Microsatellite Instability–High Metastatic Colorectal Cancer. *J. Clin. Oncol.* **2018**, *36*, 773–779. [CrossRef]
7. Lenz, H.-J.; Lonardi, S.; Zagonel, V.; Van Cutsem, E.; Limon, M.L.; Wong, K.Y.M.; Hendlisz, A.; Aglietta, M.; Garcia-Alfonso, P.; Neyns, B.; et al. Nivolumab plus Low-Dose Ipilimumab as First-Line Therapy in Microsatellite Instability-High/DNA Mismatch Repair Deficient Metastatic Colorectal Cancer: Clinical Update. *J. Clin. Oncol.* **2020**, *38*, 11. [CrossRef]
8. Lenz, H.-J.; Van Cutsem, E.; Luisa Limon, M.; Wong, K.Y.M.; Hendlisz, A.; Aglietta, M.; García-Alfonso, P.; Neyns, B.; Luppi, G.; Cardin, D.B.; et al. First-Line Nivolumab Plus Low-Dose Ipilimumab for Microsatellite Instability-High/Mismatch Repair-Deficient Metastatic Colorectal Cancer: The Phase II CheckMate 142 Study. *J. Clin. Oncol.* **2022**, *40*, 161–170. [CrossRef]
9. André, T.; Shiu, K.-K.; Kim, T.W.; Jensen, B.V.; Jensen, L.H.; Punt, C.; Smith, D.; Garcia-Carbonero, R.; Benavides, M.; Gibbs, P.; et al. Pembrolizumab in Microsatellite-Instability–High Advanced Colorectal Cancer. *N. Engl. J. Med.* **2020**, *383*, 2207–2218. [CrossRef]
10. Najafi, S.; Majidpoor, J.; Mortezaee, K. The Impact of Microbiota on PD-1/PD-L1 Inhibitor Therapy Outcomes: A Focus on Solid Tumors. *Life Sci.* **2022**, *310*, 121138. [CrossRef]
11. Di Franco, S.; Parrino, B.; Gaggianesi, M.; Pantina, V.D.; Bianca, P.; Nicotra, A.; Mangiapane, L.R.; Lo Iacono, M.; Ganduscio, G.; Veschi, V.; et al. CHK1 Inhibitor Sensitizes Resistant Colorectal Cancer Stem Cells to Nortopsentin. *IScience* **2021**, *24*, 102664. [CrossRef]
12. Ros, J.; Balconi, F.; Baraibar, I.; Saoudi Gonzalez, N.; Salva, F.; Tabernero, J.; Elez, E. Advances in Immune Checkpoint Inhibitor Combination Strategies for Microsatellite Stable Colorectal Cancer. *Front. Oncol.* **2023**, *13*, 1112276. [CrossRef] [PubMed]
13. Shulman, K.; Barnett-Griness, O.; Friedman, V.; Greenson, J.K.; Gruber, S.B.; Lejbkowicz, F.; Rennert, G. Outcomes of Chemotherapy for Microsatellite Instable–High Metastatic Colorectal Cancers. *JCO Precis. Oncol.* **2018**, *2*, 1–10. [CrossRef] [PubMed]
14. Goldstein, J.; Tran, B.; Ensor, J.; Gibbs, P.; Wong, H.L.; Wong, S.F.; Vilar, E.; Tie, J.; Broaddus, R.; Kopetz, S.; et al. Multicenter Retrospective Analysis of Metastatic Colorectal Cancer (CRC) with High-Level Microsatellite Instability (MSI-H). *Ann. Oncol.* **2014**, *25*, 1032–1038. [CrossRef] [PubMed]
15. Morse, M.A.; Overman, M.J.; Hartman, L.; Khoukaz, T.; Brutcher, E.; Lenz, H.; Atasoy, A.; Shangguan, T.; Zhao, H.; El-Rayes, B. Safety of Nivolumab plus Low-Dose Ipilimumab in Previously Treated Microsatellite Instability-High/Mismatch Repair-Deficient Metastatic Colorectal Cancer. *Oncologist* **2019**, *24*, 1453–1461. [CrossRef]
16. Lee, J.Y.; Lee, H.T.; Shin, W.; Chae, J.; Choi, J.; Kim, S.H.; Lim, H.; Won Heo, T.; Park, K.Y.; Lee, Y.J.; et al. Structural Basis of Checkpoint Blockade by Monoclonal Antibodies in Cancer Immunotherapy. *Nat. Commun.* **2016**, *7*, 13354. [CrossRef]
17. Wang, M.; Wang, J.; Wang, R.; Jiao, S.; Wang, S.; Zhang, J.; Zhang, M. Identification of a Monoclonal Antibody That Targets PD-1 in a Manner Requiring PD-1 Asn58 Glycosylation. *Commun. Biol.* **2019**, *2*, 392. [CrossRef]
18. Lepir, T.; Zaghouani, M.; Roche, S.P.; Li, Y.-Y.; Suarez, M.; Irias, M.J.; Savaraj, N. Nivolumab to Pembrolizumab Switch Induced a Durable Melanoma Response: A Case Report. *Medicine* **2019**, *98*, e13804. [CrossRef]
19. Ochoa, C.E.; Joseph, R.W. Utility of Ipilimumab in Melanoma Patients Who Progress on Anti-PD-1 Therapy. *Melanoma Manag.* **2017**, *4*, 143–145. [CrossRef]
20. Hakozaki, T.; Okuma, Y.; Kashima, J. Re-Challenging Immune Checkpoint Inhibitor in a Patient with Advanced Non-Small Cell Lung Cancer: A Case Report. *BMC Cancer* **2018**, *18*, 302. [CrossRef]
21. Martini, D.J.; Lalani, A.-K.A.; Bossé, D.; Steinharter, J.A.; Harshman, L.C.; Hodi, F.S.; Ott, P.A.; Choueiri, T.K. Response to Single Agent PD-1 Inhibitor after Progression on Previous PD-1/PD-L1 Inhibitors: A Case Series. *J. Immunother. Cancer* **2017**, *5*, 66. [CrossRef] [PubMed]
22. Perrier, A.; Didelot, A.; Laurent-Puig, P.; Blons, H.; Garinet, S. Epigenetic Mechanisms of Resistance to Immune Checkpoint Inhibitors. *Biomolecules* **2020**, *10*, 1061. [CrossRef] [PubMed]
23. Chae, Y.K.; Oh, M.S.; Giles, F.J. Molecular Biomarkers of Primary and Acquired Resistance to T-Cell-Mediated Immunotherapy in Cancer: Landscape, Clinical Implications, and Future Directions. *Oncologist* **2018**, *23*, 410–421. [CrossRef] [PubMed]

34. Nowicki, T.S.; Hu-Lieskovan, S.; Ribas, A. Mechanisms of Resistance to PD-1 and PD-L1 Blockade. *Cancer J.* **2018**, *24*, 47–53. [CrossRef] [PubMed]
35. Zimmer, L.; Apuri, S.; Eroglu, Z.; Kottschade, L.A.; Forschner, A.; Gutzmer, R.; Schlaak, M.; Heinzerling, L.; Krackhardt, A.M.; Loquai, C.; et al. Ipilimumab Alone or in Combination with Nivolumab after Progression on Anti-PD-1 Therapy in Advanced Melanoma. *Eur. J. Cancer* **2017**, *75*, 47–55. [CrossRef]
36. Reschke, R.; Ziemer, M. Rechallenge with checkpoint inhibitors in metastatic melanoma. *JDDG J. Dtsch. Dermatol. Ges.* **2020**, *18*, 429–436. [CrossRef]
37. Wong, J.S.L.; Kwok, G.G.W.; Tang, V.; Li, B.C.W.; Leung, R.; Chiu, J.; Ma, K.W.; She, W.H.; Tsang, J.; Lo, C.M.; et al. Ipilimumab and Nivolumab/Pembrolizumab in Advanced Hepatocellular Carcinoma Refractory to Prior Immune Checkpoint Inhibitors. *J. Immunother. Cancer* **2021**, *9*, e001945. [CrossRef]
38. Garon, E.B.; Spira, A.I.; Goldberg, S.B.; Chaft, J.E.; Papadimitrakopoulou, V.; Antonia, S.J.; Brahmer, J.R.; Camidge, D.R.; Powderly, J.D.; Wozniak, A.J.; et al. Safety and Activity of Durvalumab + Tremelimumab in Immunotherapy (IMT)-Pretreated Advanced NSCLC Patients. *J. Clin. Oncol.* **2018**, *36*, 9041. [CrossRef]
39. Keegan, N.M.; Funt, S.A.; Kania, B.E.; Iyer, G.; Clement, J.M.; McCoy, A.S.; Hettich, G.; Ziv, E.; Maher, C.A.; Nair, S.; et al. Durable Clinical Benefit from Combination Ipilimumab (IPI) and Nivolumab (NIVO) in Anti-PD-1 Therapy Resistant, Platinum Resistant Metastatic Urothelial Carcinoma (MUC). *J. Clin. Oncol.* **2019**, *37*, 481. [CrossRef]
40. Pathak, R.; Pharaon, R.R.; Mohanty, A.; Villaflor, V.M.; Salgia, R.; Massarelli, E. Acquired Resistance to PD-1/PD-L1 Blockade in Lung Cancer: Mechanisms and Patterns of Failure. *Cancers* **2020**, *12*, 3851. [CrossRef]
41. Prestipino, A.; Emhardt, A.J.; Aumann, K.; O'Sullivan, D.; Gorantla, S.P.; Duquesne, S.; Melchinger, W.; Braun, L.; Vuckovic, S.; Boerries, M.; et al. Oncogenic JAK2V617F Causes PD-L1 Expression, Mediating Immune Escape in Myeloproliferative Neoplasms. *Sci. Transl. Med.* **2018**, *10*, eaam7729. [CrossRef] [PubMed]
42. Hundal, J.; Lopetegui-Lia, N.; Vredenburgh, J. Discovery, Significance, and Utility of JAK2 Mutation in Squamous Cell Carcinoma of the Lung. *Cureus* **2022**, *14*, e25913. [CrossRef] [PubMed]
43. Rasmussen, M.; Durhuus, J.A.; Nilbert, M.; Andersen, O.; Therkildsen, C. Response to Immune Checkpoint Inhibitors Is Affected by Deregulations in the Antigen Presentation Machinery: A Systematic Review and Meta-Analysis. *J. Clin. Med.* **2022**, *12*, 329. [CrossRef] [PubMed]
44. Taylor, B.C.; Balko, J.M. Mechanisms of MHC-I Downregulation and Role in Immunotherapy Response. *Front. Immunol.* **2022**, *13*, 844866. [CrossRef]
45. Hazini, A.; Fisher, K.; Seymour, L. Deregulation of HLA-I in Cancer and Its Central Importance for Immunotherapy. *J. Immunother. Cancer* **2021**, *9*, e002899. [CrossRef]
46. Ivanova, M.; Shivarov, V. HLA Genotyping Meets Response to Immune Checkpoint Inhibitors Prediction: A Story Just Started. *Int. J. Immunogenet.* **2021**, *48*, 193–200. [CrossRef]
47. Chowell, D.; Morris, L.G.T.; Grigg, C.M.; Weber, J.K.; Samstein, R.M.; Makarov, V.; Kuo, F.; Kendall, S.M.; Requena, D.; Riaz, N.; et al. Patient HLA Class I Genotype Influences Cancer Response to Checkpoint Blockade Immunotherapy. *Science* **2018**, *359*, 582–587. [CrossRef]
48. Das, S.; Allen, A.; Berlin, J. Immunotherapy After Immunotherapy: Response Rescue in a Patient With Microsatellite Instability-High Colorectal Cancer Post-Pembrolizumab. *Clin. Color. Cancer* **2020**, *19*, 137–140. [CrossRef]
49. Winer, A.; Ghatalia, P.; Bubes, N.; Anari, F.; Varshavsky, A.; Kasireddy, V.; Liu, Y.; El-Deiry, W.S. Dual Checkpoint Inhibition with Ipilimumab plus Nivolumab After Progression on Sequential PD-1/PDL-1 Inhibitors Pembrolizumab and Atezolizumab in a Patient with Lynch Syndrome, Metastatic Colon, and Localized Urothelial Cancer. *Oncologist* **2019**, *24*, 1416–1419. [CrossRef]
50. Florez, M.A.; Kemnade, J.O.; Chen, N.; Du, W.; Sabichi, A.L.; Wang, D.Y.; Huang, Q.; Miller-Chism, C.N.; Jotwani, A.; Chen, A.C.; et al. Persistent Ethnicity-Associated Disparity in Antitumor Effectiveness of Immune Checkpoint Inhibitors Despite Equal Access. *Cancer Res. Commun.* **2022**, *2*, 806–813. [CrossRef]
51. Resnick, K.; Zang, P.; Larsen, T.; Ye, S.; Choi, A.; Yu, X.; Brady, K.; Angell, T.E.; Thomas, J.S.; Nieva, J.J.; et al. Impact of Ethnicity and Immune-Related Adverse Events (IRAE) on Outcomes for Non-Small Cell Lung Cancer (NSCLC) Patients Treated with Immune Checkpoint Inhibitors. *J. Clin. Oncol.* **2022**, *40*, e21115. [CrossRef]

Disclaimer/Publisher's Note: The statements, opinions and data contained in all publications are solely those of the individual author(s) and contributor(s) and not of MDPI and/or the editor(s). MDPI and/or the editor(s) disclaim responsibility for any injury to people or property resulting from any ideas, methods, instructions or products referred to in the content.

MDPI
St. Alban-Anlage 66
4052 Basel
Switzerland
www.mdpi.com

International Journal of Molecular Sciences Editorial Office
E-mail: ijms@mdpi.com
www.mdpi.com/journal/ijms

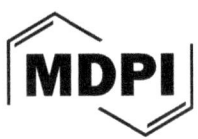

Disclaimer/Publisher's Note: The statements, opinions and data contained in all publications are solely those of the individual author(s) and contributor(s) and not of MDPI and/or the editor(s). MDPI and/or the editor(s) disclaim responsibility for any injury to people or property resulting from any ideas, methods, instructions or products referred to in the content.